BIPOLAR DISORDER

Bipolar Disorder

A Family-Focused Treatment Approach

second edition

DAVID J. MIKLOWITZ

THE GUILFORD PRESS
New York London

A Division of Guilford Publications, Inc.
72 Spring Street, New York, NY 10012
www.guilford.com

Printed in the United States of America

This book is printed on acid-free paper.

Last digit is print number: 9 8 7 6 5 4 3 2 1

The author has checked with sources believed to be reliable in his efforts to provide information that is complete and generally in accord with the standards of practice that are accepted at the time of publication. However, in view of the possibility of human error or changes in medical sciences, neither the author, nor the editor and publisher, nor any other party who has been involved in the preparation or publication of this work warrants that the information contained herein is in every respect accurate or complete, and they are not responsible for any errors or omissions or the results obtained from the use of such information. Readers are encouraged to confirm the information contained in this book with other sources.

Library of Congress Cataloging-in-Publication Data

Miklowitz, David Jay, 1957–
Bipolar disorder : a family-focused treatment approach / David J. Miklowitz.—2nd ed.
p. ; cm.
Includes bibliographical references and index.
ISBN 978-1-59385-655-7 (hard cover : alk. paper)
1. Manic–depressive illness—Treatment. 2. Family counseling. I. Title.
[DNLM: 1. Bipolar Disorder—therapy. 2. Adolescent. 3. Adult. 4. Family Therapy.
WM 207 M636b 2008]
RC516.M55 2008
616.89′506—dc22

2007049597

About the Author

David J. Miklowitz, PhD, is Professor of Psychology and Psychiatry at the University of Colorado at Boulder, and a Senior Clinical Research Fellow in the Department of Psychiatry at Oxford University. He completed his undergraduate work at Brandeis University and his doctoral and postdoctoral work at the University of California, Los Angeles (UCLA). His current research focuses on family psychoeducational treatments for childhood-onset bipolar disorder.

Dr. Miklowitz has received the Joseph Gengerelli Dissertation Award from UCLA (1986), Young Investigator Awards from the International Congress on Schizophrenia Research (1987) and the National Alliance for Research on Schizophrenia and Depression (NARSAD; 1987), a Research Faculty Award from the University of Colorado (1998), and a Distinguished Investigator Award from NARSAD (2001). Most recently he received the 2005 Mogens Schou Award for Research from the International Society for Bipolar Disorders, and the Monica Fooks lectureship from Oxford University. He has received funding for his research from the National Institute of Mental Health, the John D. and Catherine T. MacArthur Foundation, the Robert Sutherland Foundation, and the Danny Alberts Foundation.

Dr. Miklowitz has published more than 180 research articles and book chapters on bipolar disorder and schizophrenia, and four books, including *The Bipolar Disorder Survival Guide: What You and Your Family Need to Know*, a bestseller, and *The Bipolar Teen: What You Can Do to Help Your Child and Your Family* (with Elizabeth L. George). The first edition of *Bipolar Disorder: A Family-Focused Treatment Approach* won the 1998 Outstanding Research Publication Award from the American Association for Marriage and Family Therapy.

Preface

Bipolar affective disorder is a fascinating but tragic psychiatric condition. As a clinician and researcher, I often find myself marveling at the intensity with which individuals with this disorder experience life. Their creativity, energy, and artistic contributions have been well documented in the literature. But in appreciating these strengths, it is easy to overlook the severe suffering that these individuals and their families undergo. Even with the benefits of mood-stabilizing medications, persons with bipolar disorder experience intense pain, often in the form of ruined family relationships, financial problems, or lost hopes or dreams. Clearly, treatment for bipolar disorder must go beyond medication maintenance to include consideration of the familial and social–interpersonal aspects of this illness.

In the early 1980s, when I was a graduate student at the University of California, Los Angeles (UCLA), working with my colleague and mentor, the late Michael J. Goldstein, PhD, I became quite interested in the patients and families coping with this disorder. At first, this was only for the purpose of comparing their problems with those experienced by patients and families coping with schizophrenia. Goldstein had been the first to demonstrate the effectiveness of a short-term psychoeducational, crisis-oriented family intervention for schizophrenia patients (Goldstein, Rodnick, Evans, May, & Steinberg, 1978) and was enthused when I first suggested we examine the family processes—and, potentially, family treatment—in another major, recurrent psychiatric disorder.

Sometimes our best research ideas come directly from our clinical observations. While conducting a therapy group for bipolar patients, I became impressed that the patients consistently reported that their illness episodes were associated with periods of intense family conflict. But it was unclear to me, and to others at the time, whether features of the patient's family environment were somehow causally connected to bipolar affective symptoms, whether these symptoms generated a great deal of family conflict, or whether the patient's symptoms and the family's reactions were both brought about by some third variable, like a shared genetic predisposition to affective disorder. We proceeded to study these questions longitudinally: Were qualities of the family environment, if not causally related to the onset of mood disorder recurrences, at least predictive of them? A study described in Chapter 1 (Miklowitz, Goldstein, Nuechterlein, Snyder, & Mintz, 1988) verified this core hypothesis.

Based in part on these longitudinal findings, as well as on similar literature that appeared at about the same time, we felt our next step was to design and pilot a treatment for the families and married couples coping with bipolar disorder. When we began our studies, the primary treatments for bipolar disorder were exclusively medical, and in most cases limited to lithium carbonate or carbamazepine. There was little belief in the prophylactic value of psychotherapy, either by itself or combined with standard medications.

Michael Goldstein and I were fortunate to be associated with the UCLA Clinical Research Center for the Study of Schizophrenia, which had for years been conducting studies on the role of family psychoeducational treatment in combination with pharmacotherapy for schizophrenia patients. We adapted the structure provided by one of the treatments developed by the UCLA Center: behavioral family management for schizophrenia (Falloon, Boyd, & McGill, 1984; Liberman, 1988). This model consisted of four components: assessment of the functioning of the family during and following a patient's hospitalization for acute psychosis, psychoeducation for the patient and family about schizophrenia, communication skills training, and problem-solving skills training.

We found that this family treatment model for schizophrenia had to be revised substantially for bipolar patients and their families. First, bipolar patients appeared to us to be more verbally assertive, higher in social and job functioning, and more able to benefit from exploratory psychological interventions than schizophrenia patients. Second, bipolar patients were more often married and had substantial relationship conflicts related to their disorder. Third, their persistent denial of the disorder and resistance to accepting necessary medications, combined with family members' emotional reactions to these stances by the patients, stood out to us as key features of the patients' and family members' ongoing struggles.

With funding from the National Institute of Mental Health (Grant Nos. MH42556, MH43931, MH55101, and MH62555), and from the

National Alliance for Research on Schizophrenia and Depression, we were able to examine further the family processes associated with bipolar disorder and to develop and test through controlled experimental trials a new psychoeducational intervention, which we titled family-focused treatment (FFT). This treatment is designed for the bipolar patient who has had a recent manic or depressive episode (with or without hospitalization) and who returns to live with or to be in close association with caretaking family members, usually parents or spouses.

Although we retained the basic structure of Falloon's and Liberman's family treatment, we substantially revised each of the modules to address the core problems, resistances, and psychological conflicts that characterized the patients and family members coping with bipolar disorder.

Since its initial development, my colleagues and I have treated over 200 patients and families with the FFT approach. We have covered the full age range, including adolescents as young as age 13, college students with first onsets of mania, middle-aged patients in marital couples, and the elderly. We have treated lower- and upper-socioeconomic-status patients and patients of varied race and ethnicity. Our clients consistently report having benefited from the treatment, even after the 9-month treatment phase has been completed (see Chapter 1). In turn, we have learned a great deal from them: They inform us, on a relatively regular basis, as to which aspects of our treatment are helpful and which need to be improved or revised. In fact, our final treatment manual, as presented in this book, reflects revisions based not only on our own clinical judgments but on the feedback we have received from our patients and their relatives, as well as from the many clinicians we have trained over the years to administer the treatment.

This book describes the FFT approach in two major parts. In Part I, I describe the research and clinical background that led to the development of the treatment. Part II is a manual for delivering the assessment, psychoeducation, communication enhancement, and problem-solving modules of the treatment. Numerous clinical case examples are offered throughout the book. Although the examples given are based on actual patients and families, I have changed all names and other identifying information. I have also modified and edited treatment session dialogues for the sake of clarity, brevity, and additional protection of patient and family confidentiality.

This second edition differs from the first in two ways. First, it includes significant new research that has been completed since the first edition. Three randomized trials have demonstrated the efficacy of FFT in combination with drug treatment for stabilizing or preventing episodes of bipolar disorder among adults. One of the studies, the large-scale, 15-site Systematic Treatment Enhancement Program for Bipolar

Disorder (STEP-BD) showed that FFT hastened recovery from depressive episodes as compared with a psychosocial control condition (Miklowitz et al., 2007b).

Second, in 1998 my colleagues and I began to expand our work into the treatment of adolescents with the disorder. Our initial results using FFT for teens (Miklowitz, Biuckians, & Richards, 2006) indicate that it is both effective in symptom stabilization and acceptable to adolescents and parents. New case studies have been added to this second edition to illustrate the FFT approach with teens. The ways in which the core clinical techniques (e.g., communication enhancement training) can be modified to adapt to the developmental requirements of teens are discussed throughout the book.

It is my hope that the reader will come away from the book with a clearer understanding of the syndrome of bipolar disorder and the problems experienced by patients and family members during and after illness episodes. I hope it will become clear how the illness can affect families at different stages in its development. Moreover, I hope that the reader will begin to become capable of carrying out the treatment with his or her patients, whether they be young or old.

Many persons contributed to the development of the ideas reflected in this book. Margaret Rea, PhD, who served as a family clinician and family treatment supervisor at UCLA and later at the University of California, Davis, was most helpful in contributing case examples. Thanks are also due to Ellen Frank, PhD, and David Kupfer, MD, for their influential ideas on the individual–interpersonal treatment of bipolar disorder and for introducing us to the social rhythm stability interventions that we now regularly use. Robert Prien, PhD, and Joel Sherrill, PhD, of the National Institute of Mental Health, provided us with much intellectual guidance, given their substantial experience in conducting longitudinal and treatment–outcome research with mood disorders.

A wonderful team of graduate students and postdoctoral fellows served as therapists in our controlled treatment trials. At the University of Colorado, these included Elizabeth George, PhD, Dawn Taylor, PhD, Barbara Dausch, PhD, Aparna Kalbag, PhD, Kim Mullen, MA, Adrine Biuckians, MA, Jeffrey Richards, MA, Natalie Sachs-Ericsson, PhD, Teresa Simoneau, PhD, Tina Goldstein, PhD, and Eunice Kim, PhD. At UCLA, these included Jeff Ball, PhD, Jennifer Christian-Herman, PhD, Meg Racenstein, MA, Martha Tompson, PhD, Dawn Velligan, PhD, and Joseph Ventura, PhD. Thanks are also due to Shirley Glynn, PhD, Angus Strachan, PhD, and the late Gayla Blackwell, MSW, who provided family treatment supervision.

I would also like to thank the University of Colorado at Boulder for providing a 1-year Faculty Fellowship in 1995–1996, and again in 2006–

2007, during which the first and second editions of this book were written.

Special thanks are due to Kitty Moore, Executive Editor at The Guilford Press, a talented, encouraging, knowledgeable, and upbeat editor. Thanks for making the process of writing this book so much fun!

I would like to pay tribute to the contributions of Lyman Wynne, MD, and Ian Falloon, MD, both of whom passed away in 2006. Both were formative influences in my own career and encouraged me to follow my interests in the family, even when the field was becoming increasingly focused on neurobiology and genetics.

This book, like the first edition, is dedicated to Michael J. Goldstein, who passed away on March 13, 1997. His impact on me, both professionally and personally, was greater than I could have possibly imagined when we first met in 1979. It is my hope that this book will do honor to his memory and immeasurable contributions to our field.

DAVID J. MIKLOWITZ

Contents

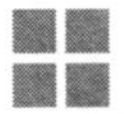

PART I. Bipolar Disorder and Families: Clinical and Research Background

BIPOLAR DISORDER

PART I

Bipolar Disorder and Families

Clinical and Research Background

chapter 1

Bipolar Disorder

Why Family Treatment?

Stewart was admitted to a city hospital for an acute episode of mania. He was extremely irritable and euphoric, pressured in his speech, and preoccupied with his "campaign" for the U.S. presidential election, for which he claimed to be a write-in candidate. The admitting physician immediately put him on a combination of lithium and antipsychotic medications, but his hospitalization lasted only 8 days. For his wife, Susan, this hospitalization seemed too short, given how ill he had been when he was admitted. In fact, in the weeks after his discharge his symptoms were still quite evident: He still slept only 4 hours per night, continued to talk of how he could "wire the presidential election," became angered easily, had trouble concentrating on conversations, and behaved in an embarrassing manner in public (talking and laughing too loudly, yelling inappropriately at waiters in restaurants). His intention to return to his computer programming job seemed to Susan like a pipe dream.

Susan tried to arrange for outpatient care with the same physician who had treated Stewart on an inpatient basis. However, Stewart refused to see this doctor, arguing heatedly, "That was the same guy who locked me up in those restraints." He finally agreed to a session at a local mental health center with a staff psychiatrist. He did not like this doctor either, describing him as "an idiot in a lab coat." Becoming desperate, Susan tried to get an appointment with a social worker at the center, only to be told there was a 3-week waiting list for such an appointment. She read everything she could get her hands on to educate herself about bipolar disorder, but everything pointed to the importance of taking medication and being under the regular care of a psychiatrist. She became quite angry with Stewart: Much of his behavior—particularly his unwillingness to consult a psychiatrist—seemed purposeful and intent upon hurting her. Stewart reacted to her criticisms by "upping the ante" and threatening to leave her.

Meanwhile, Stewart's symptoms did not abate, and the prescription given to him at the time of his discharge was starting to run out. He turned his anger upon his wife, arguing that what she was calling his symptoms of mania were really his personality and that he didn't need the medication at all. One night, after a heated argument, he revealed that he had discontinued his medications 3 days earlier to prove to her that he was healthy. "See?" he yelled triumphantly. "You said I'd have a breakdown, but here I am!"

Two days later, Stewart's behavior became increasingly disorganized. His condition resembled that which had led him into the hospital in the first place. That night, he disappeared. Early in the morning, Susan was telephoned by a police officer, who said that Stewart had been arrested while trying to break into the downtown Republican election headquarters. He was again admitted to the hospital with a recurrence of mania.

One could describe the events that occurred in this case from several different vantage points. A *biological psychiatrist* would argue (1) that Stewart's brain has genetically determined imbalances in catecholamines or other neurotransmitter or hormone systems, (2) that these must be corrected with medication, and (3) that his unwillingness to take medications has made his illness worse. In contrast, a traditional *family systems-oriented* practitioner, although perhaps not denying the presence of a biological predisposition, would argue that Stewart's disturbed behavior cannot be separated from his distressed marital relationship, which is both a cause and an effect of his symptoms and drug noncompliance. Moreover, a *community mental health-minded* professional would view Stewart and Susan's experiences as reflecting inadequacies in the delivery of mental health services to those who are most needy, and speaking to the need for better continuity of care between inpatient and outpatient services, and between different mental health subdisciplines.

Which of these views is correct? Aren't they all correct? What model might pull these different arguments together? From my perspective as a *family psychoeducational* clinician, I would agree that this patient is indeed dealing with a biologically based disorder that is likely to recur if not treated with medication. However, I would also argue that the course of his illness is influenced by the stress in his marital relationship, even if this relationship did not play a causal role in the original onset of the disorder. Likewise, Stewart's wife is suffering, rather severely, from the burden of taking care of her ill husband and from the frustration of trying to find answers. Finally, I would argue that this patient has not accepted the fact that he has a severe, recurrent psychiatric illness, a precondition for agreeing to a medication regimen. Thus, this couple needs to be educated about Stewart's illness—bipolar disorder—and taught to communicate about and solve problems related to the stress it causes for both of them. They also need coaching in how to obtain proper pharmacological care and make the mental health system work for them.

This is a book about bipolar disorder and families. In it, I recount the problems experienced by patients and their family members who are trying to adapt to this lifelong condition. I also describe how, based on both my and others' research and clinical experience, they can benefit from a psychoeducational, family-focused treatment (FFT).

How Is Bipolar Disorder a Family Problem?

Bipolar disorder is a relapsing and remitting illness. Even patients receiving optimal medication are likely to have multiple recurrences and to have trouble holding jobs, maintaining relationships, and getting along with their significant others (Perlis et al., 2006; Gitlin, Swendsen, Heller, & Hammen, 1995; Coryell et al., 1993).

The behavioral and emotional experiences of the person with bipolar disorder affect everyone—the patient's parents, spouse, siblings, and children. In fact, as hospitalizations have become shorter and shorter, and as patients are discharged in quite unstable clinical states, the burden on the family has become considerable (Perlick, Hohenstein, Clarkin, Kaczynski, & Rosenheck, 2005). In this milieu, family members need support, education, and advice in coping with the ups and downs of their relative's condition.

A second reason to view bipolar disorder as a family problem stems from the effects of the family environment on the course of this disorder. Several years ago, we examined in our research a cohort of hospitalized bipolar, manic patients whom we followed over a 9-month outpatient period (Miklowitz et al., 1988). We found something quite interesting, as well as clinically useful: A patient who returns from the hospital to a stressful family environment is at greater risk for subsequent recurrences of the disorder. When recently manic patients returned from the hospital to high-expressed-emotion (EE) homes (those in which relatives held attitudes such as criticism, hostility, or emotional overinvolvement toward the patient) or to homes characterized by negative, conflictual interactional patterns (negative *affective style* [AS]), their chances of relapsing were much higher than if they returned to low-conflict, relatively benign home situations. Further, patients from stressful environments did not function as well over time in the social–interpersonal domain as those in less stressful environments.

Interestingly, the frequent follow-ups with patients and relatives required by this study had the side effect of bringing us in close contact with the impact of a bipolar patient's disorder on his or her family, and vice versa. It became obvious to us that episodes of bipolar disorder were major life events not only for the patient, but for all who cared about him or her. Patients and relatives frequently turned to us for advice, even when our only role in the case was to conduct follow-up interviews. It appeared that no one else was available to assist them with their many problems related to dealing with the disorder.

Why FFT?

Our observations in our research and clinical work suggested we take the next step by developing a family-focused intervention program. This program, we believed, could be analogous to the psychoeducational programs that had been developed and found successful in delaying relapses for patients with schizophrenia (for a review, see Pitschel-Walz, Leucht, Bäuml, Kissling, & Engel, 2001) and should include the core components of these approaches: psychoeducation, communication skills training, and problem-solving skills training. However, we felt this program would need to address some of the unique issues relevant to bipolar patients in family contexts (described below).

This book describes our model for the family treatment of bipolar disorder. *It is not a treatment that should stand alone, but, rather, is an important component of the combined pharmacological and psychosocial treatment of the disorder.* When the model and procedures proposed here are implemented properly, they provide an organizing framework within which the goals of the pharmacological treatment can be more readily achieved. A close working relationship between the bipolar patient and his or her close family members can not only address the multiple psychological problems that emerge in the context of this disorder, but can also facilitate the patient's willingness to follow a prescribed medication regimen.

The FFT described in this book has grown out of our experience over the last 25 years in treating and conducting research with more than 300 bipolar patients—both youths and adults. These treatments have been carried out in the context of controlled clinical trials that I and my close colleagues have directed. In general, these trials have addressed the postepisode phases of a patient's bipolar disorder.

The Six Objectives of FFT

How might the symptomatic course of bipolar disorder be improved by adding a family intervention to medication maintenance? A family program has to address six important objectives if it is to have a significant impact on the stressful family relationships accompanying episodes of the disorder.

Goal 1. Assist the Patient and Relatives in Integrating the Experiences Associated with Episodes of Bipolar Disorder

Stewart and Susan began the FFT program shortly after his second hospitalization. They both were quite shaken and confused by what had occurred. Susan appeared to be experiencing a posttraumatic stress reaction, with intense, free-floating anxiety and fears that Stewart would relapse any minute. She raised the question of whether he really had bipolar disorder or some other condition—she had spoken by phone to one clinician who told her Stewart might have multiple personality disorder. Stewart, who continued to show symptoms, denied that he had even had a manic episode, arguing that he had simply been "talking too much and drinking too much coffee." He related difficult, humiliating experiences in the hospital and railed against the incompetence of the mental health system.

My colleagues and I frequently observe that patients and families have difficulty (1) recognizing the essential features of this disorder, (2) understanding the nature of the inner experience of a person who undergoes a manic or depressive episode, and (3) accepting the seriousness of the illness. Thus, a family-focused intervention must provide a theoretical structure within which patients and their relatives can gain a greater understanding of the disorder and assimilate, in a meaningful way, what has transpired in their lives. This is particularly significant for the bipolar patient who struggles to deny the seriousness of his or her disorder. But we also frequently find in the patient's relatives a struggle to accept the existence of a major psychiatric disorder in a loved one.

Goal 2. Assist the Patient and Relatives in Accepting the Notion of a Vulnerability to Future Episodes

Although there is wide variation in the clinical status of patients in the period following an acute episode of bipolar disorder, in general their most flamboyant symptoms are muted and sometimes barely evident. It is easy at this juncture to assume that the episode was a discrete event that had a beginning and is now at an end. In the absence of the most dramatic symptoms, both patients and relatives attempt to convince themselves that this was a one-time event with few implications for the future. "It won't happen again" is a frequent refrain from patients and their relatives.

The evidence I discuss in Chapter 2 strongly suggests otherwise. Thus, a major goal of FFT is to help the patient and close relatives accept that bipolar disorder is real, and that it is a chronic condition requiring long-term management. With successful management, a more benign life course can be achieved, but without it, a downward course is very likely. Of course, acceptance of an underlying vulnerability in the face of apparent recovery is a difficult challenge. For the patient, it involves a painful restructuring of his or her self-concept, and for the relatives, substantially revising their view of the loved one.

Goal 3. Assist the Patient and Relatives in Accepting a Dependency on Mood-Stabilizing Medication for Symptom Control

Stewart had already had one instance of medication nonadherence, precipitating his second manic episode. After being discharged from the hospital the second time, he agreed to a trial of lithium, Prozac, and Navane (an antipsychotic) for "3 months max." He denied having an illness and noted with an irritated tone that he was taking medication "because I have to," and "because other people say I'm better if I do, even if I feel a lot worse." Susan, in turn, argued with dismay, "You should be just taking it for yourself!" She was understandably worried that he would discontinue his medications again. When she pushed him to stay on his medications, he would mock her by sucking his thumb and saying, in a lisp, "Honey, would you get me my Prothac?"

As I discuss in Chapter 2, the evidence for the prophylactic value of mood-regulating medications is very compelling. Clinicians recognize this evidence, but it is not always easy for bipolar patients, and sometimes their relatives, to do so. Often, patients or relatives recognize the necessity of medication during the period immediately after an acute manic or depressive episode, but over time their feelings change. Why take pills, which can have some unwanted side effects, when you or your relative is doing well? This is a reasonable question to ask and is often at the root of what clinicians term *noncompliance* or *nonadherence.* About 40% of people with bipolar disorder are partially or fully nonadherent with their medications over a 2-year period, and as many as two-thirds become nonadherent over their lifetimes (Colom et al., 2005).

In my experience, problems with adherence to a recommended medication management program are often the basis of very intense conflicts between bipolar patients and their close family members. Thus, this issue must be addressed intensively and repeatedly in a family-focused program. Family psychoeducation has to address this issue at two levels: at a cognitive level, by providing important information about the risks of stopping maintenance medication; and at an affective level, by addressing significant feelings of patients and their relatives about this dependence. The FFT treatment model is designed to assist the patient and his or her close relatives in working through the emotional resistances to pharmacotherapy.

Obviously, there is a significant linkage between the second goal and this one. When the patient and close relatives can accept, despite clinical improvement following the most recent episode, that there is an underlying vulnerability to future episodes, acceptance of the need for a prophylactic medication regimen is more readily achieved.

Goal 4. Assist the Patient and Close Relatives in Distinguishing between the Patient's Personality and His or Her Bipolar Disorder

Stewart continually maintained that the behaviors other people were calling "mania" were really just exaggerations of his personality and temperament. In contrast, for Susan, everything Stewart did had become a sign of his bipolar disorder. She began labeling his reactions to even mundane daily events as signs of an impending relapse. Her hypervigilance led to great hostility on Stewart's part, who said, "You can't just hand me a tablet of lithium every time I laugh at a movie." His hostile reactions convinced Susan even further that he was relapsing again.

FFT is oriented toward assisting members of a family to accept the existence of bipolar disorder in one of them. But there can be hazards in this approach. For example, the family may come to this acceptance fairly readily and begin to see everything the patient feels or does as a sign of his or her disorder. These perhaps overgeneralized attributions cause great resentment in the patient, who may begin to lose the ability to distinguish his or her normal emotions or desires from pathological ones. Like the proverbial centipede who, when asked how he moved all 100 legs with such beautiful coordination, could not do it anymore once he thought about it, the person with bipolar disorder can be similarly paralyzed by an excessive vigilance for signs of his or her disorder.

Many patients who stop taking mood-stabilizing medication do so to distinguish their normal personality from the effects of the drugs they are taking. As one patient expressed it, "I don't know what's me and what is due to the lithium. I need to know what I'm like without it."

We have observed another, quite different side effect of education about bipolar disorder, namely, overidentification with the diagnosis by the person with the disorder. Once such patients accept the diagnosis, it explains everything. They cannot be successful in their careers because they have bipolar disorder, or relationships go sour because they have bipolar disorder, and so on. The net result is that these patients, and ironically, sometimes their relatives, no longer accept responsibility for improving their lives.

Given these hazards, it is vital that a family-focused program assist patients and their family members in finding a way to recognize the enduring qualities that define the personality of the individual with bipolar disorder (particularly those qualities that reflect positive attributes) and to distinguish them from the early warning signs of the return of the disorder. When the patient and family begin to acknowledge these continuities in the self and to challenge their assumptions that being bipolar means giving up a happy or productive life, an important impasse has been broken in their struggles to accept the disorder.

Goal 5. Assist the Patient and Family in Recognizing and Learning to Cope with Stressful Life Events That Trigger Recurrences of Bipolar Disorder

Approximately 1 month before his first manic episode, Stewart had been functioning well on a regular 9-to-5 shift at his computer programming job. However, as a result of corporate downsizing, his firm decided to redefine his job requirements and give him expanded duties and an increased salary. He was at first quite pleased with this, but the new duties required that he work well into the evening and on weekends. He tried to adapt to this new schedule by drinking excessive amounts of coffee, but found he was too "wired" and overstimulated to go to sleep at his usual time. He began to experience racing thoughts concerning new and more efficient computer programs, most of which sounded unrealistic to others.

He began to feel more agitated at work and started having run-ins with his boss and coworkers. Stewart's boss suggested he take a leave of absence and "get a handle on his nerves." Stewart reluctantly agreed, and tried to get back on a normal sleep–wake cycle. However, he continued arguing with Susan and began avoiding her by spending more and more time away from home. He found it increasingly difficult to sleep at night, and his mania escalated until he stopped sleeping altogether. When he was eventually hospitalized, he hadn't slept in several days and had developed paranoid delusions regarding plots against him initiated by his wife, boss, and coworkers.

The family-focused program described in this book is based on a vulnerability–stress model. This model emphasizes the interaction of genetic and biological factors that define the vulnerability to the disorder, and environmental stress factors that activate the underlying vulnerabilities. Our model is founded on the notion that patients and their relatives are best served when they comprehend how these two classes of factors interact with one another.

I have frequently observed that bipolar patients and their close family members do not recognize an association between life events inside or outside the family and the onset of an illness episode. As discussed in subsequent chapters, life events (such as Stewart's change in job duties) often interact with biological vulnerabilities (e.g., a central nervous system that is highly reactive to changes in the sleep–wake cycle) in producing symptoms of mania. Thus, one of the major objectives of FFT is to heighten awareness of the significance of stressful events in the life of the patient and of the family unit.

With this awareness, patients and their close relatives are more willing to examine their previous coping patterns, which may not have been effective in managing significant life events. In particular, discussions of life events open the door for patients and close relatives to examine their communication and problem-solving styles, as a prelude to developing more effective ways of dealing with stressors both inside and outside the family.

Goal 6. Assist the Family in Reestablishing Functional Relationships after the Episode

As the case of Stewart exemplifies, family relationships become quite dysfunctional in the prodromal, active, and postepisode phases of bipolar disorder. When the patient has been manic, the conflicts tend to center on his or her residual hostility, grandiosity, and denial of the disorder, as well as his or her need to reestablish independence and the often-associated rejection of a medication regimen. Family members in turn may react with criticism or overprotectiveness. In contrast, when the patient becomes depressed, family members at first try hard to help, but eventually become angry and rejecting when no amount of support seems to be enough (e.g., Coyne, Downey, & Boergers, 1992). These family conflicts cause a great deal of stress and anxiety and put a substantial burden on caretaking relatives. In turn, their negative reactions may be associated with poorer outcomes of the patient's disorder.

A major focus of FFT is to encourage the patient and family members to develop skills for open family communication and problem solving. However, unlike family psychoeducational programs for schizophrenia (e.g., Falloon et al., 1984, 1985), our focus is less on skill acquisition and more on the effects of new communication techniques on the family system. Specifically, when persons in a family are able to listen to each other and offer positive and negative feedback in constructive ways, role relationships change, power imbalances become more egalitarian, and healthier alliances develop. The result is that families who were previously critical or overprotective instead become protective influences in the course of the patient's disorder and aid his or her adaptation to a medication regimen.

The Core Assumptions and Structure of FFT

In addition to the six basic objectives outlined above, there are three core, interrelated assumptions about episodes of bipolar disorder and the need for a family-focused psychoeducational program (Table 1.1). On the basis of our clinical and research work, we have concluded that an episode of bipolar disorder is a very stressful life event for a patient and his or her family, an event that significantly disrupts the family's equilibrium. This event must be understood and accepted, but also requires the development of new coping strategies to deal with its aftermath and its likely recurrence in the future. To address these issues, we have developed three relatively distinct treatment phases or modules (after Falloon et al., 1984): *a psychoeducational phase, a communication enhancement training phase* (CET), and *a problem-solving training phase.* These treatment modules are normally delivered in 12 weekly, 6 biweekly, and 3 monthly sessions (21 total) spread over a 9-month outpatient period following a manic or depressive episode. Clinicians can also offer booster sessions after the 9-month period is over, depending on their availability and the family's needs.

The first phase—psychoeducation—involves assisting the patient and close relatives in comprehending the nature of the disorder and

TABLE 1.1. Significant Assumptions Underlying FFT

- An episode of bipolar disorder represents a disaster for the whole family system.
- Like other disasters, each episode of the disorder produces a state of disorganization in the family system.
- The overall goal of a family-focused program is to assist the family to achieve a new state of equilibrium.

its often disastrous consequences. This includes providing them with a model for understanding the origins and course of the disorder and a rationale for various components of the treatment program. Providing this information reduces guilt and mutual recrimination among family members and creates a readiness for change in family relationships.

The second phase—CET—involves assisting patients and family members to establish or reestablish effective communication patterns with one another. Many psychiatric disorders produce a deterioration in the capacity of family members and patients to communicate. This is particularly acute with a severe condition like bipolar disorder, where the symptoms of the active phase of the disorder have blocked normal communication and the residue of the episode leaves everyone unsure of how to talk to each other or reluctant to do so. Thus, an effective family-focused program needs to provide a context in which clear and effective communication can occur.

The third phase—problem solving—involves training in bringing about effective conflict resolutions. Any disaster interferes with the ability of members of a family to solve problems of daily living. Thus, a psychoeducational program needs to provide a structure in which effective problem solving can occur and to stimulate activities in which problem-solving techniques can be spontaneously implemented.

In addition to these core treatment modules, we have found that recurrent crises are expectable in the course of recovery from an episode of bipolar disorder. Most patients nowadays leave hospitals with residual symptoms—such as ongoing depression and intermittent suicidal feelings or impulses—that are difficult for them or their relatives to handle. Major or minor exacerbations of the disorder are very likely during this phase, and rarely does the course of the disorder run smoothly. Moreover, many patients develop or show a continuation of substance abuse problems that interfere with their recovery and responses to medication. Thus, a significant component of FFT is crisis intervention, provided by a clinician who knows the family well and is readily available. In our experience, this type of access to care can be extremely important in dealing with the early signs of the recurrence of the disorder and preventing full-blown relapses.

Is FFT Helpful?

There is an increasing emphasis within the research and clinical communities on empirically demonstrating the efficacy of new psychosocial treatments, usually through randomized clinical trials (RCTs) involving experimental treatment groups and comparison or control groups. As indicated above, FFT is a fairly well-operationalized treatment with a clear outline and thus lends itself to experimental evaluation.

We have evaluated the efficacy of FFT with bipolar patients in three RCTs, one at the University of Colorado at Boulder, one at the University of California, Los Angeles (UCLA), and one in a multicenter effectiveness study called the Systematic Treatment Enhancement Program for Bipolar Disorder. Much of the clinical material presented in this book is drawn from these trials. Clearly, FFT benefits patients and families coping with bipolar disorder.

Initial Pilot Work

We began with a pilot study at UCLA in 1987–1988. We treated nine patients who had been admitted to the hospital with a manic episode and offered them and their family members (parents or spouses) the 9-month, 21-session FFT protocol (psychoeducation, CET, and problem-solving training). All patients were treated with standard medications for bipolar disorder (either lithium carbonate, carbamazepine, or both, with adjunctive antipsychotic or antidepressant medications). We compared them with 23 patients consecutively admitted into a 9-month longitudinal program consisting of similar, aggressively delivered medications and active case management by our team, but no FFT (Miklowitz & Goldstein, 1990). The two groups were comparable in age, gender, and illness characteristics.

We examined proportions of manic and depressive relapses in each group over 9-month periods of follow-up. The rate of relapse was only 11% (1 of 9) in the FFT group, whereas it was 61% (14 of 23) in the comparison, no-FFT group. This finding of reduced relapse rates among patients in FFT encouraged us to evaluate the efficacy of the treatment in RCTs.

The Colorado RCT

The first RCT was conducted at the University of Colorado (Miklowitz, George, Richards, Simoneau, & Suddath, 2003; Miklowitz et al., 2000). Patients (N = 101) were recruited in a manic, depressive, or mixed affective episode and, after individual and family assessments, were randomly assigned to FFT or to a comparison treatment condition called crisis management (CM). The CM consisted of two sessions of family education and crisis intervention sessions offered as needed over the next 9 months, At minimum, patients in CM received one telephone call per month from a crisis manager. Patients in both treatment conditions received modern pharmacological treatment using mood-stabilizing medications (for details, see Miklowitz et al., 2003).

As indicated in Figure 1.1, patients who participated in FFT with their parents or spouses, and who also received medications, were much less likely to relapse during the 2-year study than patients who received CM and medications. In fact, patients in FFT were three times more likely to finish the study without relapsing and had longer periods of stability without relapse (73.5 weeks vs. 53.2 weeks). FFT was also associated with lower depression and mania severity scores over 2 years. Furthermore, patients in FFT were more likely to maintain adherence to their recommended mood-stabilizing medications than patients in CM. This enhanced level of adherence contributed to their lower mania scores over the 2-year study (Miklowitz et al., 2003).

In further analyses of this Colorado study, Simoneau, Miklowitz, Richards, Saleem, and George (1999) found that intrafamilial communication improved among patients and family members in FFT. As compared with patients in the CM condition, participants in FFT (both patients and key relatives) showed dramatic increases from pre- to posttreatment in the frequency of positive communication, as assessed in laboratory-based family problem-solving interactions. They showed increases in communication behaviors such as self-disclosures of feelings, statements of support to other members of the family, paraphrasing of each other's ideas, and statements intended to help define and solve problems. There were increases in the frequencies of positive nonverbal behaviors (e.g., smiling, helpful gesturing) as well, particularly among patients. Patients and family members in the comparison condition actually showed decreases over

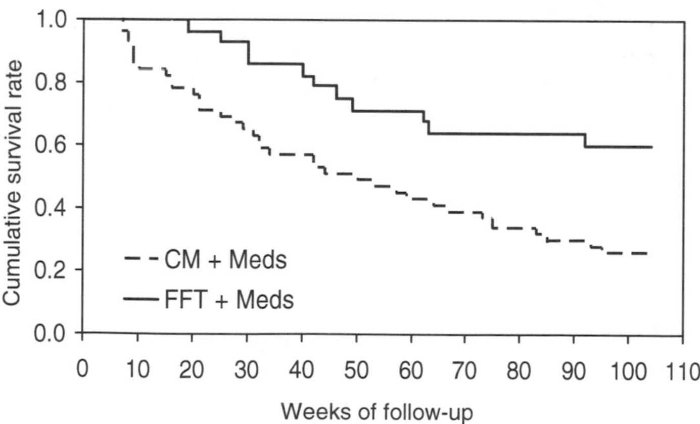

FIGURE 1.1. FFT + medication delays relapse more than crisis management and medication. $N = 101$; $p = .003$; FFT, mean survival = 73.5 weeks; CM, 53.2 weeks. From Miklowitz et al. (2003). Copyright 2003 by the American Medical Association. Reprinted by permission.

time in the frequencies of these kinds of verbal and nonverbal behaviors. When patients showed improvements in their interactions with relatives from pre- to posttreatment, they also showed greater improvements in their illness over 1 year.

The UCLA Study

The UCLA study was carried out in tandem with the Colorado study (Rea et al., 2003). In the UCLA study, patients who had been hospitalized for mania—and who returned following the hospitalization to their parents' homes—were randomly assigned as outpatients to FFT and medications or to individual therapy and medications. The individual therapy had many of the same ingredients as the FFT—psychoeducation, relapse prevention planning, and encouragement of medication adherence—but families were not involved. Like those in FFT, patients in individual therapy received 21 weekly, biweekly, and then monthly therapy sessions over 9 months, as well as the same types of medications.

The results are pictured in Figure 1.2. Patients in FFT and those in individual therapy had similar rates of relapse and rehospitalization during the first year of the study, during which they were getting the study-based psychotherapies. Once this year was over, however, patients in individual therapy relapsed (60%) and were rehospitalized (60%) at a much higher rate than patients in FFT (28% and 12%, respectively). In addition, when patients in FFT did relapse, they were less likely to require hospitalization than the patients in individual therapy who relapsed. In all likelihood, parents became skilled in identifying when their son or daughter was getting manic and called the psychiatrist for a change in medications when these prodromal signs were present. We concluded that FFT was not effective just because it was longer than other

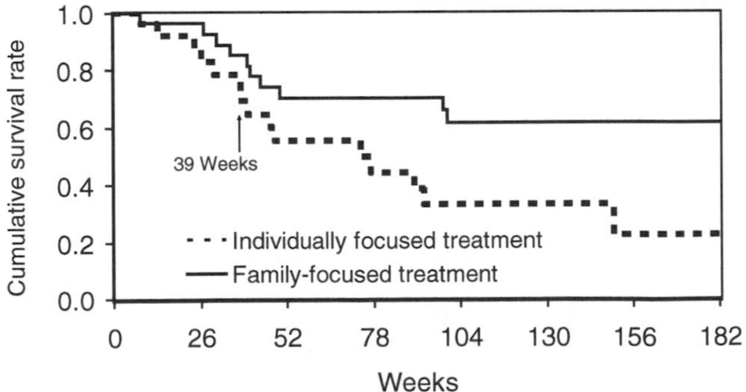

FIGURE 1.2. Greater persistence of effects of family versus individual therapy: Time to rehospitalization. UCLA FFT study. $N = 53$; $\chi^2(1) = 3.87$; $p < .05$.

comparison therapies. Instead, engaging the family, educating its members (including the patient) about the illness, and forming an alliance with them as treatment partners over the long-term course of the illness was more beneficial to the patient than psychoeducation in an individual format.

The Systematic Treatment Enhancement Program

The studies discussed above were conducted at the sites in which FFT was developed (Colorado and UCLA). How did FFT fare when tested at other sites around the country where clinicians may have had different theoretical orientations? Modern views on empirically supported treatments recommend that a treatment be tested in sites different from its origination site, as a way of minimizing the effects of theoretical allegiances to a particular program (Chambless & Hollon, 1998).

In the 15-site, NIMH-funded Systematic Treatment Enhancement Program for Bipolar Disorder, or STEP-BD (Miklowitz et al., 2007a, 2007b; Sachs et al., 2003), 293 patients with bipolar depression took part in a medication study and were randomly assigned to intensive psychotherapy (30 sessions over 9 months) or to brief psychoeducational therapy (3 sessions over 6 weeks). The intensive therapies offered varied by the site of the study and included FFT, interpersonal and social rhythm therapy (Frank, 2005), or cognitive-behavioral therapy (Newman, Leahy, Beck, Reilly-Harrington, & Gyulai, 2002. The brief therapy was called collaborative care (CC).

Over 1 year, we found that being in *any* of the three intensive psychotherapies led to higher recovery rates from bipolar depression (64.4%) than being in CC (51.5%) (p = .01) (Miklowitz et al., 2007b). Patients in intensive treatment were also 1.6 times more likely to remain well during any given month of the 1-year study than patients in the CC group. Year-end rates of recovery for the specific modalities were as follows: FFT, 77% (20/26), interpersonal therapy, 65% (40/62), and cognitive-behavioral therapy, 60% (45/75). Patients in intensive therapy also had better relationship functioning and higher life satisfaction at 1-year follow-up (Miklowitz et al., 2007a)

This study, while showing that FFT was effective when given in multiple sites around the country, also revealed one of its limitations: Many adult patients with bipolar disorder—about 46%—do not have families who are willing or able to come in for treatment. In STEP-BD we defined the family broadly, to include parents, spouses, siblings, romantic partners, and in a few cases, close friends. In cases where family members are unavailable or unwilling to take part in treatment, you can investigate these individual forms of therapy using the clinicians' manuals cited above.

Conclusion

FFT is a valuable and useful way to clinically engage patients and family members coping with bipolar disorder, and leads to better outcomes over 1- to 2-year periods than control treatments in symptomatic recovery or recurrence. Participants benefit in terms of their communication with each other and their abilities to solve family problems. Patients are also more likely to adhere to their medication regimens.

The Organization of This Book

This book is designed to orient clinicians to be capable of implementing FFT. It is organized to permit clinicians with different levels of familiarity with bipolar disorder to enter the book at different points. The first step in learning FFT is to be able to recognize the signs and symptoms of bipolar disorder, to understand its course and necessary drug treatments, and to gain an understanding of the impact of these illness factors on the family. Chapters 2 and 3 offer this background. Chapter 2 reviews the diagnostic criteria for the disorder, evidence regarding course and outcome, and the impact of medication regimens on the course of the illness. This chapter examines in detail the ways in which different symptom constellations of bipolar disorder and different patterns of the illness course affect family functioning. In turn, Chapter 3 discusses the roles of family relationships and stressful life events in influencing the course of the disorder.

Those familiar with this background material may wish to go directly to Part II (Chapters 4–13), which is devoted to the actual methods of treatment delivery. I describe our methods for connecting with and engaging families in treatment (Chapter 4), conducting initial family assessments (Chapter 5) and providing psychoeducation (Chapters 6–8), CET (Chapters 9 and 10), and problem-solving skills training (Chapter 11). Chapter 12 addresses managing clinical crises: how one deals within this treatment model with bipolar relapses, suicidality, and the crises associated with substance or alcohol abuse disorders. Finally, Chapter 13 discusses issues involved in the termination of the treatment.

In these chapters you will see some of the complexities that arise in delivering this model of treatment to the families of persons with bipolar disorder. We follow the guidelines presented in this book in providing a structure for families, but it is important to note that this structure can be useful only when delivered with a "psychotherapeutic attitude." I mean by this a sensitivity to emotional issues and resistances to change and a reliance on family and individual assessments to guide the content and focus of the sessions. Thus, these chapters outline the actual therapeutic techniques as well as our specific methods for dealing with resistances, crises, and complex emotional reactions among patients and families coping with this disorder.

Throughout the book, I give suggestions as to how to adapt the approach to the different settings in which clinicians are likely to work. For example, abbreviated versions of the treatment modules can be given in settings in which the practitioner is limited to a six-session contract. In these circumstances, one must decide which of the treatment modules is most applicable to a family under consideration: Some families may benefit most from the psychoeducation module, whereas others (particularly couples) may be better helped through the communication enhancement module.

For Whom Is This Book Intended?

FFT can be conducted with adult or adolescent patients with bipolar disorder, and examples of each are given throughout the book. This book does not target specific mental health subdisciplines. FFT can be delivered by clinicians in a variety of settings, including community mental health centers, health maintenance organizations (HMOs), hospital settings, forensic settings, and private practice. We have trained psychologists, psychology graduate students, social workers, marriage and family therapists, and psychiatric nurses to administer the treatment. We have also trained child and adult psychiatrists who desire a family-psychoeducational approach to medication management. The book is also applicable to researchers interested in treatment–outcome investigations or studies of the basic psychosocial processes associated with adult- or childhood-onset bipolar disorder. Finally, we believe that much useful information is provided for patients or family members who are coping with this disorder, who may begin to see in a different context the symptoms, life disruption, and family distress they experience.

Although I do not take a stand as to who should do this treatment, I believe that there are certain experiences that make it easier to learn the approach. They include some background and comfort in working with severely ill patients with mood disorders, training in psychotherapy, and experience in working therapeutically with groups, particularly families. These are not essential, but they are helpful. Further, some degree of familiarity with the medication management of bipolar disorder is useful, although the clinician can expect to learn some of the basics of this material in this book.

A Word about Terminology

In the forthcoming chapters, I use certain terms that require explanations. Particularly, when I refer to "family," I am including any of the various constellations the clinician is likely to encounter nowadays: (1) families with either one or two parents and an adult or underage offspring who is the patient, (2) couples in whom one member is bipolar (whether these be same- or opposite-sex pairings), (3) sibling pairs, (4) adoptive or foster families, and (5) other family constellations (e.g., grandparents raising ill grandchildren).

When I describe how the family clinician speaks with the family, I often use sentences that start with "we" rather than "I." This is because there are advantages to working in cotherapy teams, as discussed in Chapter 4. However, FFT can easily be conducted by a single therapist. I also refer to the reader as "you" rather than "the clinician," because of the unnecessary level of formality introduced by the latter term. Finally I use certain technical terms such as "vulnerability," "predispositions," "biochemical imbalances," and "psychosocial treatment." In conducting FFT, you should adapt your terminology to the educational level of the family, as well as your own style. Some clinicians prefer to use these medically based terms, and others prefer simpler language.

chapter 2

The Nature of Bipolar Disorder and Its Impact on the Family

Cathy, a 25-year-old European American woman, began to show behavioral changes approximately 2 months before her admission to a state psychiatric hospital. According to her mother, Marjorie, she became very active sexually, slept very little, and seemed easily provoked to anger. Approximately 2 weeks before her admission, she flew to Washington, D.C., to visit a boyfriend, and upon returning home was "acting strange," reciting rock music lyrics loudly, staying up until all hours of the night, cursing at her mother, charging expensive things on her credit cards, bringing different men home at night, and "telling her life story to strangers."

She was accompanied to the hospital by her mother. During the intake interview, the clinician inquired about a family history of psychopathology, including Marjorie's own history. Marjorie became quite defensive, saying, "You people always want to lay the blame on the mother!" She then refused to answer any other questions and insisted instead on talking to the head psychiatrist. Marjorie said, "I'm gonna go all the way up the ladder to get you people to cooperate!"

When the attending psychiatrist entered the interview room, Cathy was talking wildly about poetry and sex, speaking rapidly and nonsensically. Her mother frequently interrupted to correct her on facts of her recent history, and Cathy would angrily snap back, "That's your opinion. You weren't even there, as usual!" Her mother then responded defensively, saying, "You're not able to even tell your own story. How can you possibly live on your own and take care of yourself?" Cathy hammered back, "At least I have a man who wants me! Can you say the same?"

Chapter Overview

This case illustrates the behavior of a person with bipolar disorder during a manic episode. It also illustrates the way in which a close family member—in this case, a mother—can become engaged in the patient's experience and strongly affected by it. The patient's episode has been a traumatic life event for her and her mother, and the resulting family distress and conflict places Cathy at risk for future episodes.

In this chapter I offer the rationales for the first four of the six FFT goals (see Chapter 1): assisting patients and families to (1) integrate the experience of the mood disorder episode, (2) accept the vulnerability to future episodes, (3) accept the necessity of mood-stabilizing medications, and (4) learn to distinguish personality from the disorder. In explaining the basis of these goals, I review the core facts about the nature, symptoms, course, early warning signs, and drug treatment of bipolar disorder.

What are manic and depressive episodes like for the patient and family? What are the practical and psychosocial consequences of episodes? What empirical evidence exists that the patient is vulnerable to future episodes? What types of illness course patterns can the patient and his or her family members expect to see over time? Why should he or she have to accept taking medications—what is the evidence that they are effective in modifying the course of the disorder? Finally, what does the research literature say about personality and bipolar disorder—are the patient and his or her family members correct when they say that he or she has always been hyper, irritable, or grandiose? Can one identify the early warning signs of bipolar disorder on the basis of personality, temperament, or other childhood attributes?

You will be impressed by the variability in the course of the disorder and how, even with the best drug treatment, patients frequently relapse and have poor interpersonal and work functioning. In turn, families are left to pick up the pieces. It will become clear how a psychosocial treatment such as FFT can be an important supplement to the protection offered by mood-stabilizing medications. This background material—as well as the material on the psychosocial origins of the disorder presented in the next chapter—helps to clarify the underlying assumptions of our family treatment approach. These materials are critical to understanding the clinical methods articulated in Part II of this book.

What Is Bipolar Disorder?

Basic Facts

Bipolar disorder is a psychiatric disorder characterized by severe mood swings, from the highest of highs (manias) to the lowest of lows (depression). In its various forms, it affects about 4.5% of the population, or about 1 in every 22 persons (Merikangas et al., 2007). This rate breaks down into 1.0% for bipolar I disorder (at least one fully syndromal manic or mixed episode, as defined by the *Diagnostic and Statistical Manual of Mental Disorders*, fourth edition [DSM-IV]), 1.1% for bipolar II disorder (at least one major depressive episode and one hypomanic episode), and 2.4% for "subthreshold" bipolar disorder (subthreshold hypomania with major depression, or recurrent hypomanic or subthreshold hypomanic episodes without major depression). It affects men and women equally, although some studies show that women are more likely than men to have bipolar II disorder (Schneck et al., 2004). The average age at onset for bipolar I disorder is 18.2 years, and for bipolar II disorder, 20.3 years (Merikangas et al., 2007). Between 50 and 67% of these patients develop bipolar disorder by age 18, and between 15 and 28% before age 13 (Perlis et al., 2004).

Bipolar disorder is often quite debilitating, because patients usually have highly recurrent courses of illness. More than 90% of patients have recurrences of mania or depression over their lifetimes, with one study estimating that patients average three episodes and five hospitalizations over 10 years (Solomon, Keitner, Miller, Shea, & Keller, 1995; Winokur et al., 1994). Patients who have had one manic episode nearly always go on to have another, even if they are maintained on medications (Solomon et al., 2003). Bipolar I patients (those with full manic or mixed episodes) change symptom status an average of six times per year, and switch from depression to mania (or mania to depression) an average of three or more times per year. Even those who have infrequent recurrences show ongoing, significant symptoms between major episodes (Judd et al., 2002).

Researchers are finding that the depressive pole of the disorder is much more persistent and harder to treat than the manic pole. In fact, depression is now considered to reflect the largest "unmet need" of persons with the disorder. In a 13-year follow-up of 146 patients with bipolar disorder, patients spent 47% of their lives in symptomatic states, and depression accounted for three times as many weeks of illness as mania or hypomania (Judd et al., 2002). The STEP-BD study (see Chapter 1) found that among 1,469 symptomatic bipolar I and II patients followed over a 2-year period, 58% achieved a state of recovery from their symptom state, and 49% had at least one recurrence during the follow-up. About twice as many patients developed depressive episodes as those who developed manic episodes (Perlis et al., 2006).

What Are Manic and Depressive Episodes Like?

When a bipolar patient is manic, he or she experiences elated and/or irritable mood states, increased levels of energy and activity, racing thoughts, flights of ideas (i.e., jumping from one topic of conversation to another with little transition), impulsive behavior (including hypersexuality, spending sprees, foolish business decisions, or reckless driving), distractibility, and a decreased need for sleep (see the criteria of the DSM-IV; American Psychiatric Association, 2000). A manic person is like a normal person in fast-forward.

> "I walked into a real fancy restaurant with my mother and started jumping around and running, and there were these chandeliers on the ceiling. I thought I was Superman or something, and I leapt up to grab onto one of them and started swinging on it . . . [when you're manic] you think you're God . . . that the world is revolving around you, that you can change nature, and that the birds will come to you if you call them."—*A 21-year-old male bipolar patient*

Family members are perhaps most disturbed and frightened by manic episodes. Although they may find the patient's behavior exciting at first, they quickly become anxious and distressed by his or her unpredictability, impulsiveness, irritability, and grandiosity. In more severe cases, the patient may disappear for periods of time and/or engage in quite reckless behavior, and family members may begin to fear for his or her life.

On the positive side, episodes of hypomania can be associated with creativity and productivity. There is evidence that many great artists, writers, poets, and musicians had bipolar disorder or a variant of it. Kay Jamison (1993) points to the similarities between the manic and the artistic temperaments. It appears, however, that people with bipolar disorder are not particularly creative when acutely manic, only when euthymic or mildly hypomanic.

In contrast, the depressed pole of bipolar disorder is characterized by extreme sadness, the "blues," a loss of interest in activities a person would ordinarily enjoy (e.g., sexuality, friendships, sports), feelings of worthlessness, loss of energy and extreme fatigue, psychomotor retardation or agitation, an inability to sleep (despite fatigue) or needing to sleep too much, an inability to concentrate or make decisions, and suicidal preoccupations or actions.

> "[When I'm depressed] I feel like there's no hope . . . I feel like suicide is the only solution. There have been days on end where I would just stay in bed. . . . I didn't want to talk to or spend time with anybody,

not even my wife. . . . I would call in sick and just stay in bed. . . . You just give up like there's no future for you."—*A 33-year-old male bipolar patient*

Family members dealing with a severely depressed patient alternate between feelings of sympathy and frustration. Their relative's depression goes far beyond what can be helped by a supportive chat. The depressed patient may go long periods of time without functioning at work or at home, which increases the caretaking burden on family members. They may begin to fear that he or she will commit suicide and, understandably, go to great lengths to prevent this from occurring.

Generally, patients with bipolar disorder alternate between these two extremes of mood. However, some patients experience mania and depression simultaneously. During these bipolar "mixed" periods, patients experience periods of irritability, anxiety, suicidality, and feelings of worthlessness in conjunction with increased energy, activity, and impulsive behavior. These high and low states can co-occur in time or alternate across days of the week. Mixed episodes take longer to stabilize with medications than manic or depressive episodes (Kupfer et al., 2000).

What Are the Psychosocial Consequences of Bipolar Episodes?

With the help of mood-stabilizing medications, Stewart's (see Chapter 1) symptoms of mania fully remitted by the second month after his hospital discharge. However, when he returned to his computer programming job, he found he wanted to call in sick nearly every day. His work suffered; he complained that his thoughts were going slowly and that he was "bringing down the company." He found socializing with coworkers to be anxiety provoking. He was eventually given a medical leave, but it seemed clear that he would soon be replaced. After leaving his job, he spent much of his time at home watching television, smoking cigarettes, and withdrawing into his room. Susan complained that he was uninterested in sex or anything that involved more than minimal interaction with her. His friends contacted him at first, but soon became frustrated because he never returned their calls.

Stewart suffered from severe psychosocial dysfunction as well as depressive symptoms. Episodes of bipolar disorder are associated with severe decrements in interpersonal and work functioning, even when patients have been clinically stabilized on their medications. A large-scale epidemiological study found that severe role impairment (problems with functioning in work, social, or family settings) attributable to depression occurs in 90% of bipolar patients (Merikangas et al., 2007). A study involving 253 patients with bipolar I or II disorder found that only one in three worked full-time outside the home. More than half were unable to work or worked only in sheltered settings (Suppes et al., 2001).

In a 12-month follow-up of patients with bipolar I disorder hospitalized for a manic or mixed episode, 48% recovered from their initial syndrome by 12 months but only 24% were able to go back to work and socialize at their pre-episode levels of functioning (Keck et al., 1998). The effects of manic episodes on work, social, and family functioning can be observed for as many as 5 years after an episode remits (Coryell et al., 1993).

Even in the absence of any significant mood disorder symptoms, patients describe an apathetic, anergic state in which they feel unmotivated to resume work, school, or social activities. Many patients have these kinds of work and social impairments in between episodes of mania or depression, especially if they also have ongoing, subsyndromal depressive symptoms (Fagiolini et al., 2005). In this respect, bipolar disorder is like schizophrenia, which also is associated with severe psychosocial impairment.

The Impact of the Disorder on Family Members

How do family members cope? Episodes can be quite traumatic for a patient's relatives, because it is difficult for them to make sense of what has happened to their ill relative or to the family unit. It is easy to understand how the kind of stress and burden they experience can make them angry or resentful of the patient. In other cases, they may become overprotective or "enmeshed" with the ill family member.

Coping with Symptoms

A major objective of FFT is to educate patients and family members about what to expect during episodes of bipolar disorder, and what they can do to help prevent them. Learning to recognize the early warning signs of new episodes, and developing family-based plans for intervening when such signs are present, are among the many ways that families can serve a protective function in reducing the patient's risk for recurrences. We also teach patients and family members to recognize the risks associated with certain biological or social factors (e.g., drug abuse, the patient's lack of compliance with medication regimens, or intense family conflict). Once family members are able to understand the patient's experiences of the illness and develop better ways to cope with the disorder's cycling, their caretaking burden correspondingly lightens.

Coping with Psychosocial Dysfunction

Although family members are clearly distressed by the patient's acute manias or depressions (see the examples of Stewart and Cathy), family relationships often suffer more from the psychosocial consequences of such episodes. For example, during a postmanic or postdepressive phase, family members—whether these be the patient's parents, spouse, siblings, or children—must adapt to an ill relative who was once functional but now may be unable to interact with them constructively. When a man who is the primary wage earner becomes ill with bipolar disorder, his spouse may suddenly have to provide for the children and her ill husband. Likewise, the aging parents of an ill bipolar adult may find themselves in the unwelcome position of having to care for their offspring again, only now in the form of running to and from hospitals, answering late night calls from the police, bailing him or her out of jail, and paying enormous medical bills.

Medications go only so far in enabling a patient and family to cope with the rippling effects of the disorder on the patient's life functioning. Thus, a major goal of FFT is to help the patient and family to set realistic goals for the patient's work and social functioning during the post-episode period. Some patients (and often their family members) insist on the immediate resumption of previous work and social roles, but the patient's residual symptoms make the success of this endeavor unlikely. Other patients, particularly those who "overidentify" with the disorder (see Chapter 1), may set their expectations too low and accept a disabled role even though they are capable of much more. The three core modules of FFT (psychoeducation, CET, and problem-solving training) are each designed to help the patient and family to develop appropriate expectations for the patient's functioning in the aftermath of an episode, expectations that will change with different stages of recovery.

There is evidence that adding psychotherapy to medication can enhance the life functioning of the person with bipolar disorder. In the STEP-BD program (Chapter 1), patients who received up to 30 sessions of FFT, cognitive therapy, or interpersonal therapy showed better functioning after treatment—and higher satisfaction with their lives—than patients who received a three-session comparison treatment (Miklowitz et al., 2007a).

The Topography of Manic and Depressive Episodes

As you know if you work with patients with bipolar disorder, manic and depressive episodes do not just appear one day. Instead, they build over a period of days, weeks, or months. It is sometimes at the end stages of an episode's development that the patient or his or her relatives realize that anything is wrong. In this section, we describe the ways that manic and depressive episodes escalate and how the increasing severity of these symptoms affects family members.

The Manic Escalation

During the hospital intake interview, Cathy said she had for several months felt "happy, laughing about nothing, more pumped than ever before." She had become a "candy-holic," had racing thoughts, met many new people, dated and exercised more than ever before, lost weight, and slept little. She also spent money impulsively ("Instead of buying 1 soda I'd buy 50 of 'em") and bought many things for other people. None of this, however, was particularly disturbing to her or those around her. It was not until she began hearing voices and a desperate, panicky state set in that her family and friends realized something was wrong.

Carlson and Goodwin (1973) offer a template for understanding three stages by which mania progresses. Stage 1 can be thought of as a *prodromal* period of escalation (hypomania). Cathy's behavior reflects this prodromal period. Among patients having their first episode, family members may not notice anything unusual at this stage, except perhaps that "she seemed wired," "he got irritable and cranky," or that "he seemed to be doing too many things at once." This period may even be exciting: Spouses in particular feel energized by the renewed zest for life (and, often, the hypersexuality) expressed by their husbands or wives. However, as the patient has more and more episodes, Stage 1 becomes less rewarding for family members, as they become familiar with what is to come during the height of the episode.

During an *active* or *acute* period of illness (Stages 2 and 3), the patient becomes severely ill. During Stage 2, he or she may be extremely elated and grandiose, make foolish decisions (e.g., sexual indiscretions, risky or impulsive financial transactions), become motorically hyperactive, and sleep little or not at all. As Stage 3 sets in, the patient may have delusions and hallucinations, speak rapidly and nonsensically, and experience a dysphoric or panicky state in addition to manic euphoria or irritability. Family members know that something is quite wrong at this stage, and the alternative of hospitalization is considered. At this stage, family members experience a great deal of anxiety, worry, and feelings of helplessness. The manic person, however, loses insight and does not believe that anything is wrong, and can fight attempts to have his or her behavior constrained. Sometimes patients disappear at this stage, and family members do not hear from them again until they have been picked up by the police and admitted to a hospital.

> "I had thought he was calming down because he had taken one tablet before we got to the medical center. But then we made the mistake of going into a restaurant. He ordered lobster, the most expensive dish on the menu, and then he began to play with the lobster. . . . He started talking to the lobster and drinking out of the shell, and then he started crying really loudly . . . then he went into the kitchen and started screaming at the chefs. I finally went out and stopped a police car, but they said they couldn't do nothing about it."—*The mother of a 21-year-old manic patient*

Not all patients show this progression of stages, and some never become psychotic with hallucinations or delusions. In fact, bipolar II patients never move beyond Stage 1 (hypomania). However, the progression through each of these stages is fairly common among classic bipolar (bipolar I; American Psychiatric Association, 2000) patients. There is no definitive duration of these stages, although Carlson and Goodwin (1973) report that manic patients in their study were ill for an average of 4 weeks. Patients with childhood-onset disorders appear to progress through these stages very quickly, or alternate rapidly between floridly manic and depressive states (Pavuluri, Birmaher, & Naylor, 2005).

The Recovery Period

As the patient gradually begins to decelerate from a manic episode (the *recovery* or *residual* phase), he or she may reexperience Stages 2 and 1. Alternatively, he or she may cycle into a severe depressive episode, with only a short or even nonexistent period of healthy functioning in between. A number of things can happen during the recovery period. First, in today's managed care world, the patient may have been admitted to a hospital and discharged in less than a week, which is not nearly long enough for the episode to remit (see case of Stewart). In fact, the patient may not have been hospitalized at all, despite highly disorganized or dangerous behavior. Therefore, the family is likely to shoulder a greater burden of care during the recovery period. The patient, who is likely to be still manic or hypomanic, may be unduly hostile toward family members. He or she may feel humiliated by the hospitalization experience and blame family members for arranging it. Further, the recovering manic patient is likely to be easily angered by the notion that he or she cannot take care of him- or herself or make independent decisions, and instead may be full of unrealistic plans and resentful of logical counterarguments:

CATHY: I'm gonna get a recording contract. Steve said he could sign me up with a label.

MOTHER: You know that's not realistic. He was a patient there, just like you.

CATHY: (*angrily*) There you go again . . . sticking pins in all of my dreams! Why can't you just let me live my life?

The recovering manic patient may deny that he or she has been ill and exhibit high-risk behaviors (e.g., discontinuing medications; abusing alcohol or drugs) as a way of "proving I can handle it." He or she may still sleep very little and spend money to excess. Moreover, the patient is in the difficult position of having to pay the price for the mistakes made during his or her episode. The "fun" of the manic episode is over, and its aftereffects are felt quite acutely in the form of ruined relationships, massive debts, and lost work opportunities. Adolescents coming off a manic high often realize they have damaged their peer and academic relationships beyond repair.

Thus, the postmanic phase is an especially difficult time for everyone. The family tries to reorganize itself around the needs of a family member who is still quite ill. This period is often accompanied by family arguments, the blurring of boundaries between family members, and an overall decrease in the functioning of the family unit. It is during this period that family support and education can be of greatest value.

The Topography of a Depressive Episode

The stages of a depressive episode are less clear-cut. Often, the patient has been mildly or moderately depressed over a relatively long period (dysthymia), and the acute depressive episode reflects a worsening of this ongoing state ("double depression"). Alternatively, he or she may be functioning well but then gradually slip into a worsening depressive state. Depressions range in severity from mild sadness, to deep sadness with sleep disturbance and suicidal preoccupations, to emotionally deadened states with psychomotor immobility and lethargy. Although the exact sequence of these symptoms is not always clear, at least one study has shown that cognitive symptoms such as disorganized speech predate the onset of a depressive episode among bipolar patients (Altman et al., 1992).

It has been our clinical impression that a depressive episode in one family member, although stressful, burdensome, and confusing, is easier for other family members to manage than a manic episode. Less damage is done during the depression, even though this episode is extremely painful for the patient. Nevertheless, depression has its own effects on family relationships. Relatives usually try to be supportive of the depressed family member at first, but become increasingly frustrated when their suggestions and displays of empathy are rejected by or do not seem to have a positive influence on the patient (Coyne et al., 1992). Eventually, the family members may reject the patient or become quite critical of him or her. This rejection may come about in part from the relative's attribution that the patient could control these symptoms were he or she to try harder (Hooley & Gotlib, 2000). Families coping with depression often benefit from understanding the biological bases of this mood state and, particularly, that the patient is not causing this to happen through his or her faulty character attributes or moral deficiencies.

The Role of the Family in Differential Diagnosis

The physician who admitted Cathy to the inpatient unit gave her the diagnosis of "schizoaffective disorder, rule out schizophrenia." Her auditory hallucinations and thought disorder were quite salient when she was admitted, and she showed paranoid reactions within the ward milieu. She started taking antipsychotic medications. But it was not until her mother offered the treatment team a thorough history of her illness that the diagnosis was changed to bipolar disorder, manic episode, severe, with psychotic features. Marjorie laid out a chronology of Cathy's symptoms, including the fact that Cathy's hypomania had started well before any hallucinations had appeared. Marjorie also reluctantly admitted that she herself had had several episodes of depression, and that her husband's father had committed suicide. The physician introduced lithium carbonate into the treatment regimen, and Cathy began to improve.

The differential diagnosis of bipolar disorder is very difficult to make. The boundaries between bipolar and other disorders have been debated for years, and although our diagnostic criteria have improved, it is still unclear where the disorder ends and other disorders begin. For example, how do we know if the mood fluctuations we see in a presumed bipolar patient are, in fact, more clearly attributable to comorbid Axis II disorders, substance abuse, or attention-deficit/hyperactivity disorder (ADHD)?

The diagnosis is often of great concern to patients and family members. Although it may make little difference to close family members whether their ill relative has bipolar I or bipolar II disorder, they may have questions such as whether ingestion of a street drug was central to the etiology of the mood condition (which, in DSM-IV, would change the diagnosis to substance-induced mood disorder). Parents of juvenile-onset bipolar patients may be particularly concerned about the distinction between bipolar disorder and ADHD, which can influence what medications are chosen. Accurate diagnoses tell family members what treatments are likely to be effective and what may be in store for the patient's future.

You will probably be referred patients who you are told are bipolar but you suspect are not, or the reverse. If you will be involved in the initial diagnosis or the rediagnosis of patients, review the relevant diagnostic criteria of the DSM-IV (American Psychiatric Association, 2000). Chapter 5 offers guidelines for conducting psychodiagnostic interviews.

Family members can be of great help to you in making diagnostic discriminations. When initially evaluating or reevaluating a patient, we recommend conducting separate sessions with the spouse or parent to obtain a thorough history of the illness (see Chapter 5). Family members can describe prior episodes of mania, hypomania, or depression that the patient may have forgotten. For younger patients, parents generally have more reliable information than that provided by the child or his or her teachers (Youngstrom, Findling, & Calabrese, 2004). Family members are also important allies when you address the patient's denial about the validity of the diagnosis (see Chapter 8).

The Variable Life Courses of Bipolar Disorder

Soon after Cathy recovered from her manic episode, she appeared to be her normal self for a brief period. She tried to return to college, but dropped out when she found herself unable to concentrate on the course work. Blaming her attentional problems on her medications, she took herself off them. She soon swung into a depression. It was not a serious depression at first, but rather resembled the regret shown by an alcoholic the morning after a drinking binge.

Her mother tried to make her feel better by giving her "pep talks." However, Cathy said that these talks made her feel worse. Her mother would then become frustrated and accuse her of being disrespectful, at which point Cathy would leave the room, go into her own room, and pull the covers over her head. "I just have to get away to somewhere that feels safe," she explained. After she had had 6 months of prolonged, unremitting depression, her mother asked the family clinician, "Is she always going to be like this?"

I have emphasized that patients and family members must come to accept the patient's vulnerability to future episodes. What do we know about the course of the disorder that leads to this viewpoint?

Many people mistakenly think of bipolar disorder as consisting of discrete episodes of mania and depression, with periods of normality in between. In fact, it is the minority of patients who show this pattern. Bipolar disorder can follow many different course patterns, and, within any particular patient, the course may vary from one stage of life to the next. Many patients are like Cathy, cycling in and out of episodes and never fully returning to normal. This fact of the illness is particularly upsetting to relatives, who harbor the hope that once the acute episode and/or hospitalization period is over, the patient will pick up from where he or she left off.

Subtypes of Bipolar Disorder

The topographies of individual manic, mixed, and depressive episodes provide only a snapshot of what the patient and family experience over time. Not surprisingly, different subtypes of the disorder have different effects on the functioning of the family or marital unit.

Bipolar I

Cathy has the classic, textbook form of bipolar disorder, which characterizes about 35–40% of all DSM-IV fully syndromal patients (Angst, 1978; Kalbag, Miklowitz, & Richards, 1999; Merikangas et al., 2007). These patients alternate between extreme, fully syndromal depressions and manias or mixed affective episodes, with or without a return to normalcy in between (bipolar I disorder). The bipolar I form is perhaps easiest to diagnose and the most predictable in terms of its future course. Once the proper dosages of lithium, anticonvulsants, and/or atypical antipsychotics are found, and the patient decides to adhere to these dosages, the bipolar I patient often functions well in the community (Tondo, Baldessarini, & Floris, 2001).

Bipolar II

Approximately 40–45% of fully syndromal bipolar patients alternate between periods of deep depression and milder, less destructive manic states (hypomanias) (Angst, 1978). When these patients become hypomanic, they experience euphoria, irritability, flight of ideas, or other symptoms, but do not become psychotic and do not need to be hospitalized. Bipolar II patients are disproportionately women. Many relatives of bipolar II patients do not notice distinct hypomanic periods and instead describe the patient as chronically depressed. They are often accurate in their assessment; one study found that the ratio of time bipolar II patients spend depressed versus hypomanic is 37:1 (Judd et al., 2003).

Relatives of bipolar II patients may report that the patient has always been hard driving, reactive, irritable, or high in energy. However, in other cases, the hypomanic periods of the bipolar II disorder are relatively distinct and lead to disruptions in the patient's family relationships. Some relatives come to fear hypomanic episodes, knowing that these often leave full-blown depressions in their wake.

Rapid Cycling in Bipolar I or II Patients

A subgroup of patients with either bipolar I or II disorder (between 13 and 20% in most studies; Schneck et al., 2004) have quite frequent mood cycling, with more than four episodes of hypomania, mania, or depression in a single year. These patients alternate between extreme mood states with relatively short or even nonexistent periods of healthy functioning in between. Rapid cycling does not tend to be a lifelong pattern, but usually represents a phase of the illness that is gone within 2 years in most patients (Coryell et al., 2003). Nevertheless, these are the most difficult patients to treat pharmacologically, because they rarely respond to lithium or anticonvulsants alone.

Family Reactions to Different Courses of the Disorder

All of the course patterns described above disrupt the family unit and can lead to system-wide feelings of helplessness and resentment. As often occurs among the families of schizophrenia patients, families who have coped with numerous bipolar episodes begin to treat their ill family member as a "chronic mental patient" and revise their dreams and aspirations for that person's productivity or contribution to family life. The patient may, as a result, experience significant grief, guilt, and anger over his or her new role in the family and the new ways in which relatives interact with him or her.

However, not all course subtypes present the same challenges. We have observed quite variable reactions among families, depending on the patient's episode patterning. For example, some bipolar I patients do quite destructive things during their manic episodes but function at a relatively healthy level in between. Thus, their family members must cope with the unpredictability of and the damage done during the episodes, but family life returns to normal when the patient remits. Other bipolar I patients and families are not so fortunate, and each episode brings about more deterioration and a greater caretaking burden than the previous one. A goal of family treatment is to help families to recognize that recurrences of bipolar disorder are inevitable and to develop styles of coping with episodes that work well for them over the long term.

Family members face different challenges if the patient follows a bipolar II course. For the majority of these patients, the family's major challenge is the patient's unremitting states of depression (or double depressions) rather than his or her hypomanias. One cannot presume that this imposes an easier task than that faced by the family of the bipolar I patient. Often, these families need help in understanding the origins of this depression and in setting realistic goals for the future.

Families of rapid-cycling patients usually face the toughest challenges. The patient's constant variability in mood, deteriorating psychosocial functioning, and suicidal thoughts or impulses eventually make family members distance themselves from him or her. Relatives usually feel quite angry at the mental health profession, which may have promised much but delivered little. Although there is little that FFT can do to prevent rapid cycling, families may be relieved to hear that rapid cycling tends to be a temporary state rather than a lifelong pattern. They can also learn to anticipate precipitants for rapid mood swings (e.g., interpersonal conflicts) and alter their response styles to reduce the likelihood of recurrences. Moreover, one can teach patients to undertake certain behavior changes (e.g., regularizing their sleep–wake cycles) that will help them gain control over their frequent cycles.

Finally, families of patients with unremitting courses of illness (including but not limited to rapid cycling) are most vulnerable to the "personality versus disorder" disagreements described in Chapter 1. That is, if the patient's symptoms endure long enough, family members have difficulty in distinguishing symptoms from preillness character attributes. In fact, family members often report that the patient has always been moody, irritable, hyperactive, or morose, even before he or she came to the attention of the mental health profession. Sometimes these beliefs are associated with subtle innuendoes to the patient that he or she does not really need medication, or is needlessly playing the "sick role." Patients with these symptoms feel quite helpless already, and these implicit accusations can be quite painful and cause a great deal of family conflict. FFT can help patients and families to make distinctions between the disorder and the patient's personality and to identify continuities in the patient's character attributes from the pre- to the postillness period.

Developmental Precursors to Bipolar Disorder

Marjorie claimed that Cathy had always been moody. She reported that Cathy showed her first signs of disturbance when 3 years old and in day care for the first time. Marjorie and her husband had just divorced. Cathy's teachers at the day care center reported that she seemed to be rather aggressive, often pushing the other children out of the way when she wanted to get on the slide. She was also highly emotionally expressive, crying or yelling frequently. She had seemed unusually concerned about her mother's emotional state, frequently asking her, "Are you OK,

Mommy?" At the time, Marjorie attributed most of this behavior to the effects of the divorce.

As Cathy became a teen, she functioned well socially, with many female friends and a number of boyfriends. She was always "on the go." Her emotional state, however, continued to be labile. As Cathy described it, she would often have a few days of "getting hyper" followed by several days of "being really bored." By age 16 she began drinking heavily and became sexually promiscuous, frequently staying out all night. Marjorie was quite disturbed by this behavior and began to watch her more closely, which made Cathy "act out" even more. An evaluation by a school psychologist led to the not-so-helpful conclusion that Cathy was a troubled teen and that Marjorie should back off.

What does a person who develops bipolar disorder look like as a youngster? Are there ways to determine who, in a classroom of children, is most likely to develop this disorder? How can genetically vulnerable families learn to recognize the early signs of bipolarity in their offspring?

Studies of Risk for Bipolar Disorder

Researchers have used the strategy of examining children of bipolar parents and determining how these children differ from those of healthy parents. This strategy cannot fully distinguish the effects of genetic vulnerability, rearing environment, and adverse events during development, but it can give us a picture of what childhood factors may be risk markers for the onset of bipolarity, even if we cannot pin down the origins of these markers.

The Risk to Children of Bipolar Parents

Children of bipolar parents are at unquestionably higher risk for developing bipolar disorder than the children of healthy parents. The rate of mood disorders (including bipolar disorder and various types of depression) in the parents, siblings, and children of people with bipolar disorder averages 20–25%. Of this 20–25%, about 14% will develop major depressive disorder and about 9% will develop bipolar disorder (Smoller & Finn, 2003).

A meta-analysis of studies conducted before 1997 found that the offspring of bipolar parents were at a 4 times greater risk for developing a mood disorder—and at a 2.7 times higher risk for the development of *any* psychiatric disorder—than the children of parents without psychiatric illness (LaPalme, Hodgins, & LaRoche, 1997). There is quite a bit of variability in different studies: Rates of bipolar "spectrum" disorders (bipolar I,

II, bipolar not otherwise specified, or cyclothymic) in offspring range from 14 to 50% across studies, and rates of major depressive disorder range from 7 to 43% (Chang, Steiner, & Ketter, 2003).

The children of bipolar parents do not develop only bipolar disorder. Hammen, Burge, Burney, and Adrian (1990) found in a 3-year follow-up that 72% of the children (ages 8–16) of bipolar mothers had had at least one lifetime psychiatric diagnosis (i.e., affective disorders, behavior disorders, or significant anxiety disorders), a rate higher than that seen in the children of medically ill mothers (43%) and more than twice as high as that in the children of healthy mothers (32%). Interestingly, the highest rates of psychiatric diagnosis, and the most severe diagnoses, were seen in the children of unipolar depressed mothers (82%). Thus, having a bipolar parent increases the risk that a child will develop a psychiatric disorder, just as does having a parent with other recurrent forms of psychiatric illness.

Childhood Indicators of Risk

Mood swings are often observable from early childhood. Several early investigations found higher levels of aggressiveness and affective expressiveness among the young children of bipolar parents (e.g., Decina et al., 1983). One study found evidence among high-risk children—as young as age 2—of increased aggressiveness, difficulty with empathy for other children, and overconcern about the emotional discomfort of their parents (Zahn-Waxler, McKnew, Cummings, Davenport, & Radke-Yarrow, 1984). Thus, in addition to being emotionally labile, children who are genetically at risk for bipolar disorder may learn to become caretakers of their ill parents from a very young age (see the example of Cathy). Interestingly, Mayo, O'Connell, and O'Brien (1979) found that those children of bipolar patients who were functioning at the lowest levels were those who had become intertwined with the parent's illness and symptoms, whereas children with better outcomes had been better able to separate and to develop more friendships outside the family.

Among those genetically predisposed children who do develop bipolar disorder, severe and disabling symptoms are often seen by late childhood or the early teen years. Often, these children are first diagnosed with ADHD, oppositional defiant disorder, or just depression. Girls are particularly likely to show mood disturbances after puberty, whereas boys may show aggression, externalizing behavior, and impulsiveness even before puberty. Clinicians may or may not recognize the subsyndromal signs of mania or hypomania, which may present as outbursts of rage or aggressiveness, impulsive suicide attempts, self-cutting, decreased need for sleep, or substance abuse. If they do observe these symptoms, they often chalk them up to a difficult transition to adolescence or to other disorders.

One study (Findling et al., 2005) with 400 children ages 5–17 found that the children of bipolar parents were more likely to show symptoms of mania or hypomania than were children without a bipolar parent, but were not at higher risk for ADHD or disruptive behavior disorders. The combination of elevated mood with irritability and rapid mood fluctuations—along with social dysfunction—identified a high-risk group, which the authors referred to as "cyclotaxic." A similar cluster of early indicators was identified by Shaw, Egeland, Endicott, Allen, and Hostetter (2005) among children in the Amish community. In their 10-year follow-up study, children with a bipolar parent, as compared with children without a bipolar parent, were distinguished by mood lability, high energy, anxiousness, hyperalertness, distractibility, easy excitability, poor school performance, decreased sleep, problems in thinking and concentration, oversensitivity, somatic complaints, and "excessive and loud talking."

Not all children with these early features become bipolar, of course. A team at the National Institute of Mental Health (Rich et al., 2007) found that children with early-onset bipolar disorder were distinguishable from children with "severe mood dysregulation"—children with intense, highly reactive changes in mood—on a number of psychophysiological measures, including a measure of executive attention. So, having a genetic predisposition to bipolar disorder—or showing severe mood dysregulation—does not mean that a child will grow up to be bipolar.

Parents with a child showing early mood dysregulation are in a very difficult position. They know something is wrong and may even have read about bipolar disorder and know that it runs in the family. But they also want to believe their child is normal, like everyone else's. They may feel guilty about the genes they may have passed on (see "Gene Guilt" in Chapter 7). Unfortunately, parents often feel unsupported by mental health professionals, who give them a variety of inconsistent opinions about diagnosis or treatment, or worse yet, imply that there is something wrong with their parenting.

Personality Predispositional Factors

Are there distinct personality features that predispose people to bipolar disorder? Akiskal et al. (2000) have shown that patients with bipolar disorder often have "core temperamental disturbances" that presage the onset of the disorder and persist between major episodes. For example, some patients (like Cathy), have *cyclothymic* temperaments (frequent mood shifts from unexplained tearfulness to buoyant jocularity, variable sleeping patterns, shifting patterns of self-esteem) before they first become ill. Others have *hyperthymic* (chronically cheerful, exuberant, overoptimistic, extraverted, stimulus-seeking, and meddlesome styles) or *subsyndromal mixed* (pessimistic, depressive, anxious, and irritable) predispositional temperaments.

There is evidence to support the view of Akiskal and colleagues. For example, the children of bipolar parents are more likely to show clinically diagnosable cyclothymia than the children of parents without bipolar disorder (Klein, Depue, & Slater, 1986). Likewise, young adults with cyclothymic temperaments have been found to have a high familial loading for affective disorder (Akiskal et al., 2000). Bipolar adults report that, as children, they experienced depressions and hypomanias—and symptoms of anxiety and attention deficit disorders—well before the onset of their first manic episode (Lish, Dime-Meenan, Whybrow, Price, & Hirschfeld, 1994).

Longer-Term Follow-Up Studies of Children at Risk

What happens to children with early signs of mood disturbance over time? Few studies of these children have been done, and the periods of follow-up have not been long enough. Nonetheless, a 2-year prospective study in France examined 80 children and adolescents (ages 7–17 years) with DSM-IV major depressive disorder (Kochman et al., 2005). Of the 80, 35 (43%) converted to bipolar I or II disorder within 2 years. Youths with cyclothymic temperaments ($N = 47$) were highly likely (64%) to experience at least one full-blown hypomanic or manic episode within 2 years, as compared with only 15% without a cyclothymic temperament ($N = 33$). The cyclothymic children also had more depressive episodes at follow-up, more psychotic symptoms, and more suicidal ideation and attempts. Cyclothymic children were described at baseline as highly mood labile and emotionally overactive, explosively angry, impulsive, aggressive, and emotionally hypersensitive.

Leibenluft, Cohen, Gorrindo, Brook, and Pine (2006) analyzed longitudinal data on 776 youth who were assessed at three time points: mean age 13.8, mean age 16.2, and mean age 22.1. The best predictor of the onset of new manic episodes by the second and third time points was "episodic irritability" at time 1, meaning intervals of rage and anger that were clearly distinct from the child's usual state. Depression in early adolescence also predicted later mania onset. Interestingly, chronic, non-episodic irritability predicted the later onset of ADHD and major depression, but not bipolar disorder. Thus, the *cyclicity* of mood symptoms seems an important variable to consider in defining the risk for bipolar onsets.

The Course and Outcome of Bipolar Youth study most clearly documents that children with well-defined early subsyndromal signs of bipolar disorder are at high risk to progress to bipolar I or II disorder (Birmaher et al., 2006). In a study of 131 children with bipolar disorder, not otherwise specified (manic episodes that fell short of the DSM-IV duration criteria, or the required number of symptoms), 24% "converted" to bipolar I or II disorder within 1.5 years. Those with a first- or second-degree relative with mania or hypomania were significantly more likely to develop bipolar I or II disorder than were those without (30.6 vs. 17.4%). Children with bipolar disorder, not otherwise specified, were at high risk for a variety of adverse outcomes at follow-up, including rapid mood changes, suicidality, and psychosocial dysfunction.

Implications for the Family Coping with Bipolar Disorder

The literature on children at high risk suggests that the children of bipolar parents, especially those with subthreshold mood disturbances or core temperamental disturbances, are at high risk for developing fully syndromal bipolar disorder.

It is easy to understand why patients, and sometimes family members, would be confused about the distinction between the patient's premorbid personality and his or her diagnosed disorder. In some cases, the disorder appears "out of the blue," and in others it seems to reflect a continuation or perhaps exaggeration of the patient's premorbid temperament. In FFT, it is helpful for patients and family members to see the continuities between who the patient used to be and who he or she is now, and to recognize that these preexisting temperamental attributes, although troublesome, may also have positive features (for example, heightened energy or creativity).

When attempting to understand the genesis of the disorder, the families of bipolar persons have other significant questions on their minds: Will other members of my family get the disorder? Should my young son, who is showing signs of aggressiveness in school, be put on lithium? Should we risk having more children? Can the disorder be prevented?

In the next 10–20 years we may see new research on DNA markers or magnetic resonance scan abnormalities that can be used to identify high-risk youth. In the meantime, however, we have to rely on early warning signs to tell us whether a child is likely to develop bipolar disorder. In FFT, you can help parents by sharing information about the actual risks to their nonbipolar children, and about the various forms of counseling and other services available to children showing high-risk behavior. Furthermore, acquainting parents with the prodromal signs of new episodes (see "The Relapse Drill" in Chapter 7) can lead to the development of contingency plans should any of their children show these signs.

The Interface between Drug Treatment and FFT

So far, I have discussed the nature of bipolar disorder, its course over time, its developmental precursors, and its impact on the functioning of the family. In so doing, I have emphasized that families need to make sense of the current episode (FFT Goal 1), accept the patient's vulnerability to future episodes (Goal 2), and come to distinguish between the patient's personality and his or her disorder (Goal 4). Another major goal of FFT is to assist the patient and relatives to accept the patient's ongoing need for mood-stabilizing and/or atypical antipsychotic medications (Goal 3). But why should a patient or family be willing to accept this necessity?

Bipolar disorder is unquestionably a disorder of genetic and biological origin, and it cannot be treated with psychotherapy alone. It nearly always runs in families; identical twins have higher concordances for the disorder than fraternal twins; and the biological parents of bipolar adoptees have higher rates of affective disorder than the adoptive parents (for a review, see Smoller & Finn, 2003). There is also a substantial literature suggesting that dysregulations in dopamine, norepinephrine, serotonin, neurohormone, and gamma-aminobutyric acid systems underlie the symptoms of the disorder (for a review, see Manji et al., 2003). Moreover, as discussed below, medications targeting these dysregulations are effective in ameliorating the course of the disorder. Thus, medications must be a part of the standard inpatient and outpatient treatment of this disorder.

Standard Drug Treatments

Currently, the pharmacological treatment for bipolar disorder almost always includes a mood stabilizer (most typically lithium carbonate, divalproex sodium [Depakote, Depakene], or lamotrigine [Lamictal], and less frequently carbamazepine [Tegretol, Carbitrol]). Depending on the clinical condition of the patient and the stage of the disorder, the physician may prescribe an atypical antipsychotic (olanzapine [Zyprexa], risperidone [Risperdal], quetiapine [Seroquel], ziprasidone [Geodon], or aripiprazole [Abilify]) as a primary or adjunctive treatment. The physician may also prescribe adjunctive antidepressants, benzodiazepines, or other mood-regulating agents such as topiramate [Topamax] or thyroid supplements. If you wish to learn more about the drug treatment of this disorder, we recommend reading several up-to-date treatment guidelines (National Institute for Health and Clinical Excellence, 2006; Suppes et al., 2005; Yatham et al., 2005).

As will become clearer in subsequent chapters, family treatment can be a vehicle for organizing the various pharmacological treatments in the patient's recommended regimen and in encouraging his or her adherence to this regimen. To accomplish this goal, FFT is designed to parallel the various stages of drug treatment, each of which poses special issues for the patient and family.

The Stages of Drug and Psychotherapeutic Interventions

Treatment of bipolar disorder can be thought of as a phasic process (Prien, 1993). In forthcoming chapters, I refer to an *acute treatment phase,* a *stabilization phase* (also referred to as *continuation therapy),* and a *maintenance phase* (also referred to as *preventive treatment).* Table 2.1 lists these stages and the critical issues for pharmacological and psychosocial care that accompany them.

The first is the *acute* stage, consisting of those medical and psychosocial interventions designed to control the worst stages of the manic or depressive episode. The lithium and antipsychotic regimen recommended for Stewart (Chapter 1) during his inpatient phase is an example of acute treatment. The acute stage can involve but does not always require hospitalization. During this stage, families, particularly those in which the patient is having his or her first or second episode, experience trauma and shock. They need assistance in making sense of what has transpired and in dealing with the practical and emotional problems brought about by the hospitalization.

TABLE 2.1. Critical Challenges in the Stages of Pharmacological and Psychosocial Treatment

Stage	Goals of treatment	Issues for patient/family
Acute	Gain control over severe symptoms	Trauma and shock, dealing with police and/or hospitalization (in some cases), making sense of what has happened
Stabilization	Hasten recovery from the acute episode, address residual symptoms/ impairment, encourage medication adherence	Adapting to postepisode symptoms and social–occupational deficits, financial stress, accepting a regular medication regimen, uncomfortable discussions about medication and illness, denial about the realities of the disorder
Maintenance	Prevent recurrences, alleviate residual affective symptoms, continue to encourage medication adherence	Fears about the future, accepting the illness and the vulnerability to future episodes, coping with ongoing deficits in social–occupational functioning, issues surrounding long-term medication adherence

During the stabilization stage, the core objective of drug and psychosocial treatment is to alleviate the manic or depressive symptoms that remain after the worst of the acute episode is over. For example, were Cathy to have continued treatment with a psychiatrist during the months after her hospital discharge, this physician would likely have reevaluated her regimen and possibly prescribed new medications or dosage schedules. During this stage, families need help in adjusting to the patient's residual symptoms and psychosocial impairment, and, often, his or her irritability, denial about the disorder, or reluctance to take medications.

Once the acute episode has resolved, the gains from drug treatment must be maintained over the long term. The goal of the *maintenance* stage, an ongoing, sometimes permanent period of treatment, is to support a relatively remitted patient in the community for as long as possible and to prevent recurrences of the disorder. Patients have less severe symptoms at this stage, but many have lingering states of depression that remain long after the manic symptoms have been stabilized. Patients with bipolar disorder spend about three times as many weeks in their lives in states of depression as in states of mania or hypomania (Judd et al., 2002, 2003). Unfortunately, having residual depressive symptoms means that the patient is at risk for earlier recurrences of the disorder (Perlis et al., 2006). As a result, the bipolar patient often must be maintained on complex combinations of mood stabilizers, atypical antipsychotics, and often antidepressants as well (Thase, 2006).

During the maintenance phase, families frequently need help with uncomfortable issues such as when the patient is likely to have another episode, the distress and worry caused by his or her subsyndromal symptoms (e.g., dysthymia, irritability, pessimistic thinking, or mild grandiosity), whether he or she will ever fully return to work or school, and whether the patient can agree to regular, long-term maintenance medication. For many families of bipolar patients, the maintenance stage feels like a long period of being on an emotional roller coaster.

Medications: How Well Do They Work?

As in Cathy's and Stewart's cases, many patients leave the hospital and enter the stabilization phase only partially remitted from their acute episodes. Drug treatment and family treatment are therefore oriented toward symptom alleviation and relapse prevention, or maintaining the patient's longer-term stability in the community. But what are the actual odds that a bipolar patient taking medication will have a relapse or recurrence of the disorder? When in the maintenance phase is this likely to occur? What can the family expect if the patient is treated with medication? What if the patient refuses medication?

The Naturalistic Course of Untreated Bipolar Disorder

Without psychiatric medicine, the outlook for bipolar patients is bleak. Several investigators studied the course of what was called manic–depressive illness in the prepharmacological era, when patients were often hospitalized for decades and treated with hydrotherapy, seclusion, or hemodialysis. Kraepelin (1921) studied more than 900 mood-cycling patients and observed that some patients experienced depressive episodes that lasted 10 years or more. Examining the hospital records of bipolar patients from the prelithium era, Cutler and Post (1982) found that episodes became more frequent and intervals of wellness shorter as the illness progressed (the "kindling effect"). Thus, in the absence of interventions that arrested this process, parents and spouses had to cope with longer periods of illness and fewer periods of healthy functioning in their ill relative, which meant increasing financial and emotional strain over time. Perhaps for these reasons, many families in the prelithium era, out of desperation, eventually abandoned the patient.

The Course of Medically Treated Bipolar Disorder

The introduction of lithium in the early 1970s gave hope to many patients and families. People with bipolar disorder who were formerly living as chronic psychiatric patients were suddenly able to work, socialize, and have family relationships again. Between 50 and 70% of bipolar patients respond to lithium during the acute manic phase (Thase, 2006; Tondo et al., 2001).

The drug is less impressive as a prophylactic agent in long-term maintenance. About 40% of patients who receive standard dosages of lithium (with appropriate blood level monitoring) have recurrences of mania or depression in 1-year follow-ups, about 60% over 2–3 years, and about 75% over 5 years (see, e.g., Gitlin et al., 1995). One review of lithium effectiveness from studies in the 1970s through the 1990s concluded that about 33% of patients remain episode-free while on lithium and that the drug reduces hospitalization rates by 82%. However, patients still have an average of about one manic or depressive episode per year (Tondo et al., 2001). Thus, lithium significantly improves the course of bipolar disorder, but patients continue to have "breakthrough" recurrences.

There are fewer effectiveness data on the anticonvulsant medications, particularly for the long-term prevention of recurrence. It appears that divalproex (Depakote) and carbamazepine (Tegretol) are about as effective as lithium in controlling acute manic episodes, with at least a 50% response rate (for a review, see Goldberg, 2004). Lamotrigine appears to be more robust than lithium in stabilizing depressive episodes, whereas lithium may be stronger than lamotrigine in stabilizing manic episodes (Goodwin et al., 2004). The atypical antipsychotics, notably quetiapine, olanzapine, and the combination of olanzapine and fluoxetine (Symbiax), have strong antimanic and antidepressive properties and are often the first choice for patients in acute periods of illness. However, these drugs, particularly olanzapine, can cause considerable weight gain (Tohen et al., 2003, 2005; DelBello et al., 2006).

Many clinicians no longer use antidepressants (for example, selective serotonin reuptake inhibitors [SSRIs]) with bipolar patients because of the possibility that these drugs will provoke mania or rapid cycling. It is not clear that antidepressants cause cycling when they are dosed correctly and given alongside mood stabilizers like lithium or divalproex. However, it is not clear that they add anything either (Sachs et al., 2007).

The data from controlled pharmaceutical trials carry the clear implication that we need to give patients more than just medications. Psychosocial intervention, delivered as a maintenance treatment in combination with medication, may be a way of reducing relapse rates further, reducing the severity of those episodes that do occur, improving between-episode symptoms and social functioning, and, as discussed below, keeping patients on their medications.

The Problem of Medication Nonadherence

Despite the fact that lithium clearly controlled her acute symptoms, Cathy was never convinced that she really needed it. She agreed to a trial of lithium only to appease her mother, who threatened to kick her out of the house if she did not. However, she hated the side effects, and she disliked telling friends and prospective boyfriends that she was taking it and the "feeling of being a mental patient" that it caused. She took herself off lithium only 2 months after her hospitalization. She soon developed a severe, prolonged depression, and then rebounded into another manic episode requiring rehospitalization. But when she went back on lithium the second time, it became apparent that she was no longer responding as well as she had at first.

Although few patients and family members would yearn for the days when bipolar patients were not treated with medication, a different problem is raised by the necessity of long-term medication treatment: the fact that patients, particularly early in the stages of their disorder, are loath to take it. Most bipolar patients experiment with discontinuing their medications at some point in their lives. In our 9-month follow-up of first- and second-episode bipolar patients, 70% (16 of 23) showed noncompliance with lithium, ranging from missing at least one dose per week to discontinuing all medications against medical advice (Miklowitz et al., 1988). One study found that when patients in an outpatient health maintenance organization were treated with lithium, they took it for an average of only 76 days! (Johnson & McFarland, 1996). Medication nonadherence is also a problem among young patients. One longitudinal study found that only 35% of bipolar teens took all their medications during the first year of treatment, and almost 25% did not take their medications at all (DelBello, Hanseman, Adler, Fleck, & Strakowski, 2007).

The outlook for this disorder significantly worsens when patients stop their medications suddenly: Relapses come sooner and are more severe, and suicide is more likely (e.g., Suppes, Baldessarini, Faedda, Tondo, & Tohen, 1993; Tondo & Baldessarini, 2000)). Some patients, like Cathy, may be less likely to respond to lithium when it is reintroduced after a discontinuation period (Post, 1993). We do not know the long-term implications of "start–stop" medication taking among child patients, but data from studies on adults certainly do not bode well.

Family Treatment as a Means of Reestablishing Drug Adherence

Family treatment can be an important adjunct to medication if it addresses the issue of adherence (also called compliance). In a family setting, patients can be encouraged to explore their resistances to taking medication. Sometimes, the issues revolve around the patient's denial of the disorder. In other cases, the patient's nonadherence can be tied to the belief among family members that the patient is not ill or could control his or her symptoms if he or she really wanted to. Patients like Cathy have strong reactions to the side effects of their medications or the required blood tests, and the associated feelings of being a sick person. In still other cases, patients reveal that taking pills limits their autonomy and makes them feel like a child again.

In FFT, we guide patients and family members, through a combination of psychoeducational and exploratory interventions, toward a greater understanding of the purposes of medication and the ways in which adhering to medications increases the patient's control over his or her own fate. We educate participants about the nature and side effects of the medications prescribed and encourage regular, clear communication between the patient and his or her physician. We label the patient's resistance to taking medication, and the family's hypervigilance, as normal and understandable reactions to the process of learning to accept an illness. Eventually, patients and family members come to accept the necessity of medication, and to mutual agreements about how to discuss and negotiate the problems that arise from the patients' drug treatments.

Concluding Comments

Bipolar disorder is a recurrent, disruptive disorder that emerges in the late teens to early 20s, although early warning signs may be present much earlier. It takes a huge toll on the patient and family. Patients are highly likely to have recurrences, and most experience residual depressive and manic symptoms during the postepisode recovery and long-term maintenance phases. Although persons with bipolar disorder are often highly creative, socially skilled persons, their illnesses frequently force them to function at a level lower than their capabilities. Like many psychiatric disorders, bipolar disorder places a great deal of practical, financial, and emotional burden on the caretaking parents or spouse.

Pharmacological treatments, although bringing about dramatic improvements in many patients' and families' lives, are simply not enough by themselves to combat the disastrous effects of this disorder. Family treatment can advance the goals of pharmacological treatments by helping patients and family members to accept the realities of the disorder and recognize that long-term medication is probably going to be necessary. Involving the family in treatment increases the chances that patients will stay on their medications.

As I discuss in Chapter 3, stress factors, including those within the family milieu, may elicit episodes of bipolar disorder when they operate against the background of the patient's preexisting biological vulnerabilities. As you will see, psychosocial interventions targeting the family have the potential to augment the efficacy of drug treatments if they reduce the level of stress in the family environment and promote the use of the skills necessary for coping with stressful life events.

chapter 3

Family and Social Factors in the Course of Bipolar Disorder

Wes was a 39-year-old European American man who lived with his mother, Helen, and two sisters, ages 35 and 37. His first manic episode occurred at 20, and he had undergone 14 hospitalizations since then. The episode that precipitated his entry into the FFT program was a psychotic depression. Owing to the severity and chronicity of his illness, he was unemployed and collecting disability income.

Wes's mother had long believed that his illness could be treated only with Chinese herbal remedies. For more than a decade she had devoted her life to pursuing these treatments for him. She had sold some of her belongings to fund her travels abroad to seek remedies that were unavailable or not recommended in the United States. She had become very angry with and distrustful of the mental health system.

Helen was seldom overtly critical of her three children, but her apparent emotional overinvolvement with them had been long-standing. Moreover, it appeared quite difficult for them to separate from her: None of them had ever lived independently. The family members seemed united by their joint distrust of the mental health system.

Shortly after his episode, Wes expressed an interest in living on his own and made arrangements to move into a state-subsidized apartment. But once his plans were in place, his mother circumvented them by arranging for the whole family to move to a new house and insisting that Wes move with them. Wes acquiesced, but his clinical state worsened following this event.

Chapter Overview

The difficult course of bipolar disorder clearly affects the functioning of families. However, as the case of Wes illustrates, family functioning also affects the course of bipolar disorder. What psychosocial factors—either within or outside the family—act as *contextual risk factors* that provoke or at least influence recurrences of the disorder?

This chapter is dedicated to reviewing the research on contextual risk factors. The discussion is limited to two classes of variables that we target in FFT: *family environmental factors* and *stressful life events.* I first describe early, clinically oriented approaches to the family, and then a series of empirical studies by our group that demonstrate the role of the family in the longitudinal course of the disorder. I then review studies suggesting that stressful life events can precipitate episodes of mania and depression. Life events cannot usually be prevented with a psychosocial intervention, but some can be anticipated, and the patient and family can develop coping mechanisms for dealing with these events when they do occur.

In reviewing the research on psychosocial risk factors, it will become even clearer that the long-term treatment plans for patients with this disorder should be broadened beyond strict pharmacological approaches to more comprehensive biopsychosocial programs that augment the protective effects of the patient's environment. This view is the basis for the final two goals of FFT: *restoring functional family relationships after a mood disorder episode* (Goal 6), and *assisting patients and family members in recognizing and coping with stressful life events that trigger recurrences of the disorder* (Goal 5).

The Vulnerability–Stress Model

Psychosocial influences on this disorder do not operate independently of an individual's genetic and biological predispositions. Instead, genetic, biological, and social factors interact in bringing about episodes of mood disorder or in protecting against their occurrence. The vulnerability–stress model (Figure 3.1; Zubin & Spring, 1977) offers a framework for understanding this biological–psychological interface.

In this model, if a person's genetic and/or biological vulnerability is high (e.g., many members of the family tree are diagnosed with mood disorder, or the patient has certain structural or functional brain abnormalities), the level of stress sufficient to elicit an episode of bipolar disorder in that person is low. That is, for a patient with high vulnerability, stressors as minimal as missing a paycheck or having a family argument may serve as environmental provoking agents. Likewise, for a patient

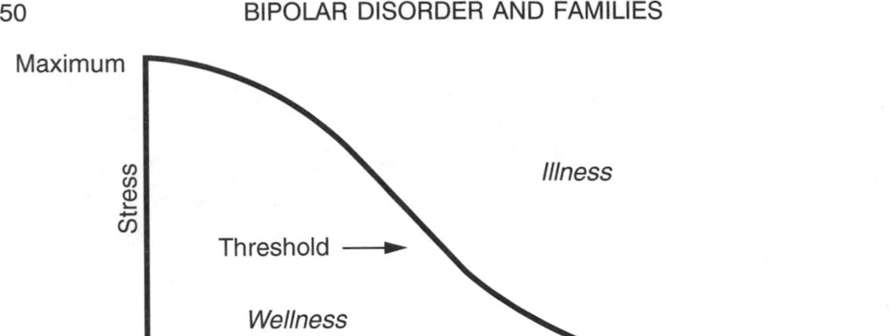

FIGURE 3.1. The vulnerability–stress model. *Source:* Adapted by permission from Zubin and Spring (1977). Copyright 1977 by the American Psychological Association.

with low genetic and/or biological vulnerability, stress must be quite severe (e.g., divorce; death in the family; severe, unexpected family conflicts) before an episode will occur. Thus, low levels of environmental stress protect against recurrences of mood disorder that may have been expected based on a patient's biological vulnerabilities. The nature of these vulnerability–stress interactions, and the relative roles of risk and protective factors, change at different phases of a bipolar person's development (Miklowitz & Cicchetti, 2006).

The vulnerability–stress model is a useful way to think about episodes of bipolar disorder. In the following review of psychosocial provoking agents, I frequently point out the ways in which these agents interact with underlying biological predispositions. Toward the end of the chapter, I present an integrated vulnerability–stress model that is relatively specific to this disorder and show how our biopsychosocial, family-oriented program derives from this model.

Family Environmental Factors in Bipolar Disorder

Shortly after his episode, Wes and his mother and sisters were brought into a laboratory to allow the family clinicians to observe their interactional styles, as a means of planning for their treatment. When asked to talk about and try to solve a series of self-identified family problems, their discussions were at first low-key. However, as the session progressed the clinicians observed that Wes's mother and sisters often spoke about him in the third person, as if he weren't there. Wes's mother frequently completed his sentences and often interpreted his underlying feelings or motives. In general, the discussions were rambling, unfocused, difficult to follow, and not oriented toward solving the original problem. They clearly had a disorganizing effect on Wes: Toward the end, he became angry, agitated, and argumentative, and his speech became more tangential.

What family attributes provide a context for understanding recurrences of bipolar disorder? Consider first the *attitudes* of family members toward each other, such as whether they think the spouse, parent, or offspring has primarily positive versus negative attributes; whether they feel close to this relative; whether they feel irritated or annoyed by certain of his or her behaviors or attributes; or whether they feel protective of him or her. The protective attitudes of Wes's mother are reflected in her preoccupation with his treatment, anger at the mental health system, and difficulty with his attempts at independence.

The attitudes of family members are to be distinguished from their *interactional behaviors*, which are the ways in which members communicate with each other (both verbally and nonverbally) in face-to-face discussions. The interactions in Wes's family could be understood in regard to *affective qualities* (How critical, domineering, or aggressive is one family member toward others? How supportive or nurturing?) or in regard to communication *clarity* or *efficiency* (Does each member of the family make sense when he or she talks? Do members of the family share a focus of attention? Do problems get solved?).

Throughout these discussions of family attitudes and interactional behaviors, keep in mind two operating principles. First, the cause-and-effect relationships between mood disorder symptoms and family environmental factors are bidirectional: Families are affected by bipolar disorder as much as they affect it. That is, parents or other relatives are not to be blamed for their emotional reactions, which usually come about from trying to help an offspring or spouse who has a very difficult illness and, often, a difficult personality. Second, there is no convincing evidence that disturbed family relationships *cause* the onset of bipolar disorder. High levels of family stress may play a role in precipitating recurrences of bipolar disorder, but one cannot assume that this same stress brought about the illness in the first place.

Early Family Environment Studies

Family dysfunction has long been described in relation to bipolar disorder. Back in the early phases of the psychoanalytic era, Cohen, Baker,

Cohen, Fromm-Reichmann, and Weigert (1954) described the families of manic–depressive persons as highly driven, socially climbing, highly conventional, and competitive. Mothers in these families were described as cold, domineering, and impersonal, but highly reliable; and fathers as weak, inept, and unreliable. Similarly, Gibson (1958) found in a retrospective questionnaire study that manic–depressive patients reported coming from highly conventional families and were often subjected to the envy of their siblings. Gibson concluded that patients used self-defeating behaviors in adulthood to cope with this perceived threat from real or symbolic sibling figures (e.g., coworkers or spouses).

Psychoanalysts believed, as many also believed of schizophrenia at the time (e.g., Fromm-Reichmann, 1950), that disturbed family dynamics played a causal role in the onset of bipolar disorder. However, the nature of this causal relationship was never made clear. They based their conclusions on case studies with no comparison groups or other experimental controls, and all of the patients they observed already had bipolar disorder. Moreover, disturbed family dynamics were inferred from the patient's retrospective recall. Although these investigators offered some intriguing insights, there is little direct empirical support for their claims.

In the 1970s, a separate spate of studies concerned the role of parental loss or deprivation. Parental loss (death or separation) during or before the adolescent years has been reported in 27–43% of adult bipolar patients, as compared with 10–28% of adults with unipolar depression (Brodie & Leff, 1971; Carlson, Kotin, Davenport, & Adland, 1974; Perris, 1966; Roy, 1980). However, it is not clear how an early loss experience would cause the severe mood swings characteristic of bipolar disorder. In fact, in these studies many of the early parental losses were probably due to suicides associated with major affective disorders in these parents, illustrating how psychosocial events in a person's developmental history can sometimes reflect genetic predispositional mechanisms.

Thus, early clinical–observational studies suggested the presence of significant familial stressors in the backgrounds of persons later diagnosed with bipolar disorder. However, in the absence of longitudinal studies of children at risk for bipolar disorder, we cannot establish causal connections between these features of the childhood family environment and the eventual onset of bipolar disorder in adulthood.

The Family and Recurrence Risk: Expressed Emotion Studies

More germane to our core topic—family treatment as a means of delaying, minimizing, or preventing recurrences of bipolar disorder—is the role of the family environment in the disorder's course and outcome. To what degree do stressful family environments predict the extremely variable courses of illness we observe in persons with the disorder?

Much of our thinking about family factors in bipolar disorder arose from our own and other investigators' research showing that stressful family environments were associated with high rates of relapse in schizophrenia, and correspondingly, that successfully modifying these environments through family treatment reduced relapse rates (for a review, see Miklowitz, 2004). To put our research on bipolar disorder in context, I briefly review the literature on expressed emotion (EE) and outcome in schizophrenia.

EE is a measure of emotional attitudes among relatives (usually parents or spouses) of a psychiatric patient. EE is based on a 1- to 1½-hour audiotaped, semistructured interview conducted with a close, caretaking relative (Vaughn & Leff, 1976). EE is usually assessed when the patient is in an acute phase of the disorder and may reflect family functioning when stress is at its highest.

Families are classified as high in EE if one or more relatives (1) express many (six or more) critical comments, (2) show evidence of hostility, or (3) show evidence of emotional overinvolvement or overconcern regarding the patient (see examples in Table 3.1). Some parents (e.g., Cathy's mother, Chapter 2) mainly show evidence of critical or hostile attitudes. Others (such as Wes's mother) are primarily characterized by emotional overinvolvement. Families in which no caretaking relative has these attitudes are called low in EE.

When a schizophrenic patient returns from a hospital to a high-EE family, his or her chances of relapsing in the 9 months to 1 year following this hospitalization are two to three times higher than if he or she returns

TABLE 3.1. Examples of High-EE Attitudes among Caretaking Relatives

Type	Example
Critical	"I'm annoyed about how he keeps his room." "I don't like the hours he keeps."
Hostile	"I can't stand talking to him." "I like nothing about him."
Emotionally overinvolved	"When I know she hasn't eaten, I can't eat anything myself." "I don't invite people to the house 'cause Allen [son] doesn't like it." "I am scared to death about his trip to California. I don't think he should go on a plane by himself."

to a low-EE (noncritical, nonhostile, normally involved) family. The fact that this prospective relationship has been replicated in 23 of 26 studies qualifies EE as an important risk factor in schizophrenia (Butzlaff & Hooley, 1998).

Is family EE a construct relevant to bipolar disorder? We have conducted two studies on this question. In the first, we evaluated 23 acutely ill manic patients who had been hospitalized at the UCLA Medical Center. We observed that the attitudes of criticism and emotional overinvolvement were just as common among these patients' parents as among the parents of hospitalized schizophrenic patients (Miklowitz, Goldstein, Nuechterlein, Snyder, & Doane, 1987). Moreover, the manic patients who were discharged from the hospital to high-EE parents had recurrences at 9-month follow-up at almost twice the rate (90%) of patients with low-EE parents (54%; Miklowitz et al., 1988).

We recently replicated this result in the Colorado Treatment–Outcome study (N = 101), which, being a controlled treatment study, had lower overall rates of relapse (Miklowitz et al., 2000; Figure 3.2). In that study, patients in high-EE parental homes relapsed at a rate of 45% over 1 year, whereas patients in low-EE homes relapsed at a rate of 19%. Our findings have also been replicated by several other groups of investigators, one in Berlin, Germany (Priebe, Wildgrube, & Muller-Oerlinghausen, 1989), one in New York (O'Connell, Mayo, Flatow, Cuthbertson, & O'Brien, 1991), and one in Los Angeles (Yan, Hammen, Cohen, Daley, & Henry, 2004). This last study found that EE was a significant predictor of relapses into depression, but not mania.

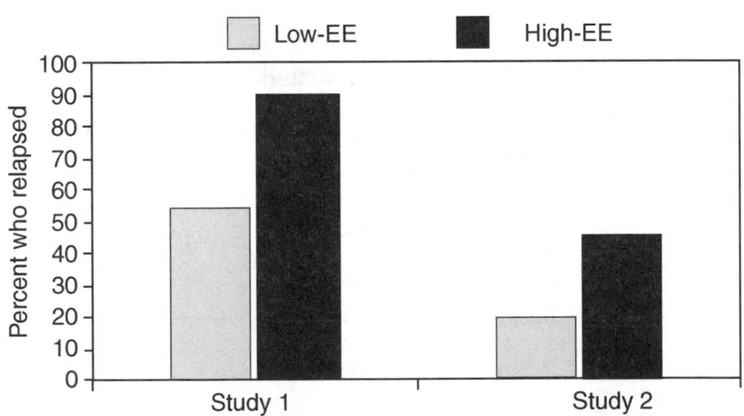

FIGURE 3.2. EE and follow-up relapse rates in two studies of patients with bipolar disorder. *Sources:* Miklowitz et al. (1988); Miklowitz et al. (2000).

We suspect that the impact of EE attitudes depends to a large extent on how biologically vulnerable the patient is; for example, a patient with a strong genetic history of bipolar disorder, or certain biological imbalances associated with frequent cycling (e.g., hypothyroidism, high cortisol production), may be most vulnerable to relapses in the presence of high-EE family attitudes. EE by caregivers may also intensify at different phases of the person's development: Relatives appear to become more critical over time, for example (Hooley & Richters, 1995). Thus, highly critical, hostile, or emotionally overinvolved attitudes among close relatives, although not necessarily causing relapses, are risk factors that should be assessed and, when possible, targeted for modification in psychoeducational treatment approaches.

Affective Style and Coping Style

EE construct is only one way of understanding how a family organizes itself around an acute episode of psychiatric disorder in one of its members. Another way is to examine the interactional behaviors—direct, face-to-face communication between members—that accompany episodes of the disorder. The case study of Wes illustrates how family interaction patterns, although at first hidden, can become salient when one observes how family members try to solve a problem.

We have focused in our research on two measures of family interaction, both drawn from laboratory-based problem-solving discussions like those undertaken with Wes and his family: affective style (AS; Doane, West, Goldstein, Rodnick, & Jones, 1981) and coping style (CS; Strachan, Feingold, Goldstein, Miklowitz, & Nuechterlein, 1989). AS refers to the emotional–verbal behavior of relatives during interactions with their ill family member (i.e., how verbally supportive, critical, guilt-inducing, or intrusive is the relative?). CS refers to the emotional–verbal behavior of the patient in the same interactions (i.e., how defensive, oppositional, self-critical, critical of the relative, or supportive of the relative is the patient?).

In our first UCLA bipolar study (Miklowitz et al., 1988), the best prediction of relapsing versus nonrelapsing outcomes at 9-month follow-up was achieved by combining data on parental attitudes (EE) during the acute inpatient phase with data on parental interactional behaviors (AS) during the outpatient stabilization phase. Bipolar patients from families who were high in EE and/or negative in AS (i.e., the parents were severely critical, guilt inducing, and/or highly intrusive toward the patient in stated attitudes *or* face-to-face verbal interactions) had recurrences of mania or depression at a rate of 94%. Of those from low-EE and benign-AS homes (those in which neither parent showed these negative attitudes or interactional behaviors), only 17% had recurrences. Furthermore, bipolar patients with parents who had high rates of negative AS showed poorer social–interpersonal functioning at follow-up than those whose parents showed low rates of negative AS.

Clearly, there are disturbances in the relationships of families coping with the episode and postepisode phases of bipolar disorder. When designing FFT, we predicted that by reducing negativity in these relationships, perhaps by augmenting the frequency of positive interactions, we would be able to reduce relapse risk in the affected patient. But in order to do so, we first wanted to know more about what actually happened in these families. What family interaction patterns or communication styles are encompassed by terms like "high EE" and "negative AS"? To what degree are patients provoking these attitudes or behaviors in their relatives?

Verbal Interactions in the Families of Bipolar Patients

One way to examine these questions is to conduct detailed analyses of the interactional processes that accompany episodes of bipolar disorder, and to compare these processes to those of families coping with other recurrent forms of psychiatric illness. In so doing, we can begin to understand how to intervene.

The contrast between the family processes associated with bipolar versus schizophrenic disorders is quite an interesting one. Both disorders are recurrent and often require hospitalization; both require long-term maintenance medications; both impair social and occupational functioning; and both disrupt the functioning of the family or marital unit. Furthermore, family interventions for schizophrenic patients have been implemented with much success. Do the same family processes that characterize schizophrenia—and that have been successfully modified by various psychoeducational programs—also characterize bipolar disorder?

In the late 1980s, my colleagues and I conducted a series of studies comparing bipolar and schizophrenic patients—all studied during the postepisode stabilization phase—on various measures of family interaction. We found dramatic differences between these groups in levels of AS (see Figure 3.3). Compared with the parents of bipolar patients, the parents of schizophrenic patients expressed more statements of AS intrusiveness (i.e., statements that indicated a knowledge of the patient's internal states, beyond what he or she actually stated; e.g., "You enjoy being hurt") and, to a lesser extent, of criticism (e.g., "You have a bad attitude about working"). In contrast, both groups of parents expressed AS support statements (e.g., "We know you're really trying hard to be friendly") with equal frequency (Miklowitz, Goldstein, & Nuechterlein, 1995).

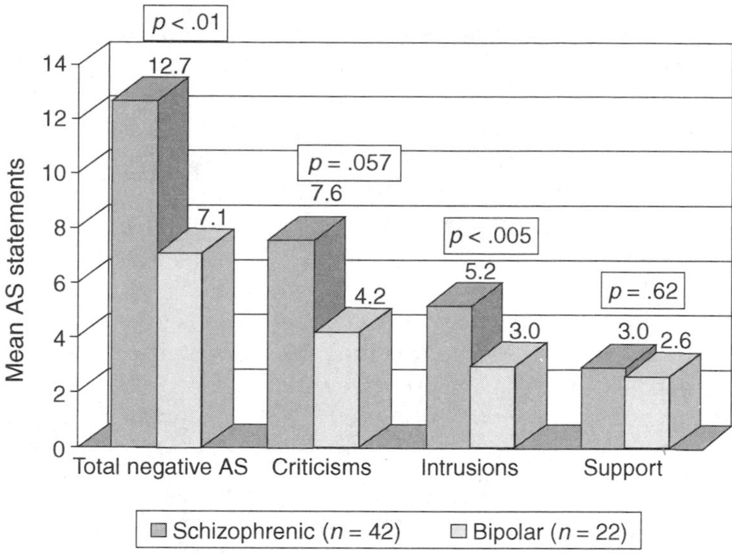

FIGURE 3.3. Levels of AS behavior in parents of patients with bipolar disorder and schizophrenia. *Source:* Miklowitz et al. (1995).

What were the patients doing during these interactions? Were bipolar patients somehow easier to interact with or more mollifying toward their relatives, and therefore elicited less criticism or intrusiveness? Actually, bipolar patients were more verbally active and "feisty" during these discussions, speaking nearly twice as often as the patients with schizophrenia. But even more important, when parents were high in negative AS (i.e., they frequently criticized or made intrusive statements to the patient), bipolar patients were most likely to *externalize*, making many CS "refusal" statements such as "I don't agree with you" or "I won't do what you're suggesting." We suspect that this style of interacting among patients was intimidating to some relatives, and perhaps inhibited the amount of negative AS expressed by these relatives. In contrast, schizophrenic patients were more likely to *internalize* or self-criticize when with high-AS relatives (e.g., "I know I don't deserve any of your help").

A second study clarified these family processes further. Simoneau, Miklowitz, and Saleem (1998) examined the family interaction patterns of parents and their adult bipolar offsprings, or spouses with their bipolar partners, shortly after resolution of an acute episode of the patient's illness. In a laboratory-based interaction task, high-EE families were found to be locked into "attack/counterattack" cycles of communication that neither the patient nor the relative was able to interrupt. The members of low-EE patient/relative dyads also had arguments during the task, but these were short-lived and usually were derailed by one or both members. The high-EE and low-EE families were best distinguished by the frequency of the "three-volley sequence": a negative statement from a relative, followed by a negative statement from the patient, and continued by a negative statement from the relative. In general, in high-EE families, patients and relatives were more likely to reciprocate negative affect.

Finally, a reanalysis of the original UCLA sample by Rosenfarb et al. (2001) found that relapses over a 9-month follow-up could be predicted from the patient's behavior during the interactions. Patients often showed grandiose or mildly delusional thinking during these interactions. Patients who became more thought disordered during the family interactions and whose relatives made frequent statements of harsh criticism (negative AS) were more likely to relapse than patients whose relatives were low in AS and who did not become thought disordered during the interactions. So, combining data on patients' and relatives' behavior provided the best prediction of patients' relapses over the subsequent 9-month period.

What are the implications of these findings for new family interventions? For the bipolar patient, one goal of FFT must be to help him or her tone down and respond less defensively when interacting with relatives. Relatives, in turn, may need to be aware that their critical or intrusive statements are likely to generate opposition or argumentativeness in the patient, or even a mild exacerbation of his or her symptoms. These goals may be achievable through structured interventions that modify specific aspects of the family's communication and problem-solving styles.

More generally, our results suggest that relatives need to recognize the importance of the family milieu to the patient's process of post-episode recovery, and modify their expectations for his or her immediate adaptation during the postepisode period. In turn, patients need to recognize the significant emotional impact that their episodes have had on close relatives and to acknowledge that the behavioral responses of these relatives—even if sometimes offensive—are often the result of a desire to help.

The Clarity of Family Communication

Family communication can also be disordered in the domain of communication clarity. If family members have difficulty communicating their ideas in a coherent fashion, little effective problem solving can be achieved. Fortunately, clarity of communication is something one can teach to families through role playing and rehearsal of effective communication strategies.

For years, families of schizophrenic patients have been described as high in communication deviance (CD), meaning that their verbal interactions are characterized by difficulties in sharing a focus of attention, communicating messages clearly, or bringing about closure when discussing their ideas (Wynne, Singer, Bartko, & Toohey, 1977). Numerous studies suggest that the parents of schizophrenic patients have higher levels of CD—as assessed by their responses to projective tests like the Thematic Apperception Test (TAT)—than the parents of patients with nonpsychotic disorders or of normal persons (Miklowitz & Stackman, 1992). But do families having a bipolar member show CD?

In our research, we found that overall levels of CD are similar in the families of bipolar and schizophrenic patients (Miklowitz et al., 1991). That is, parents in both groups occasionally make unintelligible remarks, speak tangentially, or do not complete their sentences. However, the parents of bipolar patients are more likely to exhibit a specific form of CD, that is, "contorted, peculiar language." For example, when making up a story about a TAT card, a parent of a bipolar patient is more likely to use phrases such as "This man is in *the process of thinking of the process* of being a doctor."

Patients and parents coping with bipolar disorder also show this form of CD in face-to-face discussions with each other. For example, a patient said to his mother, *"It's gonna be up and downwards along the process to go through something like this."* Their messages are understandable but jumbled, with many unnecessary words or words used out of order.

We suspect that these kinds of speech errors occur when family members or patients are anxious, hurried, or perhaps ambivalent about the message they are conveying. Problems are discussed in a somewhat disorganized way, irrelevant topics are introduced, and the meaning of certain messages is lost. Consistent with this pattern, one study found that communication clarity worsened when relatives discussed the patient's difficulty or inability to uphold the family's ethnic and cultural values (Kymalainen, Weisman, Rosales, & Armesto, 2006). These findings argue for culturally sensitive interventions that encourage the communicating of clear messages and that introduce an external structure when families attempt to solve important conflicts.

Summary

Our family-focused intervention for bipolar disorder was guided by our research observations regarding how families of bipolar patients cope with episodes of the disorder. Several conclusions can be drawn, as listed in Table 3.2.

Many of the negative emotional attitudes and communication patterns we observed are probably the result of the caretaking burden on

TABLE 3.2. Research Observations about the Families of Bipolar Patients

- Their face-to-face communication is characterized by emotionally charged interchanges.
- The speech of family members and patients can become disordered and unclear when they try to solve emotionally charged family problems.
- Negative affective relationships between the patient and relatives are associated with a poorer course of illness and poorer social functioning for the patient.

family members during the stabilization phase, when most of these assessments are undertaken. Relatives must deal on a day-to-day basis with the patient's mood swings, disorganized thinking, and social or work impairment. We suspect that beneath the high-EE attitudes and negative interactional behaviors of relatives is a great deal of disappointment, anger, and anxiety. Nevertheless, these family processes bode poorly for the disorder's outcome, particularly when biological and genetic risk factors are also present. FFT, particularly if administered with medications during or shortly after a patient's illness episode, may help the patient and relatives to adopt new styles of communication and conflict resolution that will help them adjust to the demands imposed by the patient's illness.

Life Events Stress

Approximately 1 year after his depressive episode, Wes obtained a job at a sheltered workshop in a community mental health center. He seemed healthy for a time and became more and more involved in the activities at the workshop. Then, news came that representatives of a state agency were going to visit and evaluate the functioning of the community center. Wes became convinced that the real purpose of the visit was to fire him. As the evaluation visit approached, his behavior became more agitated and disorganized and his mood more irritable. The day before the agency's visit, he flooded the basement of the center and destroyed much of its property. He lost his job and was hospitalized again.

There is substantial evidence that the periods prior to manic or depressive episodes contain more stressful life events than other periods in patients' lives (for reviews, see Johnson, 2005a, 2005b). Some of these life events seem to be the direct result of the disorder's escalating symptom (e.g., Wes's loss of his job), and others occur quite independently of the patient's behavior (e.g., the visit of the state agency to Wes's community center). An understanding of what forms of life stress are associated with recurrences is crucial to the development of psychosocial treatment plans for the postepisode period.

Life Events Research

The difficulties of conducting life events research are well documented (e.g., Dohrenwend, Dohrenwend, Dodson, & Shrout, 1984). Nevertheless, the most carefully crafted studies show the influence of life stress on the course of bipolar disorder, even when events that could have been caused by the person's behavior are excluded from consideration (Johnson, 2005a).

Of particular interest are studies that use longitudinal designs. For example, Ellicott, Hammen, Gitlin, Brown, and Jamison (1990), in a 2-year follow-up of 61 bipolar outpatients, found that those patients with high life events stress scores had a 4.5 times greater chance of having a bipolar relapse during the follow-up than those with medium or low life events stress scores. These results could not be accounted for by patients' medication regimens or compliance with these regimens. Johnson and Miller (1997) found that negative life events increased the amount of time it took bipolar patients to recover from a depressive episode, and were associated with increases in depressive symptoms over several months, even when patients were taking medications.

Several theories have been proposed for the linkage between life stress and recurrences of bipolar disorder. One particularly promising model is the social rhythm stability hypothesis (Ehlers, Frank, & Kupfer, 1988; Ehlers, Kupfer, Frank, &. Monk, 1993; Frank, 2005). This model postulates that the core dysfunction in bipolar disorder is one of instability. Specifically, people maintain certain patterns of daily social activity and social stimulation, or "social rhythms" (i.e., when they go to work, when they socialize, how many people they usually interact with, and the level of social stimulation provided by these people). People also have daily sleep–wake cycles and patterns of neuroendocrine regulation, or biologically driven "circadian rhythms."

The stability of social rhythms is believed to be in part due to the presence of "social zeitgebers," which provide an external clock to regulate a person's daily habits. A parent or spouse can be a zeitgeber for a patient, in that close relatives usually help organize the patient's eating and sleeping schedules and probably modulate patterns of social stimulation. Similarly, a job with regular hours is a zeitgeber. Other external factors may serve as "zeitstorers," which disrupt daily rhythms. A new romantic relationship and the birth of a baby are examples of zeitstorers. A job that requires frequent air travel and changes in time zones is also a zeitstorer (Ehlers et al., 1988, 1993).

The social rhythm stability model postulates that certain life events provoke changes in social rhythms (via introducing zeitstorers or removing existing zeitgebers), which in turn alter circadian rhythms and influence the onset of affective symptoms. A series of studies at the University of Pittsburgh School of Medicine found that bipolar patients were more likely to have had a social rhythm-disruptive life event in the 8 weeks prior to a manic episode than at other points in the course of their illness (Malkoff-Schwartz et al., 1998, 2000). These events were not necessarily of emotional significance (e.g., needing to stay up late to study for an exam) but had the effect of throwing off the patient's sleep–wake cycles.

How else can we understand the role of life events in bipolar episodes? Another model with comparable empirical support emphasizes the role of "goal dysregulation" in the onset of mania (Johnson, 2005b). In this framework, mania results from an excessive focus on goals resulting from increased sensitivity of the dopaminergic reward pathways. Excess reward sensitivity may heighten a patient's reactivity to success experiences, such that manic symptoms are more likely to worsen after life events involving goal attainment. Results of a longitudinal study indicating that goal-attainment life events (e.g., getting a job promotion, starting a new relationship) predicted increases in manic symptoms over 6 months, but not depressive symptoms (Johnson et al., 2000). In other words, people with bipolar disorder can become manic after something good happens, just as they can become depressed after negative events.

Implications of Stressful Life Events for Family Functioning

The life events and family literatures share some common assumptions, but there has been little attempt to examine how life events, family dysfunction, and changes in daily rhythms may be linked. In the case of Stewart (Chapter 1), his change in work shift hours led to changes in his sleep–wake cycles, which may have contributed to his manic state. His increasing irritability as a result of sleep disturbance and hypomania caused conflict in his relationship with Susan, whose sleep and mood were probably also disturbed by these schedule changes. In turn, the couple's escalating conflicts contributed to Stewart's rhythm instability and symptoms. Likewise, Wes's move to a new home with his family, in addition to generating emotional conflicts about his attempts at independence, probably shifted his daily routines and sleep habits. Thus, life events may provoke family conflicts, particularly those that existed in more attenuated form prior to the occurrence of an event. Family conflicts, in turn, may contribute to the stress and daily rhythm instability introduced by life changes.

Under most circumstances, the family is a source of social support to a psychiatric patient, and the absence of social supports at times of high life stress increases the probability of a mood disorder episode (Brown & Harris, 1978). Thus, a family intervention needs to take into account the life events that may have precipitated a patient's most recent manic or depressive episode. Specifically, one can (1) educate the family about the reciprocal interactions between life stress, family conflicts, and affective episodes; (2) encourage open communication about the emotional significance of painful life events; (3) encourage the family to anticipate future life stressors; and (4) teach new ways of adapting to stress, such as regularizing social routines and sleep–wake cycles when disruptive influences occur (Frank et al., 2005). Finally, although a clinician would want to celebrate a patient's successes, it may be useful to reacquaint him or her—and family members—with the early warning signs of mania when positive, goal attainment life events occur.

The Vulnerability–Stress Model Revisited

Genetic vulnerabilities, biological vulnerabilities, and socioenvironmental stressors interact in influencing episodes of mood disorder. But how can we put these diverse elements together into one comprehensive model? Moreover, what are the treatment implications of such a model?

Figure 3.4 presents our conceptualization of vulnerability–stress interactions in episodes of bipolar disorder. This model has been adapted from the "instability model" of Goodwin and Jamison (1990; Miklowitz, 2008). First, episodes of bipolar disorder occur against a background of genetic and biological vulnerability. Second, stresses in the domains of life events and family dysfunction represent separate but possibly interlinked provoking agents. Life stress appears to exert its effects, at least in part, through changing social and circadian rhythms, but almost certainly has effects on other biological systems as well, such as dopaminergic reward pathways. It also affects the patient's psychological state, such as when a death in the family occurs and the patient enters a period of mourning.

Family stress has been repeatedly linked to mood disorder episodes, but its mechanisms of action are unclear. It is possible, for example, that family stress is overstimulating to the patient, causing certain stress reactions that affect the functioning of biobehavioral systems (e.g., the behavioral inhibition or facilitation systems). Family stress may also augment the negative impact of changes in daily rhythms, as discussed above. Moreover, family stress affects the patient psychologically, such as by engaging his or her defensive coping systems (e.g., oppositionality or

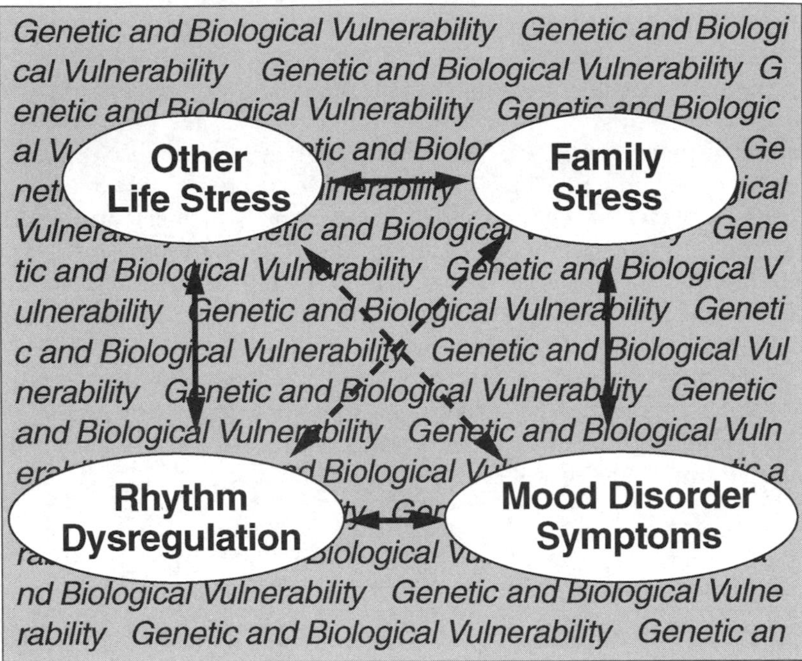

FIGURE 3.4. A vulnerability–stress instability model of bipolar disorder episodes. *Sources:* Goodwin and Jamison (1990); Miklowitz (2008).

withdrawal). Finally, dysfunction in the family milieu may mean that the social supports the patient normally counts on to protect him- or herself from life stress are absent.

This vulnerability–stress model, although in need of more supporting empirical work, directs us to a certain model of outpatient treatment. This model contends that drug treatment—even though essential to the bipolar patient—will be less effective in cases where stress is high. Rather, a more comprehensive biopsychosocial program goes beyond pharmacotherapy to reduce directly the risks associated with environmental stress. We have focused our model on family relationships. Others (e.g., Frank, 2005) focus on intervening with the individual bipolar patient to alter interpersonal stress and regularize social rhythms.

Concluding Comments

Reestablishing functional family relationships after an episode of bipolar disorder is a very challenging endeavor. For some families, the high-EE attitudes and disturbed patterns of interaction described here reflect the traumatic impact of the patient's episode or hospitalization, as well as any antecedent life events. For others, these attitudes or patterns are longstanding, and they predate, or at least persist independently of, the disorder.

Beyond educating families about how to understand and cope with bipolar disorder, there is a strong focus in FFT on the learning of new communication and problem-solving skills through behavioral techniques such as modeling, role-playing, and rehearsal. When members of a family practice new ways of listening or giving positive and negative feedback to each other, new alliances develop, a feeling of collaboration becomes more salient (i.e., "we're all in this together"), and family relationships begin to change. These improvements in the structure or function of family relationships have the potential to reduce the risks associated with high levels of EE, AS, and unexpected life events.

PART II

Conducting Family-Focused Treatment

chapter 4

Planning the First Encounter

During her inpatient stay, a family clinician approached Maryann, a 29-year-old African American woman, about participating in an outpatient family psychoeducational program with her mother, Geena. Maryann was at first quite suspicious, fearing that she would be forced to confront her mother about issues that would be too difficult to talk about. However, the clinician seemed genuinely concerned about her, taking time to ask Maryann about her interests, her future goals, and other matters that did not involve her illness. The interchange with the family clinician was the first she'd had since her hospital admission in which she didn't feel like a mental patient. She said she would think about it.

With Maryann's consent, the clinician held a conjoint family meeting with Maryann and Geena. Maryann was impressed that the clinician seemed to be interested in getting to know her and her mother as people, often joking with them while at the same time gathering information. The clinician explained that they would receive educational information about bipolar disorder and that they would be exposed to different and perhaps more effective ways to communicate and solve problems. However, after these explanations, Geena said, "You know, Maryann has been in the hospital a couple of times now, and after each one, everyone says they have a new therapy to offer, and everyone says that theirs will work. We've been through all this stuff. Why should we believe this will be the cure-all?"

Maryann was a bipolar patient who might be able to benefit from family-focused treatment (FFT). She had had a recent episode of bipolar disorder, she was confused about the new ways that people related to her now that she had the diagnosis, she had a mother who was regularly involved in her care, and there was conflict in the mother–daughter relationship. However, the clinician quickly encountered resistance to the family program from both the patient and her mother. This resistance was understandable: Why should they immediately jump at this opportunity, when in the past they had been offered other therapies—often at great cost—that didn't help? Why shouldn't they view a new therapist, with a new approach, as nothing but another snake oil salesman? The manner in which the first encounter is planned and, particularly, the way that FFT is initially presented to patients and families, have much to do with its successful implementation.

Chapter Overview

This and the next chapter describe the initial phases of FFT: planning and carrying out the first encounter (this chapter) and administering the individual and family assessments that inform the treatment (Chapter 5). This chapter is concerned with three issues. First, who is an appropriate candidate for FFT, and at what stage of the disorder? Second, what are the specifics of conducting the treatment—the appropriate treatment frequency, duration, and clinical setting? Third, how do you, as the FFT clinician, connect with the patient, the family, and the treating physician in introducing and encouraging participation in the program?

Particular attention is given to addressing the expectable doubts and resistances expressed by patients, family members, and treating physicians as they are asked to participate in or at least support the program. There are good and bad ways to address these resistances, and your strategies during the initial connecting phases often make or break the treatment.

For Whom Is FFT Appropriate?

Attributes of the Patient

The FFT program, although designed within the context of controlled experimental trials, is intended for a broad population of bipolar patients. Clinicians implementing FFT in the community will likely obtain referrals from a wide variety of sources (e.g., hospitals, day hospital programs, HMOs, private referral). However, as discussed in this section, there are difficulties that arise in implementing FFT with certain subpopulations. Although these difficulties do not necessarily rule out a patient's participation, they raise issues that may require modification of the program or the introduction of ancillary treatments.

First, we usually administer FFT to patients who have just had an episode of bipolar disorder, although there is no requirement that this episode involve a hospitalization. There are no age limitations (e.g., the affected patient can be an elderly person or an adolescent, or, with appropriate modifications of the reproducible handouts that follow, a child). In our research we have targeted recently manic, mixed-phase, and depressed patients. Patients who have been remitted for some time may also benefit from the program, but in our experience neither they nor their family members are as motivated to participate. Generally, families are most motivated when there has been some kind of crisis, whether this be a first onset or a recurrence of the patient's disorder, severe family or marital conflicts, or a stressful life event. Thus, assess in your initial meetings with the family members their motivation to take part in the program (e.g., ask, "What has been your experience with therapy before?" "Could you imagine yourself committing to this program over the next 9 months?").

Acutely ill patients who are located on inpatient units, and for whom the program will continue once they are outpatients, are usually those most in need of it. However, you should consider the nature of the inpatient setting in organizing your treatment plans. For example, if you work in an inpatient care facility or day treatment program, you may be able to connect with the patient and family and initiate the program while the patient is still in the hospital. In this day and age you may only be able to meet once with the patient and/or family to discuss the program and set up a first outpatient visit before the patient is discharged.

Different clinical settings cater to different kinds of patients. Specifically, patients who are located in state hospital inpatient units are often quite severely and chronically ill. In contrast, those in private hospitals are, on average, less severely ill. Patients referred from outpatient private practitioners are usually the least severely ill. Thus, you may choose to "pitch" the treatment at a more intensive level (i.e., using more sophisticated explanations of the educational materials, allowing for more exploration of potentially explosive family issues) if your eligible patient comes from an outpatient referral, and at a less intensive level if your patient originates from a state hospital.

Patients with comorbid developmental disabilities (e.g., pervasive developmental disorders) or *neurological conditions* (e.g., severe strokes, brain lesions, dementia) may have cognitive limitations that interfere with the processing of the educational materials or the learning of new communication skills. These are not reasons to exclude such patients, but rather suggest tailoring the treatment to the patient's functional level. For example, a creative therapist may be able to convey the educational information using visual rather than reading materials.

Patients who are unwilling to take medication from the outset pose special problems. Such patients are likely to be symptomatic and at high risk for recurrences. Family treatment, if well delivered, may be a means of getting the patient back on a medication regimen, particularly if the decision not to take medication is due to misunderstandings about the disorder or a direct reaction to another family member's controlling behavior (see Chapter 8). However, the patient and family should not be led to believe that family treatment is a substitute for medications. Our position has been to accept patients into FFT who are not currently taking mood-stabilizing medications, but to make clear that beginning a medication regimen is a condition of remaining in the program. Furthermore, we specify a date by which the patient must have initiated medications in order to continue in the program (i.e., after six or seven sessions, or the typical length of the psychoeducation module).

Finally, evaluate *patients with substance or alcohol abuse or dependence disorders* carefully before admitting them to FFT. An assumption of FFT is that the primary diagnosis is bipolar disorder and that substance abuse problems, if present, are secondary. There is no point in conducting a thorough family education about the signs and symptoms of bipolar disorder if the real diagnosis is alcohol-induced psychotic disorder, substance-induced mood disorder, or Korsakoff's psychosis. In fact, as discussed in Chapter 5, a careful diagnostic evaluation should precede the introduction of FFT.

Nonetheless, if the primary diagnosis is bipolar disorder, patients with comorbid substance or alcohol abuse or dependence are candidates for FFT. Educational information about the influences of alcohol or substances may supplement the didactic material provided about the disorder (see Chapters 6 and 7). Encourage the patient to attend substance abuse programs (e.g., Alcoholics Anonymous [AA] or Narcotics Anonymous [NA]; outpatient drug rehabilitation services) while also participating in FFT. Chapter 12, which addresses managing crises within FFT, discusses ways to prevent or minimize the effects of relapses of substance or alcohol abuse.

Attributes of the Family

Family structures are quite variable, and FFT can be adapted to most of these constellations. Thus, workable constellations include single- or two-parent families in which the diagnosed patient is an adult or adolescent offspring; couples in which one member is bipolar, including those with young children; or parent–offspring dyads wherein the offspring is a primary caretaker of his or her bipolar parent. Often more important than the actual composition of the family is the presence of a caretaking family member who considers it part of his or her role to monitor the health of the bipolar family member. The absence of such a person may render much of the psychoeducational material, as well as the skill-training procedures, irrelevant. In most families, this person is a parent or a spouse, but we have also included siblings, adult offspring, romantic partners, close friends, and even roommates.

A separate issue concerns the frequency of contact and the living situation. There is no requirement that the family members and patient share living quarters. In fact, we have conducted FFT with families in which various members drive in from opposite sides of town. But what is considered enough "face-to-face contact" to warrant family treatment? There are no hard and fast rules, but we generally find that family members with less than four face-to-face weekly contact hours with the patient view family intervention as irrelevant to them. These family members are often trying to dissociate themselves from the patient and see family treatment as an attempt to draw them back into a game they wish to stop playing.

The Mechanics of FFT

This section addresses three issues: the structure and frequency of FFT, the setting of FFT sessions (in the family's home vs. the clinic), and qualities of the clinical treatment team.

Treatment Structure and Session Frequency

In Chapter 1, I briefly describe the structure of the 21-session FFT program. Table 4.1 describes this structure further, as a function of the stages of the patient's disorder. Although these illness phases vary in duration and may not be fully distinct from each other, there are certain therapeutic objectives associated with each phase.

The focus of treatment during the acute episode stage and the immediate postepisode stabilization period is on connecting and developing an initial alliance with the patient and family and on carrying out the functional assessment (Chapter 5). Although there is no specific number of contact hours recommended for this initial phase, it has three objectives: to introduce the program to the patient and family and (if necessary) conduct a diagnostic evaluation with the patient; to gain information about the history of the disorder from the patient and relatives; and to assess the family's emotional atmosphere, communication styles, and problem-solving abilities.

Most bipolar patients are clinically stabilized (although not necessarily symptom-free) by 3 months after a hospital discharge (or after the onset of an illness episode that did not require hospitalization). During this 12-week stabilization phase, you can usually complete the psychoeducation module and begin training the patient and family in communication skills (12 weekly sessions).

TABLE 4.1. Structure of the FFT Program

Illness phase	Treatment goals	Frequency of sessions
Acute	Connect, assess, develop a treatment alliance	As needed
Stabilization	Finish assessments, conduct psychoeducation module (7 sessions), begin CET module (5 sessions)	Weekly for 3 months (12 sessions)
Maintenance	Finish CET module (about 2 more sessions), conduct problem-solving skills module (4–5 sessions), terminate (2–3 sessions), and plan maintenance sessions as necessary	Biweekly for 3 months, then monthly for 3 months (9 sessions)

Once the patient has achieved a degree of clinical stability, he or she enters a maintenance treatment phase, in which the focus is on resolving current family conflicts and preventing future ones. During this nine-session, 6-month phase, complete the communication enhancement module and the problem-solving training module. The first six sessions of this phase are biweekly, and the last three are monthly. Spend the final two to three sessions (or more if necessary) on practicing problem solving and termination of the treatment. Maintenance or "tune-up" sessions, and sessions concerning the resolution of specific family crises (e.g., relapses), can be given at any time during or following the 9-month treatment period.

This structure is for the prototypical case. Some families, for example, may benefit from weekly sessions that continue throughout the maintenance phase. Some patients need longer than 3 months to stabilize, and communication training may need to be delayed until they are able to handle the interpersonal discomfort that may be associated with role-playing exercises. For other families, you may decide to begin with the communication enhancement module (e.g., a couple presenting with severe marital disturbance, for whom learning about bipolar disorder is of secondary importance). Finally, if your clinical setting limits you to a few outpatient sessions, you may be able to deliver only part of the program (e.g., the psychoeducation module). Thus, be flexible in the timing and delivery of these treatment modules.

Setting

Falloon et al.'s (1984) behavioral family treatment of schizophrenia was conducted in families' homes. However, the results of several controlled treatment–outcome studies suggest that family psychoeducational treatments for schizophrenia are also effective if delivered in a clinic setting (for a review, see Pitschel-Walz et al., 2001). In today's managed care world, most community practitioners are unable to conduct regular home visits, and the clinic is likely to be the only option. Other managed care settings support home visits if they are carefully justified in the patient's treatment plan (e.g., if one argues that the home is a more ecologically valid setting for addressing family conflicts).

If you are free to make a choice, there are certain advantages and disadvantages of home- versus clinic-based treatments. In most cases, home-based treatment is more convenient for the family than clinic-based treatment (particularly for those families with young children, or when a large number of family members are coming from different places). It will usually, although not invariably, ensure better attendance at sessions. Home sessions also make the generalization of certain communication skills more likely. For example, couples who have learned to listen to each other while sitting in comfortable chairs in their living room may return to this setting when practicing the skills.

However, in some cases, family members may regard inviting therapists into their home as a shaming experience. They worry that neighbors will find out who the clinicians are, and that the "family secret" (often the son's or daughter's illness) will become public. In other cases, families participating in home treatment may begin to take the clinicians' visits for granted. In fact, home visits sometimes engender in families the belief that "you need us more than we need you." Families who repeatedly arrive late to home sessions, or allow sessions to be interrupted by telephone calls, children's demands, doorbells, or other distractions, may secretly hold this belief.

Other factors to be weighed in deciding on home versus clinic visits include the time availability of the clinician, the duties for which he or she can be compensated, and, most important, the possibility that the choice of one setting over another will increase the likely success of the treatment. Thus, the decision about where to conduct FFT should be made on a case-by-case basis.

The Clinicians

FFT can be provided by any trained clinician who is comfortable in working with families. There are no restrictions as to degree status. Clinicians who administer FFT should preferably have a minimum of 2 years of therapy experience, including some work with families. Knowledge of bipolar disorder—its symptoms, diagnosis, course, and treatment—is a must.

Although FFT can be easily conducted by a single therapist, there are times when a cotherapy team is advantageous. Each clinician can monitor the other's behavior within sessions and identify issues or themes that the other clinician may have missed. In some cases, the two clinicians can develop alliances with different subsystems of the family. For example, if a single clinician errs in directing too many of the interventions toward the more verbal members of the family, a second clinician can balance the session by drawing out the less verbal members. Finally, because this treatment is best learned "on the job," the pairing of a trained therapist with a therapist-in-training can be cost-effective.

Getting Started: The Initial Contacts

Once you have identified a patient who you think may benefit from FFT, make contact with three persons or groups of persons: the patient's physician (and the individual therapist, if there is one), the patient, and the family members. As discussed below, special issues come up in introducing the program to each of these persons. Chapter 6 discusses the more thorough introduction to the program given to families once the psychoeducation module begins.

In your initial contacts with these persons, point out that your initial assessments may reveal that the program is not right for the patient or the family. For example, you may learn that family members do not have enough weekly contact with the patient to make skills training worthwhile. Make clear that your initial purpose is to set up appointments for the initial assessments (discussed in Chapter 5), to determine if the program is a good fit.

Coordinating Family Treatment with Drug Treatment

Maryann was suspicious of her physician. He seemed to be a rather harried "pill pusher" who wasn't much interested in her life history. He expressed annoyance at her questions about the nature and causes of bipolar disorder, saying simply, "It's not as big a deal as you think. It's kind of like having diabetes. You just have to take your medication." He accused her of being "passive–aggressive" when she stated that she didn't want to take her medications. When she asked him about the family program she had been offered, he said simply, "Yeah, I heard about it, and that's up to you. But most therapies don't work for this sort of problem." Maryann then became doubtful about what the family clinician had told her.

As this case vignette illustrates, coordinating treatment plans with the physician is an issue of substantial importance. Of course, FFT and medication maintenance can be provided by the same person, but in our experience this is rare. More frequently, family treatments are provided by clinicians who have close connections with community psychiatrists in their own or nearby settings, with whom they coordinate treatments for a variety of different patients. Clinicians working within HMOs or community mental health centers, for example, may be more easily able to integrate FFT into the patient's ongoing pharmacological plan.

The first step after identifying a potential patient is usually to call the treating psychiatrist or general practitioner. In most cases, the physician can pave the way for you to initiate contact with the patient and family, which usually requires that the physician first discuss the matter with the patient. Of course, the physician must obtain written release-of-information from the patient before discussing the details of the case with you.

In other cases, it may make sense to contact the patient before contacting the physician. For example, if a patient or family member calls you and expresses interest in the treatment, or if a colleague refers the patient to you, you may decide to explain the program briefly to the caller first and then obtain release-of-information for further contacts with the physician.

Most psychiatrists and general practitioners are more than happy to hear about the availability of an outpatient family psychoeducational program and to discuss it with the patient, especially if the physician's plan is only to manage the patient's medications. Occasionally, however, one runs into the problem of "patient ownership." This is a very real issue in private practice settings, where the number of paying patients may be few and competition for them high. Alternatively, as in Maryann's case, the physician may not believe in family or other forms of therapy for bipolar patients. In such cases, the physician may decline even to discuss the matter with the patient.

There are a number of ways to approach a physician to increase his or her willingness to collaborate. First, point out that (and give examples of how) the patient's participation in the program will enhance rather than detract from the goals of the drug treatment. For example, the focus within psychoeducation on drug adherence may help ensure the success of the pharmacological plan. In one of our randomized trials, patients in FFT were more adherent with their medications than patients receiving minimal family psychoeducation (Miklowitz et al., 2003). Second, you will be able to provide the physician with ongoing information (e.g., the presence of previously undocumented psychotic symptoms) or historical facts that may help resolve diagnostic ambiguities and inform medical treatment decisions. Third, you may recognize drug side effects, drug toxicity, or symptomatic relapse earlier than the physician because of the greater frequency of family sessions. Fourth, you can provide additional crisis intervention and backup in the patient's community maintenance.

Of course, it should be up to the patient and his or her family to decide whether they wish to participate in a psychosocial treatment program, and the physician who does not inform a patient or family of the program's availability is being irresponsible. Nevertheless, coordinating treatment plans with and obtaining the support of the physician is crucial to the success of FFT. I revisit this issue in later chapters.

Engaging the Patient

It is likely that your first contact will be with the patient rather than with his or her relatives. This is not invariably the case, but there are risks involved in contacting the family first. The patient may feel that plans are being made for treatment without his or her input, or worse yet, that the clinician has already bought into the family's ways of thinking. Contacting the parents or spouse first may even imply that the clinician feels the patient is not competent to make independent decisions. Of course, if the patient has residual psychotic symptoms (e.g., paranoid ideation), his or her interpretations of such events will be distorted.

Your first contact with the patient may be on an inpatient ward, at an outpatient clinic, or by telephone. We recommended approaching the patient—particularly one who is manic and irritable—in a low-key and nonaggressive, but persistent way. Consider the following interchange:

CLINICIAN: Hi, I'm Dr./Mr./Ms. ____________. I'd like to talk to you about a family program you might find interesting. Do you have a few minutes?

PATIENT: What's this about? Who are you?

CLINICIAN: I'm from the Mood Disorders Clinic. I'm a clinical psychologist [psychiatrist, social worker, nurse practitioner, etc.], and I work in a program that provides help to people who've had an episode of mood disorder. We work with people on improving their family relationships and in dealing with the period after they get out of the hospital, which tends to be hard on everybody in the family. Can I tell you more about this now?

PATIENT: Go ahead, but make it quick.

CLINICIAN: Well, we know that people who've had an episode of mood disorder often have difficulty returning to live with their spouses [or parents], and that this is a time when support from outside professionals can be quite valuable.

PATIENT: (*irritable*) Yeah, my wife and I've been fighting more recently. But that's because of this damn medication I'm on.

CLINICIAN: Well, we would be working in close coordination with your physician. But our main focus is on working with family relationships and in getting people to learn as much as they can about their mood disorders. For example, we help people to learn new ways to communicate and solve problems within the family. Does it sound like this might be useful to you? I don't know you well, so I'd like your input.

PATIENT: It might. But my wife and I are real busy, and besides, I may be moving out of town once I get outta here. I can't commit to anything right now.

CLINICIAN: That sounds fine. All I'm asking now is that you think about it and discuss it with your wife and your doctor. We'll want to see if this program is right for you. In the meantime, should I give your wife a call and see if she'd be interested?

In this interchange, the clinician gives the patient plenty of room. There is no pressure, yet the necessary information is imparted. For example, the clinician does not challenge dubious claims such as the patient's plans to move away. This low-key approach helps the patient feel he or she has some control over the treatment process.

Engaging the Family

Because of the extreme stress and caretaking burden associated with being a parent or spouse of a psychiatrically ill person, most family members will be happy to hear that a support program exists. In fact, many will report having felt ignored by mental health professionals treating their patient-relative, and that attempts to get their questions answered have been unsatisfying. Thus, when initially contacting the family, you are likely to get an interested, if not immediately acquiescent, response.

In other cases, family members will be resistant to being introduced to or evaluated for the FFT program. They may feel that they've had enough of therapists (a reaction common among the relatives of more chronically ill patients); angry about their recent dealings with the patient's nurse or physician; and skeptical about the efficacy of any form of therapy, either medical or psychological. They may be confused about why a psychotherapeutic program would be helpful for a disorder that, they've been told, is entirely biological in nature.

Perhaps most insidious is the feeling among some relatives that having a mental illness in the family is stigmatizing and sets them apart from their surrounding community. This negative "upward social comparison" may make relatives particularly resistant to becoming involved in a program that will remind them of this negative stigma.

In your initial contact with the relatives, the goal is simply to engage their interest. Briefly describe the program and try to set up an initial appointment. The section that follows applies primarily to initial telephone contacts but, with minimal modification, could apply to face-to-face contacts as well. Consider the following interchange:

CLINICIAN: Hi, Mrs. Gutierrez. I'm Dr. ___________, and I'm from the Mood Disorders Program. I've been working with your son, Emilio. Has he mentioned to you that I might be contacting you?

MOTHER: No, he hasn't.

CLINICIAN: I work in a program that specializes in the family care of bipolar mood disorder, which is the disorder that Emilio appears to have. Our clinic involves families in the outpatient treatment of our patients. Can I tell you more about our program?

MOTHER: Um, well, I guess so.

CLINICIAN: We offer family members an educational program for dealing with the period just after an illness episode (or hospitalization), when their ill family member comes back home. This tends to be a stressful time for everyone, particularly for family members who are trying to cope with the illness. The program is oriented around stress management. It consists of sessions in which we'll give you information about the nature of bipolar disorder, what causes it, and how it's treated. Later on, we work more directly with families to improve the way they communicate and solve problems. Does this sound like it would be of interest to you?

The clinician normalizes the need for stress-management skills, never implying that this particular family is having a tougher time than others in the same situation. Note that the term "family therapy" is not used. First, this term can be threatening as it may imply the family is at fault for causing the disorder. Second, the program itself is oriented toward psychoeducation, skill training, and stress management, rather than the domains typically targeted in family therapies. Thus, the terms "psychosocial treatment" and "psychoeducational program" are better.

Addressing Initial Resistances

Geena, Maryann's mother, expressed a lot of skepticism about the usefulness of family treatment in Maryann's outpatient plans. She noted that Maryann's physician had told her the disorder was entirely biological, and that there wasn't much she as a parent could do to help control it. She also said, "I read somewhere that a lot of psychologists still think that parents make people mentally ill. Is that what you people think?"

Like Geena, many relatives immediately express their reluctance to participate in a family program. In this section, we discuss the specific resistances often voiced (or implied) during the initial encounters and how you can obtain an agreement from relatives and patients to meet, learn about the program, and participate in the initial assessment sessions.

You may wonder why you should need to do such a selling job for a therapeutic program that is likely to benefit the family. It's a reasonable question. As is true of all forms of treatment, people mistrust what they don't know. They may view an offer of family psychoeducation as they would view a new medication: It might prove helpful or it might not, but there might also be side effects that could make things worse. So, try to be patient with family members who initially refuse treatment or who seem mistrustful of you.

Schedule Conflicts

The logistics of arranging many people's schedules can be quite challenging. A parent may say he or she does not know when another parent is available, a spouse may be concerned about the availability of child care, an adolescent patient may have conflicting after-school activities, or there may be only minimal overlap between the work hours of one family member and another. Often, these are very real issues, and a certain amount of flexibility in scheduling is usually in order.

However, scheduling conflicts often mask resistances to the program itself. Rather than arguing with family members about time availability, you are more likely to gain cooperation through statements such as the following:

> "I think it is difficult to arrange a session with many people, and we often run into this difficulty. We'll be as flexible as our own schedules permit in working out an agreeable time. But you may also have questions about whether this program is for you, and that is entirely understandable. I want to assure you that you're not signing up for anything at this point. We don't know yet whether this program is right for you or for him (or her)—it may not be. All we want is an initial meeting to tell you more about the program and find out more about you as people."

Here, the clinician interprets the schedule conflicts as masking doubts about committing to a new treatment program. She makes it clear to the family members that she is not expecting any guarantees from them, only their willingness to discuss the program further.

Disbelief in the Value of Psychotherapy

Some relatives immediately raise the question of how a psychosocial program fits into the patient's overall treatment plan. In some cases this question reflects the belief that psychological factors are irrelevant to the disorder. However, this question is often motivated by a fear that the family clinicians will place blame on the family for causing the disorder in the first place. Much has been written about the history of the relations between mental health professionals and family members, which in the past have involved the implicit or explicit blaming of parents and a lack of recognition of the caretaking burden they face (Hatfield, Spaniol, & Zipple, 1987; Perlick et al., 2007). Although it is most often parents for whom this issue is salient, spouses may also fear that the marital relationship somehow played an etiological role in the disorder.

It is unlikely that family members will raise these issues directly. Instead, they may simply ask how therapy can help, whether events from the patient's childhood will be raised in the treatment sessions, and what psychotherapy has to offer someone with a presumed medical illness. You can begin to address these questions by responding the way the clinician does in the following vignette:

GEENA: We've been through all this stuff. Why should we believe this will be the cure-all?

CLINICIAN: Geena, many family members are understandably skeptical about beginning a new treatment program. I know you've been promised a lot in the past, and a lot hasn't been delivered. You may wonder how it can be helpful, and this is an important question to ask. Our goal is really to make the period after a hospitalization as manageable for everyone in the family as possible. Our program is not designed to place blame on anybody. In fact, we view family members as allies in the treatment process, and we feel your input is essential to the success of Maryann's outpatient care (*joins with mother and normalizes her resistance*).

GEENA: Well, I appreciate that, but I still don't see how therapy for this will help.

CLINICIAN: I think the ways in which family treatment sessions can be helpful will become clearer as we proceed, but for now, all we're asking for is an initial meeting so we can more fully address your questions and find out about your views on Maryann's history. You are not making any commitment at this point.

These initial "joining" statements can help you get your foot in the door. Of course, you may have to go further before family members will agree to an initial session. If at all possible, avoid exploring in-depth issues during the initial encounter, especially if it is via a phone call. Relatives' or patients' emotional reactions to the disorder, feelings about the mental health system, or distrust of psychotherapy can all be addressed during the family psychoeducation module, once an initial therapeutic alliance has begun to develop. In the meantime, normalize their reactions with responses of the form "That's understandable" or "Yes, I think many people feel that way."

Desires to Disengage from the Patient

A somewhat less workable issue is the desire on the part of family members to distance themselves from the patient and his or her problems. This issue is particularly salient in marital couples, in which the spouse may be considering a separation or divorce. It may also surface in parents who have "survived" many of the patient's prior episodes and who do not wish to continue in the caretaker role. Statements to the clinician such as "We've heard all this before. He's got to start taking care of himself," reveal this position.

Some family members may be motivated by the notion that, through participating, they may learn concrete skills for coping with the patient's disorder and future episodes. However, if the overriding desire of key family members is to disengage from the patient, alternative treatment recommendations may be in order. Finally, whether or not family members choose to participate in FFT, they will probably benefit from attending mutual support groups for parents of psychiatric patients, such as those offered by the National Alliance on Mental Illness (800-950-NAMI; *www.nami.org*) or the Depressive and Bipolar Support Alliance (800-826-3632; *www.dbsalliance.org*).

Concluding Comments

FFT should be undertaken with careful consideration of the clinical characteristics of the patient, the training of the clinician, and the nature of the local clinical setting. Furthermore, developing a contract with a family for FFT involves careful engagement of each caregiving relative and other relevant members of the treatment team.

If you succeed in arranging a first appointment, you will probably want to spend some time assessing the patient and family to determine whether the program is appropriate for them: How much do they already know about bipolar disorder? What level of family conflict is present? What are the various attitudes of family members toward each other? What level of communication and problem-solving skill do they already possess, and what do they need to learn? These "functional assessments" are the topic of the next chapter.

chapter 5

The Functional Assessment

The family clinician interviewed Geena, Maryann's mother, to help determine the family's eligibility for the FFT program. She asked Geena about the development of Maryann's most recent episode, her prior episodes, and the impact of her illness on the functioning of the family unit. Geena painted a much different picture than had Maryann of the development and course of the illness, pointing to a relatively young onset (age 16) and the occurrence of several prior episodes that Maryann had not reported. Geena discussed these issues calmly at first, but then became angry, saying, "I don't know why I've put up with this so long!" She noted the burden that the illness had imposed on her; that she had given up many friends, lovers, and even a job because of Maryann's illness; and that, despite all this, she and Maryann were scarcely talking.

Chapter Overview

Before FFT commences, it is essential to conduct a series of assessments to help determine whether FFT is appropriate, and if so, to develop an individualized treatment plan that targets specific areas for change (after Falloon et al., 1984). There are several goals of the functional assessment, as outlined in Table 5.1. These goals can be achieved in a series of individual and family interviews conducted prior to or in the beginning phases of FFT. Some of the goals involve learning more about the illness and its history, and others, about the functioning of the family unit.

Keep in mind that FFT is geared toward improving a family's functioning during the period following a major affective episode. Its focus is

TABLE 5.1. Goals of the Functional Assessment

- Develop an initial therapeutic alliance with each family member. Establish that bipolar disorder is the correct diagnosis.
- Obtain a thorough psychiatric history, from the vantage point of the patient and key relatives.
- Evaluate the distress level of the family.
- Determine how existing individual and family resources or skills can be enhanced, in the domains of managing the disorder effectively, communicating productively, and solving problems.

on enhancing patients' and family members' knowledge of the disorder and their communication and problem-solving skills, and in developing strategies for effectively managing the disorder. Thus, the assessments should identify the skill assets of family members (e.g., their current strengths in communicating) as well as their skill or knowledge deficits (e.g., problem solving that deteriorates into negatively escalating arguments, or the tendency to view signs of depression in the patient as laziness).

This chapter describes the assessment methods related to these goals. The assessments you choose to undertake with any given family will vary according to your setting, your history with the patient, and the length of your treatment contract with the family. However, in some cases you may feel that introducing intensive assessments during the beginning phases of FFT will interfere with engaging a new patient or family. In these cases, conduct only those assessments that determine eligibility for the program (i.e., Is the primary diagnosis bipolar disorder? Is the primary problem one of substance or alcohol abuse? Are family members engaged in the patient's care?). Then, skip directly to the psychoeducation phase, where the program is more fully introduced and the treatment begins. Assessments may be introduced later, once you have developed a stronger alliance with the family.

Assessing the History of the Patient's Disorder

The Diagnostic Interview

If you work in a setting in which diagnostic evaluations are part of the ordinary intake procedures, a standard diagnostic interview may not be necessary. But if diagnoses within your setting are often in question, become familiar with instruments such as the Structured Clinical Interview for DSM-IV Axis I Disorders (First, Spitzer, Gibbon, & Williams, 1995) or the MINI International Neuropsychiatric Interview (Sheehan et al., 1998). If the patient is a child or teenager, use the Kiddie Schedule for

Affective Disorders and Schizophrenia, Present and Lifetime Version (KSADS-PL; Chambers et al., 1985; Kaufman et al., 1997) or the Washington University KSADS (Geller, Warner, Williams, & Zimerman, 1998). When establishing the diagnosis of children and teens, it is essential to administer the KSADS-PL to at least one parent as well, changing the format of the questions to "Has he ever had a period of depression . . . ?" or "When she gets elevated, does she also need to sleep less?" Structured diagnostic interviews, when administered properly, can yield reliable diagnoses, documentation of previously unrecognized comorbid disorders, and identification of previously undetected episodes. We recommend conducting these interviews during the second meeting with the patient (or, if the patient is a minor, the patient and parents), after giving a brief introduction to the program in the first meeting (see Chapter 4). The material gathered in the diagnostic interview will be of use in the psychoeducational phases of FFT. For example, the patient's descriptions of the prodromal and active phases of the recent episode can be revisited during the "relapse drill," when family members become acquainted with ways to intervene at the first signs of a recurrence (see Chapter 7).

Developing a rapport with the patient prior to conducting the interview is crucial to obtaining reliable diagnostic information. In introducing the interview, a good rationale is, "We would like to offer you a program for coping with bipolar disorder. Before we do that, we want to know if that is really an accurate diagnosis. If we're assuming you have that disorder and we're wrong, then we'll want to consider other programs." Be aware that the patient may have been asked many of these diagnostic questions before. A simple statement to the patient such as, "Please bear with me even if this is at times tedious" is usually enough to gain his or her cooperation.

Patients who are psychotic may not be able to tolerate a full diagnostic interview conducted in a single session. Specifically, questions about delusions or hallucinations, although important to determining the diagnosis, are often threatening to the patient, especially if he or she believes that admitting to such disturbances will place him or her at risk for a lengthier treatment or hospitalization. Therefore, preface questions with phrases such as, "Many of the people I've worked with have experienced [delusional beliefs, voices, etc.]. I wonder if this has been true of you?" Be prepared to discontinue the interview if the patient shows signs of agitation.

In conducting the interview, always consider "rule-out" diagnoses. Pay particular attention to the distinctions between bipolar and unipolar, schizophrenic, attention deficit, schizoaffective, or substance-induced mood disorders (see Miklowitz, 2002, *The Bipolar Disorder Survival Guide*, for an extensive discussion of the differential diagnosis of bipolar disorder). If the diagnostic interview proves inconclusive, detailed life history information (see the next section) from the patient and relatives may help resolve ambiguities.

Assessing the Prior Course of Illness

When the family clinician interviewed Maryann about her prior history, a number of important facts emerged. First, she had had at least two manic episodes prior to the current hospitalized manic episode. Neither of these episodes had been treated, but they had taken their toll on her functioning: In one case, she had dropped out of school, and in another, she had been fired from a job. She hadn't labeled these episodes as periods of illness, but instead reported being "stressed out" and having little emotional support from her family and friends. In fact, her conflicts with her mother had escalated prior to and during these episodes.

More detailed questioning revealed that both prior episodes, as well as the most recent episode, were precipitated by beginning new romantic relationships. In all three cases, she reported falling deeply in love with a man and giving up all other activities to be with him. She also reported radical changes in her sleep habits during these phases. She noted that her mother had objected to each of these relationships and had tried to interfere, which had precipitated overt conflict between Maryann and Geena.

In the most recent case, Maryann had "skipped town" following an argument with Geena and had flown with her lover down to Puerto Vallarta. However, her manic symptoms escalated there, and she had had to fly back to the United States to be hospitalized. Her relationship broke up shortly after she was admitted to the hospital. Geena was left to "pick up the pieces" in the aftermath of the episode and to resume a caretaker role with which, sadly, she was all too familiar.

Collecting prior course of illness data is crucial for establishing the correct diagnosis, determining prognosis, and planning the FFT intervention. For example, Maryann's evaluation revealed the frequent co-occurrence of new romantic relationships, family conflict, and sleep disturbance prior to each of her episodes. In turn, the psychoeducation focused on helping Maryann and Geena to clarify the nature of her particular risk factors (e.g., irregular sleep patterns) and develop plans for intervening should these factors reappear. As another example, consider the contrasting needs of patients who have had only one prior episode versus many. For such patients, those parts of FFT dealing with accepting the reality of the disorder may be the most salient. In contrast, an older patient who has lived with the disorder for most of his or her life may prefer a greater focus on ways to improve family relationships, how to succeed in his or her job, and how to find the right balance of medications and stress management tools.

Be aware that collecting illness history information may require several interview sessions involving the patient and family members. If so, begin the FFT sessions before completing this full evaluation, so that the patient and family members do not feel they are being tested rather than treated.

Prior Course of Illness from the Patient's Viewpoint

Different clinical settings rely on different instruments for collecting prior illness information from patients. Some use detailed timelines such as the Life Chart (Post & Leverich, 2006), whereas others rely primarily on a simple episode history form, such as that available in the Structured Clinical Interview for DSM-IV Axis I Disorders. There are several basic pieces of information that should be obtained about each prior episode, as outlined in Table 5.2. Of course, many patients, particularly those who are psychotic, will not be able to provide this information. For these, the reports of family members (see below) and physicians, or the medical records, are quite helpful.

Perhaps most germane to the FFT program is the role of stressors in precipitating prior episodes, as exemplified by Maryann's case. Do major family conflicts co-occur with the prodromal or active phases of illness? What life events or other stressors have preceded—if not necessarily caused—prior episodes, particularly the most recent episode? Do life transitions (e.g., relationship initiations or terminations, job losses, promotions, or changing schools) often precede episodes? What about events that alter

TABLE 5.2. Questions about Prior Episodes of Illness

- When did the episode occur?
- What manic, depressive, or psychotic symptoms dominated the picture?
- How long did it take for the episode to resolve?
- Did the episode require hospitalization? How did the patient and family cope with the hospitalization?
- What medications was the patient taking prior to and during the episode, and were they effective? Was he or she compliant with them?
- Was the episode precipitated by drug or alcohol abuse?
- Did the patient receive any psychotherapy? In what ways was it helpful or unhelpful?
- What family conflicts or life events precipitated the episode or occurred during the recovery period? Did any life events disrupt the patient's sleep–wake cycle (e.g., losing or gaining a new relationship; changing job hours; transatlantic flights; finals week)?
- How did the patient and his or her family members cope with these conflicts or events?

the patient's daily rhythms, such as transcontinental flights or starting a new school year? To what degree do these events appear to be influential in the onset of episodes, and to what degree were they apparently caused by the patient's escalating symptoms? For example, in Maryann's case, new romantic relationships may not have caused her manic symptoms, but the accompanying family conflicts and attendant changes in her sleep–wake habits may have contributed. The termination of these relationships, in contrast, may have been the direct result of her escalating mood disorder symptoms, and may have contributed to the depressive episodes she often developed after her manic episodes had crested.

Prior Course of Illness from the Relative's Point of View

Maryann's mother gave a rather thorough history of Maryann's disorder. Geena noted that Maryann's father, from whom she was now divorced, had been an alcohol and drug abuser and, during Maryann's childhood, had disappeared from the home for weeks at a time. She described Maryann as a quiet, somewhat isolated child and noted that they had lived in a dangerous neighborhood where "going outside and playing in the street was a big risk." She described Maryann's two prior manic periods as the direct results of getting involved with "stupid men." She felt that Maryann had a yen for men who were like her father: angry, rebellious, exciting, and irresponsible. She vowed that "the next time she gets involved with a guy who's not good for her, I'm just gonna take over and throw him right out of the house, whether she likes it or not."

The information provided about prior illness history is sometimes best obtained from a relative, particularly a parent who has had consistent contact with the patient. In a one-to-one session with the relative, you can obtain his or her perspective on a number of issues, including the development of the most recent affective episode and the presence of prior episodes the patient may not have acknowledged. You can also obtain important information about the patient's genetic background (i.e., Have any first- or second-degree relatives had bipolar or unipolar affective disorders?) or significant facts about the patient's developmental history (i.e., Are there any significant early life events, such as long periods of separation from a parent, instances of physical or sexual abuse, or deprived economic conditions? Was the patient's childhood chaotic or unpredictable?). An early history of adversity is predictive of a younger age at onset of bipolar disorder and a more difficult and treatment-refractory course of illness (Post & Leverich, 2006).

In conducting these interviews, be attuned to the relative's emotional reactions while recounting the patient's history. These reactions often give clues as to what issues will be salient during the FFT sessions, as well as to whether the postepisode family climate is likely to be protective against recurrences of bipolar disorder.

In research settings, the Camberwell Family Interview (Vaughn & Leff, 1976; Leff & Vaughn, 1985) provides a useful format to follow in eliciting illness history information from a relative, particularly the development of the most recent episode. This interview provides the data source from which ratings of EE (criticism, hostility, and emotional overinvolvement) are made. However, reliable coding of the Camberwell Interview requires months of training, and rating each interview takes 2–3 hours. For most clinicians working outside a research setting, this is a prohibitive amount of effort. Administering a brief, open-ended interview with questions similar to those posed in the Camberwell Interview (see Table 5.3) can nonetheless be helpful in obtaining information about the emotional effects of the disorder on family members.

In conducting this or a similar interview, be vigilant about certain nuances in the relative's response style, particularly those nuances that indicate a critical or hostile attitude toward the patient. What topics generate affect? At what point does the relative's voice tone change? Does he or she become more serious, talk more slowly, or get an irritated tone when discussing certain events that have affected the family? Alternatively, does the voice speed up or is it accompanied by an ironic, sarcastic tone? Are there many instances of statements that begin with phrases like "I don't like it that . . . " or "I resent it when . . . "? Does he or she make global, sweeping statements such as "He's a loser" or "She's never going to amount to anything" (Leff & Vaughn, 1985)?

TABLE 5.3. Interview Questions for Obtaining Illness History Information from Relatives

- When did his or her illness first begin?
- When did the most recent episode begin? How did it come about?
- How did he or she end up going to the hospital?
- What were his or her symptoms? How did you or others in your family react to these symptoms?
- How did he or she spend a typical day prior to the episode? What time did he or she get up, eat, go to work or school, come home, and so forth? Who was there with him or her at the time?
- Were there family arguments during this time? How did they start? How were they resolved?
- How would you describe him or her as a person?
- How well do the two of you typically get along together?
- What about him or her do you find attractive/enjoyable?
- What aspects of his or her behavior do you find most disturbing?

Note. Sources: Leff and Vaughn (1985); Magana et al. (1986).

Be equally attuned to signs of emotional overinvolvement. In the case vignette above, Geena stated that she would usher any inappropriate man out of the house without consulting Maryann, an example of overprotectiveness. Other examples include self-sacrificing behaviors (e.g., "That's when I quit my job and started staying home so I could be there in case he needed me"), exaggerated emotional displays (e.g., "I just broke down and cried when I heard that she'd gone and consulted a psychiatrist"), or an excessive use of positive remarks (e.g., "He's just a wonderful, lovable, incredibly talented person"). Emotionally overinvolved attitudes are more likely to occur among parental than spousal relatives (Miklowitz et al., 2000).

Premorbid Functioning

Premorbid adjustment, or the level of social–occupational functioning in the adolescent, preillness years, is a strong predictor of outcome and treatment response in a number of psychiatric disorders. Although bipolar patients tend to have better premorbid adjustment than patients with schizophrenic disorders (Cannon et al., 1997), there is nevertheless variability in this attribute.

Usually, patients are the best source of this information, but verify questionable responses (e.g., "I had more friends than I could possibly count") by consulting relatives. Assessing premorbid adjustment entails asking questions about whether the patient was able to function in social environments and/or develop attachments to others in the preillness years, his or her number of friendships and activities during high school, the duration and quality of any romantic relationships, and the prior occupational history. Ask the patient questions like "Some people had close friends in high school, and others did not. How was it for you?" "Some people dated when they were teenagers, others didn't. What about you?" Patients who had at least two or three close friends and one or more romantic partners, and who participated in social or club activities during school, are usually classified as having good premorbid adjustment.

Use of Illness History Information in Treatment Planning

After the interview, assemble the information obtained from the patient and his or her key relatives and consider its implications for planning FFT. First, what has been learned about the history of the disorder and the role of life stress in the occurrences of episodes? From this background data, what pattern of illness course would be expected during the course of the treatment? How would one know if the patient was getting better? How can the patient and family more effectively cope with the life stressors that appear to contribute to episodes?

Second, are there significant facts about or events in the history of the family that may be important for understanding the onset or course of the disorder? What are the implications of these historical facts for treatment? For example, an interpersonal loss during the course of treatment may place a bipolar patient at high recurrence risk if he or she has an early history of separation experiences. If so, how can the skill-training modules of FFT be adapted to help the patient anticipate and cope with future loss events (e.g., the anticipated breakup of a romantic relationship)?

Third, what level of social and job functioning can the patient, family, and treatment team reasonably expect during the postepisode period? It is unlikely that the patient will be able to immediately regain his or her premorbid level of social or job functioning after an episode, but this level may be set as a goal for the patient's future functioning. However, discourage the patient and family from expecting a higher level of functioning during the postepisode period than was evident during the preillness period.

Fourth, and perhaps most important, how have family members coped with the cycling of the disorder? Is this a high-stress, high-EE family, signaling a heightened short-term risk of recurrence for the patient? What family conflicts can be anticipated during the postepisode period? How can FFT help relatives who are suffering from the emotional strain of taking care of a psychiatrically ill person?

Assessing Family Interactions

About 2 weeks after Maryann left the hospital, the clinician treating her undertook a family interactional assessment, in which she asked Maryann and Geena to discuss a series of family problems while she observed through a one-way mirror. The clinician was skeptical about conducting this assessment, fearing that she would be opening a Pandora's box. After all, her individual discussions with each of them had revealed the presence of significant, long-standing conflicts in their relationship.

Surprisingly, the destructive, counterproductive dyadic discussions she expected never materialized. Maryann and Geena were quite respectful of each other. They avoided expressing hostility, and let each other finish speaking before responding. Although Geena was prone to giving advice, she delivered her advice in a rather mild, supportive way (e.g., "You need to stop getting involved with men who hurt you"). Maryann, in turn, expressed dismay about the effects of her disorder on Geena's life, saying that she wanted her mother to be able to have friends, lovers, and a rewarding career despite Maryann's illness.

The clinician did note, however, that the concrete problems Maryann and Geena discussed were never solved. For example, when Maryann raised the issue of going back to school, the discussion became unfocused, and the topic was eventually dropped. A similar process occurred when they discussed household chores.

The individual assessments should give you a sense of each family member's experiences of the disorder, his or her interpersonal skills or deficits, and, perhaps, his or her goals for treatment. However, skill deficits identified in individual interviews may not appear as deficits when a person interacts with the rest of the family, and, likewise, he or she may show difficulties in the family context that did not appear in the individual interviews (Miklowitz et al., 1995). Moreover, the family as a unit will almost certainly have styles of coping and interacting—adaptive or maladaptive—that cannot be identified through individual interviews. Thus, often most informative for the planning of FFT are structured family interaction tasks that give a sample of the family's communication and problem-solving behavior.

From watching how members of a family or a couple define, discuss, and attempt to solve problems in their current milieu, you can develop hypotheses about where best to intervene. In our experience, assessments of family interactional styles are best undertaken during the stabilization period (a few weeks after the height of the episode) when the patient is at least partially remitted. Interactional assessments conducted with a highly symptomatic (or, especially, a psychotic) patient may be destructive rather than constructive and will not clarify how the family behaves when the patient is well. Further, the family interactional behaviors accompanying the stabilization period appear to be the most relevant in predicting the subsequent course of psychiatric disorders (for a review, see Miklowitz, 2004).

Setting the Stage for a Family Interaction

We use a guided protocol for assessing family interactional behavior (Doane, Goldstein, Miklowitz, & Falloon, 1986; Miklowitz, Goldstein, Falloon, & Doane, 1984). This protocol involves a series of individual interviews of each member of the family or couple, followed by two 10-minute, directed problem-solving discussions with the clinicians absent from the room, or present but not intervening. These assessments can be conducted in a relatively straightforward manner by interviewing the family or couple about its current concerns and conflicts and requesting that members discuss some of these issues without your interruption. If you have available an interview room with a one-way observation mirror, leave the room and watch the interaction as it progresses. The following interchange illustrates setting the stage for a family interaction.

CLINICIAN: Let's see if you can agree on something that's a problem within the family, something you'd like to see solved during our treatment sessions.

GEENA: (*Laughs.*) Well, I'd sure like to see her clean her room!

MARYANN: (*Half smiles.*) It's not my room that's the problem, it's the whole house. Your room's a mess, too.

GEENA: If someone came into our house and looked at your room and mine, whose do you think they would want to clean first?

CLINICIAN: Let me stop you there. You're doing just what I'm going to ask you to do in a minute. Let's use your example of "getting the house clean" as a topic for discussion. Would you both agree this is a problem?

GEENA: We've discussed it a million times.

CLINICIAN: Well, that tells me it's probably not getting solved. So would you be willing to discuss it one more time, while I'm watching? Maybe then we could put this problem on our agenda for the treatment sessions.

GEENA: Yeah, but I'm not optimistic about it.

CLINICIAN: OK, I hear that, but let's give it a try. Part of what I'm interested in is the process by which you go about discussing and trying to solve a problem, rather than the actual solution. So what I'd like you to do now, while I'm watching [or behind the mirror], is to discuss between yourselves this problem of getting the house clean. Tell each other why you think this is a problem, say how each of you feels about the issue, and try to reach a solution. I'm not going to interrupt you while you're discussing it—just pretend I'm not here. OK? Do you have any questions?

You can then leave the room (or remain in the room without interrupting) and allow the family up to 10 minutes to discuss the problem. If necessary, a second problem can be introduced for another discussion, perhaps a topic generated by the family member who did not generate the first topic.

Determining Communication Assets and Deficits

There are several domains to assess while observing these family or couple interactions. First, the family's *structure* or *hierarchy*: Who speaks first, and who follows? Does the discussion have a leader? Do one family member's opinions tend to dominate? Who is allied with whom, and what members are disengaged from each other? In a couple, does the husband or the wife do most of the talking? Alternatively, is there a constructive sense of mutuality in the discussions?

Second, what is the *affective tone* of the family's or couple's interactions? Are many criticisms expressed by one member toward the other? Are criticisms constructive, or do they tend toward the personal and the accusatory (e.g., "You're a lousy roommate")? Do parents attempt to "mind read" when discussing problems with their patient-offspring? Does the couple or family engage in negatively escalating cycles, consisting of back-and-forth volleys of nonconstructive communication? Alternatively, who supports whom? Do various family members express empathy for each other, or praise each other's efforts to cope? Do they "mirror" or paraphrase each other's statements before offering their own?

Third, how does the family *solve its problems?* Does a problem get well defined before members attempt to solve it? Do members throw out viable solutions? Are solutions cut off and discounted by other family members before they get realistically evaluated? Do problems get bigger and more personal as they are discussed? Do members "cross-complain" or bring in other problems not germane to the issue at hand (e.g., "I didn't clean the living room because you didn't loan me your car")? Finally, does the discussion yield a plan of action for solving the problem, or is the problem left hanging?

Finally, how *clear* is the family's communication? Do all participants seem to be talking about the same topic? Do family members sometimes not make sense? How much of the discussion is tangential, vague, or even incomprehensible? Are ideas expressed incompletely (e.g., "I wish you would just . . . whatever")? Are there frequent uses of words like "him" or "that thing," without clear referents? Do participants jump from topic to topic?

A tape recording of the family's discussions may help you to identify areas in need of remediation, as well as those communication assets that can be built upon. For the research-minded, there are several well-validated systems for coding family interactions (see Chapter 3), such as the AS system for coding relatives' behaviors (Doane et al., 1981), the CS system for patients' behaviors (Strachan et al., 1989), the Category System for Coding Partner Interactions (Hahlweg et al., 1989), the Marital Interactional Coding System (Floyd, O'Farrell, & Goldberg, 1987), and the Interactional Communication Deviance system (Velligan, Goldstein, Nuechterlein, Miklowitz, & Ranlett, 1990).

Assessing Prior Knowledge of Bipolar Disorder

A primary objective of FFT is to encourage a full understanding of bipolar disorder and its nature, course, etiology, and treatment. Thus, before the psychoeducational module is introduced, assess the patient's and family's current understanding of the disorder. Some participants in FFT—

although, in our experience, a minority—come to the treatment sessions already quite knowledgeable (e.g., one family member began a first session by asking, "What is the latest thinking about the kindling effect?"). They may also come in with strong preexisting, although not necessarily accurate, opinions (e.g., one parent argued that the most effective treatment for all psychiatric disorders was kidney dialysis; another believed that any change of the patient's mood was rapid cycling). Thus, begin by asking yourself, "How much new information will they need to learn?"

Table 5.4 offers a brief Knowledge of Bipolar Disorder interview. This interview can tell you about specific holes in the family's knowledge base, as well as what coping strategies have been utilized, and which have succeeded or failed, in family members' prior attempts to manage the disorder. Administer the interview in a conjoint session with the patient and his or her parents or spouse. Begin by asking each participant

TABLE 5.4. Knowledge of Bipolar Disorder Interview

Question	Possible answers
• What do you understand to be the symptoms of a manic episode?	• Elation, irritability, racing thoughts, grandiosity, hyperactivity
• A depressive episode?	• Sad mood, insomnia, fatigue, suicidality
• What do you think has caused him or her (you) to be this way?	• Chemical imbalance, genetics, stress in combination with biological imbalances
• What do you think is the course of this disorder? What will happen in the future?	• The disorder cycles over time, manic or depressive symptoms will probably recur
• What are the treatments for this disorder? What do you think has been (or could be) helpful?	• Medications (i.e., lithium, anticonvulsants, antipsychotics, antidepressants), psychotherapy, hospitalization
• What behaviors would indicate to you that he or she (or you) were getting manic again? Depressed?	• Lists two or more prodromal symptoms (e.g., inflated self-esteem, decreased need for sleep, rumination)
• What would you do if he or she (or you) were getting manic again? Depressed? How would you handle things next time?	• Go in for a medical evaluation, test blood levels, have a crisis therapy session
• What is the role of the family in helping manage the disorder?	• Assisting patient in following through on appointments and remembering medications; being supportive and encouraging; learning to recognize early warning signs of recurrence; communicating and solving problems effectively

an open-ended question like "What is your understanding of bipolar mood disorder?" Then, follow up with the more specific questions detailed in Table 5.4. In evaluating their answers, try to determine the gap between what you would like them to know and what they already know. Be prepared, however, to cut off the discussion if the patient begins to feel scapegoated or if he or she argues that the disorder is irrelevant to him or her (see Chapter 8).

Concluding Comments

This chapter has emphasized the importance of evaluating the preexisting knowledge base, the coping strategies, and the interpersonal strengths and weaknesses of each patient and family member, and the entire family unit, before proceeding with the core FFT treatment modules. Depending on your clinical setting and the needs of the patient or family, you may choose to skip some of these assessments or conduct them in more abbreviated fashion. But as is true of any psychosocial treatment, obtaining comprehensive background information and observational data is crucial to developing a "theory of the case" and an organized plan for treatment delivery. Thus, conducting assessments early saves time in the later phases of the treatment.

chapter 6

Family Psychoeducation

The Initial Sessions

William was a 21-year-old European American man who was hospitalized for a manic episode while in college on the west coast of the United States. He had become increasingly irritable and his behavior was bizarre in the classroom; he had become convinced that certain of his professors were "long-lost relatives" who were "connected to me in a series of web-like forms, like cells in the body of a huge organism."

After his hospital discharge, he went home to live with his parents, Stan and Alyssia. Both parents had their own psychiatric history, Stan with periods of hypomania and drug abuse and Alyssia with depression and suicidal preoccupations. However, both parents were employed and able to support William financially through his episode and posthospital recovery period.

William and his parents began a series of psychoeducational sessions offered by a clinician who had approached William while he was in the hospital. The first sessions were quite difficult; William felt he was being pidgeonholed as a psychiatric patient and felt annoyed by his mother's protectiveness. As he and his parents learned more about the disorder, William became intrigued by, if not entirely in agreement with, the content of the sessions. Although he never went as far as to admit he had a psychiatric disorder, he did agree to continue taking divalproex sodium (Depakote) as a result of what he had learned about the likely causes of his episode.

Overview of the Psychoeducation Module

There are two primary goals of the first FFT module, psychoeducation. The first is to give specific information to the patient and family about bipolar disorder. This information can tremendously relieve, enlighten, and resolve the many confusions and misconceptions held by family members. Didactic information is also an essential basis on which to build a rationale for the involvement of the family in the later communication enhancement and problem-solving FFT modules. For example, knowing that patients with bipolar disorder benefit from low-stress family environments helps convince family members of the value of learning new speaking and listening skills.

Family members often immediately put this information to work. For example, they may learn not to assign blame to the patient for emotional reactions or other behaviors beyond his or her control (Miklowitz, Wendel, & Simoneau, 1998). They may begin to realize that the patient's inability to hold a job is a sign of his or her illness rather than of laziness. In addition, the patient may learn to keep a regular schedule of sleeping and waking as a way of modulating his or her mood states.

Psychoeducation also offers an opportunity to talk about the difficult truth that the patient has a psychiatric disorder that is probably going to be recurrent over the lifespan. Resistances expressed by patients and family members to the psychoeducational materials often signal the presence of unresolved feelings about this core issue. We have observed these resistances in families of patients who have had multiple episodes as well as those of patients experiencing their first episode.

This chapter describes the initial psychoeducational sessions, during which you will develop a therapeutic alliance with the patient and his or her relatives, acquaint the participants with the signs and symptoms of the disorder, review the development and identify the psychosocial precipitants of the most recent mood episode, and discuss the long-term course of the disorder. Chapter 7 describes the crucial information given to the family about the etiology, treatment, and self-management of the disorder.

Chapter 8, in contrast, is a troubleshooting chapter. It discusses the ways that the FFT clinician addresses the expectable resistances on the part of patients and family members to accepting the reality of the disorder, the patient's vulnerability to future episodes, and the necessity of long-term medication treatment. The didactic information imparted in the psychoeducation module has a much stronger impact if these emotional reactions are addressed. Thus, the three psychoeducational chapters should be considered as a unit.

A Word about Terminology

You will notice that, in the clinical vignettes that follow, the therapist refers to him- or herself as "we" rather than "I." This reflects the possibility that he or she is working with a cotherapist. As discussed in Chapter 4, working in cotherapy teams has advantages, but FFT can be just as easily administered by a single therapist. Moreover, you'll find that we refer to "the family" when we may just be treating a couple. Feel free to substitute "your relationship" for "your family" where appropriate.

The Therapeutic Stance

Your therapeutic stance will help the family to accept the realities of the disorder and put the communication and problem-solving skills to use in their everyday lives. First, as is true of any good therapy, it's important to be as human as possible: approachable, friendly, open, and emotionally accessible. Use humor frequently, allow for a certain amount of chitchat, and self-disclose when it might aid the therapeutic process (e.g., acknowledging your own discomfort with blood tests when the patient admits to his or her fears). Whereas you may disagree with certain beliefs or attitudes held by the patient or family members, show acceptance by attempting to understand these different points of view.

Second, carry on a "Socratic dialogue" with the family, rather than reviewing the psychoeducational materials in a rote way. There should be a constant give and take between you and the patient and family members, and among the participants themselves. For example, frequently ask questions of the form "What do you think about this material?" "How did you experience this life event?" "How are you reacting to what we're saying?" Encourage all family members, even those who are very quiet, to offer input, opinions, or personal experiences within a nonjudgmental atmosphere.

Third, avoid the trap of thinking that FFT is a classroom course rather than a psychosocial treatment. Although much of the psychoeducation involves the use of written handouts, you should depart from this agenda if more pressing issues present themselves (e.g., the patient needing a place to live, recurrence of symptoms, severe family disagreements, or a death in the family). Furthermore, the psychoeducational materials frequently arouse anger, fear, and sadness in participants (see Chapter 8). When these reactions are in evidence, stop presenting the materials and explore with the participants these emotional responses. Where appropriate, normalize emotions and label them as healthy and understandable (e.g., "I can understand why this would upset you. Most people react this way to the notion that they have to deal with a chronic illness").

Fourth, avoid technical jargon. Use terms like "your brain" instead of "your central nervous system;" "ways to cope" instead of "defense mechanisms." Explain yourself further when participants do not seem to understand the words used or the concepts conveyed. Keep checking in with them, especially if they seem to be "spacing out." Pace the sessions according to the abilities of family members to assimilate the materials, which may vary according to their educational levels.

Finally, be optimistic about what is to come. Avoid painting a rosy picture of the future (which could alienate patients and family members who have been through multiple episodes), but point out that if the patient remains on medication, and the patient and family members use the skills learned in FFT, there is every reason to expect the patient will achieve an optimum recovery and be at reduced risk for recurrences. Comment that many individuals lead creative, productive, and happy lives despite having the disorder (Jamison, 1993).

"Setting the Stage" for the Psychoeducation Module

On average, you can expect the psychoeducational module to last about seven sessions. More or less time may be required, depending on the existing knowledge base of the family, their levels of resistance, and other issues. The first meetings with the family or couple are primarily "get acquainted" sessions in which the treatment program is explained, a contract for a certain number of sessions is developed, and an initial therapeutic alliance is developed.

Remember that these initial sessions may reveal other problems that must be addressed before the psychoeducational materials are introduced. Therefore, the order of the treatment modules should be viewed as a guideline rather than a rigid structure. For example, if you are treating a couple with severe marital problems, it may be more appropriate to begin with communication enhancement or problem-solving skills training rather than psychoeducation.

Getting Acquainted and Joining

As indicated in Chapter 4, you need to "join" and develop a therapeutic alliance with the family or couple. Before introducing any therapeutic tasks, get to know each family member as a person and promote a safe, nonthreatening atmosphere. Optimally, you will have had at least one prior contact with each family member through the functional assessment phase, but the initial alliances developed through these contacts need to be solidified and strengthened. If you have done little or no family or marital treatment before, you may wish to consult several books that discuss joining and connecting techniques, including Anderson and Stewart (1983), Anderson, Reiss, and Hogarty (1986), or Haley (1987).

At the beginning of each psychoeducation session, check in with each family member and the patient before moving on to the general agenda for the session. In so doing, you will communicate an interest in each participant above and beyond your interest in the patient's disorder. For example, ask a patient's spouse how her new job is going; joke with a patient's father about a recent football game (if you and he are so inclined); express interest in how a new mother is adapting to the demands of infant care.

If the family is a couple, it is helpful to begin the first psychoeducation session with "How did you two meet?" (after Jacobson & Margolin, 1979). Laughing with them about the events early in their relationship can help in developing a therapeutic alliance. Showing an appreciation for the history of their relationship communicates an optimism about the future and the couple's abilities to work through their current problems.

Introducing the Treatment Program

During the first and, sometimes, the second psychoeducation session, you should more fully explain the nature of the FFT program. Although you will have described the program to a degree during the initial phone contacts and functional assessment sessions, assume that the patient and family are still unclear as to the program's purposes. Give details as to the actual content of the sessions, what participants can expect from you, and what you expect from the participants.

The Reentry Model

During the first or second session, explain the "reentry model": that the patient has just been discharged from the hospital and may only be partially recovered, and that families coping with this stage of the disorder are often in a state of emotional crisis. In this model, family treatment is seen as an important addition to medication in helping the patient and family cope with the highly stressful, posthospital recovery period:

> "As we discussed with you earlier, there are some good reasons why we think this program might help you. We believe you, William, have just had an episode of what we call 'bipolar' or 'manic–depressive' disorder. Bipolar disorder is a psychiatric illness involving high and low moods. When people get manic, they feel on top of

the world and full of energy. When they're depressed, everything feels bad and they have very little energy or will to do things. Of course, William, you may not agree that this is what happened to you, but we think this is a reasonable guess, given what we understand about your episode."

At this point, you may already be deluged with comments, questions, and arguments from the patient or his or her relatives about the term "bipolar disorder." This is particularly true for first-episode adolescent or young adult patients, who may perceive the episode and/or hospitalization as a fluke that will never occur again. For example, the patient may argue that he or she was just under stress and the symptoms will never occur again. In turn, family members may express concern about the patient's denial of the disorder, particularly if he or she is still symptomatic. You may feel quickly drawn into the family system and pushed to ally with one member of the family against another.

I recommend underlining the importance of the participants' questions about the validity of the disorder, but asking the family to hold off on discussing these issues until some of the didactic materials have been presented. Chapter 8 discusses in detail the various ways to address resistances to the illness notion and the family conflicts that arise from these resistances:

"It's understandable that you'd have these questions at this point, as well as questions about whether our program applies to you. Sometimes the person who's had an episode of mood disorder (or, been in the hospital) doesn't want to be a part of this program and learn the facts about the disorder, even though his relatives may want to. Sometimes it's the person's relatives who resist. We know you may not all be in the same place with this, and we'll be discussing these disagreements later. Most people have ideas about what psychiatric disorders are, and we'll certainly want to hear yours. But for now, let us give you a better sense of what we're doing here, and then I think things will get much clearer."

You can then describe the problems encountered when a recently ill patient reenters the family and community. Emphasize that FFT is time-limited and that its objectives pertain primarily to the year after the patient has either been discharged from the hospital or treated on an outpatient basis for an acute episode:

"We know that when someone is just getting over an episode of bipolar disorder, that person may feel and look better but he or she is not really fully recovered. In fact, this is a very critical time, in which the person is quite vulnerable to having another episode. The reason we want to involve you, William, in the program for this year after your hospitalization is to help you get assimilated back into the life you had before you became ill and achieve the best recovery you can. Likewise, we want to involve your family members because they have had their own stress to deal with in the last few months, and because we think they can help support you in your recovery during this year."

In this passage, the clinician acquaints the patient and family with the concept of a recovery/reentry period. The FFT is cast not as a therapy for disturbed, dysfunctional families but rather as a support for patients and families undergoing the difficult process of reintegration following the episode.

The Rationale for Involving the Family

The clinician in the preceding examples made clear that he views family members as allies in the treatment/recovery process. Nonetheless, a likely question from relatives at this point is "What does this have to do with us?"

The aftermath of a manic or depressive episode can be associated with a family-wide form of posttraumatic stress. Specifically, family members, and often the patient, feel that the episode is still occurring (which it may be) or will recur at any minute, members avoid each other or feel emotionally distanced and disconnected ("emotional numbing"), or emotions become labile or are expressed impulsively. A statement that acknowledges this trauma, and further explains the role of the family in the patient's treatment, is most useful at this point:

"An episode of illness in one family member can be quite traumatic to all members of the family, whether the illness is medical or psychiatric. William, if you had been hospitalized for a medical disorder like diabetes, I think your family would also be experiencing stress and worrying about the future, and they might very well benefit from an educational, stress-management treatment after you got out of the hospital.

"In bipolar disorder, when the person returns home and begins to recover, there is a 'getting reacquainted' period in which everyone has to get to know everyone else again, and when everyone tries to make sense of what happened. This is a tough time for any family, and part of our purpose here is to make the 'reacquaintance period' less disturbing to all of you. We'd like during this year to get you, as a family, back to where you were before William became ill. We want to give you some tools to deal with this recovery period."

A statement of this sort, delivered in the early sessions, communicates to the family members that their emotional reactions to the episode, although often unstated at this point, are normal, expectable reactions to dealing with an illness in one member of the family. It also implies that the psychoeducational treatment will not be all information giving with no exploration of emotions, a worry they may harbor but are unlikely to be able to verbalize.

The Recurrent Patient

If you are explaining the program to a patient and family members who have coped with multiple, severe episodes, tailor the introduction differently:

> "We know you've recently had an episode of bipolar disorder and we know from your history that this is not the first time this has happened. I think you've all learned that it's not an easy thing to deal with these episodes—they are very painful and costly to the person with the disorder and to the family. I'm sure if you had your choice, neither you [patient] nor your family would ever want this to happen again.
>
> "We'd like during this year to help you achieve a better recovery from your illness and develop some strategies for preventing future episodes from occurring. You've tried a number of different treatments, and we know that many things that have been promised have not been delivered. We're not going to promise a cure-all, but it may be that learning to manage the stress in your life better, and helping your family members learn to manage the stress they face, is the missing piece that would keep you from having more of these episodes."

In this passage, the clinician acknowledges that the patient and family have been through this before. He does not oversell the family treatment. However, he does encourage the patient and family members to consider the importance of the psychosocial component of the disorder, a component that may have received short shrift in the family's earlier treatment experiences.

Previewing the Treatment

Once the rationale for the program has been presented, acquaint the family with the more specific goals, format, and expectations of the family program. Distribute Handout 1 to all participants. Introducing and explaining this handout puts family members at ease, because it makes

Family-Focused Treatment: Goals and Expectations

Role of clinician

- Coordinate, guide, and assist

Goals

- Reduce tension in family relationships
- Improve family's internal communication
- Increase family's understanding and acceptance of illness
- Assist family in developing problem-solving strategies that are more satisfactory

Format

- Assessment of each member individually
- Education regarding nature of illness and treatment prescribed, specifically medication
- Communication skills
- Problem solving
- Strategies for specific problems

Expectations of family members

- Quality attendance and participation
- Active role playing
- Completion of all homework assignments
- Cooperation

Family can expect clinician to provide

- Thoughtful, systematic intervention
- Strict confidentiality
- A comfortable working environment
- Homework materials
- Telephone or e-mail consultations

HANDOUT 1. *Source*: Adapted by permission from Mueser and Glynn (1995).

clear that you have a definite agenda and that a predictable treatment structure will be provided.

When reviewing this handout, give specifics about what will transpire during the treatment sessions. For example, in referring to "goals," you can say:

> "We're going to work with you on two different levels. One is encouraging William's ongoing work with his psychiatrist so that he can get himself stabilized on medications. The second is how you as a family can minimize stress, particularly stress within your family. We think there are several ways to do this, including acquainting you with the facts about bipolar disorder, and working with you on improving your communication and problem-solving skills with each other. These strategies should increase William's chances of making a good recovery and help you as a family cope with the disorder. How does this sound to you?"

In referring to "expectations of family members," the following is a useful approach:

> "We'll be expecting you to come regularly and let us know at least 24 hours in advance if you have to reschedule. We'll be giving you homework assignments—not like those you had in school—but tasks like practicing new ways to talk to each other or going through the steps of solving a family problem. In and out of sessions, we'll be asking you to 'role-play' new ways of talking to each other, which involves turning your chairs toward each other and practicing, for example, how to listen better when someone else is speaking. Have you ever done these sorts of things before?"

Describing the Role of the Clinician

The family will probably be curious as to what you will do during the sessions to help them. Describe your role as much like a coach, and underline some of the differences between psychoeducational treatment and traditional psychotherapy. For example, you can say:

> "This will probably be a bit different from the other treatments or psychotherapies you've had. We'll be active and directive with you at some times, and we'll sit on the sidelines at others. We may talk about ourselves from time to time. We'll coach you on some new skills that should help in your day-to-day dealings with each other. We'll offer concrete suggestions about what you can *do* to make your

situation better. Also, we're going to encourage you to tell us if these sessions are not meeting your needs—there may be things we can do to make them more useful."

Assessing Goals for the Treatment

Once the agenda has been presented, step back and gain a greater sense of the patient's and family members' goals for treatment. Families have an easier time with this question after the FFT agenda (Handout 1) has been presented. Few family members come into FFT with a clear sense of how to proceed, and previewing the structure of the treatment makes them review their personal goals, those pertaining both to the patient's disorder and to their own lives. The following is a useful lead-in:

"In a minute, we'll be getting into talking about the signs and symptoms of bipolar disorder. But before we do, why don't we focus a little more on how this program fits in with your goals? We do have our own agenda, but that doesn't mean it can't be modified to fit what you think you need. Why don't we start with you, William? Where do you want to be in, say, 6 months?"

We prefer asking participants to discuss "Where do you want to be in *X* months?" to "What do you want to get out of these sessions?" Most participants have more difficulty answering the latter than the former question, especially if they have never been in any form of psychosocial treatment before. Furthermore, the former question opens up areas of concern that can be addressed later through problem solving. For example, the healthy spouse in a couple may comment that she wants to go back to school, raising the question of how this could be accomplished during the year following her husband's hospitalization. Thus, assessing each participant's goals for the period of treatment informs the immediate as well as the later phases of the program.

It is usually best to address these questions to the patient first. An adolescent offspring in a parental family may enter family treatment believing that the sessions are really for his or her parents. Similarly, a married bipolar patient may worry that his or her spouse—who may be threatening to leave—is the real target of the program. Addressing these questions to the patient underlines the notion that he or she will have some control over what transpires in the sessions. However, the questions should be separately addressed to each participating parent, spouse, or sibling, and their answers summarized by the clinician. The patient may be relieved to learn that, independent of the impact of his or her disorder, family members have their own worries, anxieties, unmet needs, or challenges in their lives.

If your patient is a teen, you may get answers of the form "to get my parents off my back" or "to get money for a car." Although these may not seem like helpful therapeutic goals, praise the patient for his or her attempts to contribute and think in terms of the future. For example, say, "Good idea. I don't know if I can help you get a car, but I can certainly help you think through the steps of how you might work toward getting one."

Presenting the Didactic Material: Reviewing the Index Episode

Table 6.1 presents the core content areas that are covered in the psychoeducation module. More or less time will be spent on certain of these areas depending on their emotional significance to the family, as well as the family's existing knowledge about the topic.

Introducing the Review of the Most Recent Episode

When William was asked to discuss the symptoms associated with his most recent episode, he balked at first. He said, "I've told this story already." The clinician empathized with this, noting that the episode was probably painful to talk about. The clinician also pointed out that discuss-

TABLE 6.1. Issues in Psychoeducation

The symptoms and course of the disorder

- The signs and symptoms of bipolar disorder
- The development of the most recent episode
- The Recent Life Events survey
- Discussing the hospitalization experience
- Variations in prognosis: The course of the disorder

The etiology of bipolar disorder

- The vulnerability–stress model
- The roles of stress and life events
- Genetic and biological predispositions
- Risk and protective factors

Intervening within the vulnerability–stress model

- Types of medications and what they do
- Psychosocial treatments
- How the family can help
- The self-management of the disorder
- The relapse drill

ing the episode might help resolve some of the "unfinished business" to which William had alluded in regard to his parents' behavior during the episode. As William began to experience the treatment environment as safe and nonjudgmental, he became more willing to share the details of his episode.

William recalled his feelings of being quite powerful and on top of the world, and that he had begun to understand the science of the universe. His mother, Alyssia, focused more on his degree of activity; lack of sleep; and angry, often provocative, behavior. A fact about William's history that hadn't been clear from the earlier diagnostic interviews surfaced during this discussion: He had come down with the flu just 2 weeks prior to the onset of his manic symptoms. He had spent several days in bed recovering from this flu, and, because this put him behind in his course work, he had decided to "pull several all-nighters" to catch up. His symptoms began to escalate after the third night without sleep.

In many ways, the most important component of the psychoeducation module involves helping the patient and family to integrate and make sense of the most recent episode of illness (FFT Goal 1). Proceed in a gentle way to (1) review with the family the presenting symptoms of the index (i.e., the most recent) episode, (2) review the symptoms the patient showed during the prodromal period, (3) facilitate an open discussion of the life events and family conflicts that precipitated the episode, and (4) explore the course of the hospitalization (if one occurred) and the patient's and family's reactions to it. In so doing, keep in mind a basic rule in conducting FFT: The more material that comes from the participants, the better.

Reviewing the most recent episode can introduce an "approach–avoidance" conflict in the family. The patient and family want to understand what happened yet are reluctant to let reemerge the feelings and conflicts associated with the episode. Thus, a useful opening statement to the family is the following:

> "We're going to start by discussing your most recent episode, with a special emphasis on the symptoms William experienced. We'll then share with you a model for understanding what causes the disorder and how it's treated.
>
> "If feelings come up for you when we're discussing this material, please bring them up. We're not only interested in the facts—we want to know how this material applies to you and your own experiences. You may or may not agree with some of the material we present here. We know you've all been through a tough time, and the purpose of focusing on this material is to put your own experiences into a context that will make sense."

Thus, the clinician gives the patient and family permission to raise emotional reactions that may on the surface appear to run counter to the didactic tenor of the sessions.

It is often helpful to describe the patient as the "expert" in the disorder and to give him or her special status in the discussions of the episode. For example, say, "____________, we're going to depend on you to educate us about what this disorder is really all about. Although we know a lot about the science of this disorder, you're the one who's been through it, and you have a perspective that neither we nor your parents (spouse) may share." Nonetheless, family members should be strongly encouraged to chime in as they see fit. It is critical to review not only areas of shared perception about the disorder, but also areas about which the patient and his or her family members have substantial disagreement. Exploring and resolving disagreements about the most recent episode can contribute to restoring healthy family functioning (FFT Goal 6).

Acquainting Family Members with the Symptoms of Bipolar Disorder

Begin by presenting the diagnostic criteria for episodes of mania, depression, and psychosis, any of which may be relevant to the patient's most recent episode or its prodromal period of development. Handout 2 helps organize these discussions. Avoid getting caught up in the details of DSM-IV criteria; instead, give the participants a general idea of the key symptoms of mania and depression.

There are several reasons to acquaint the participants with the symptoms of bipolar disorder. First, in learning this material, patients and family members become able to identify the prodromal symptoms of new episodes and can more aggressively intervene (e.g., by arranging an emergency appointment with the psychiatrist) when such symptoms occur. For example, in reviewing the list, one family member said, "I remember when you got depressed the last time. You got very guilty about not having gone to church often enough. I think that's when things really got started—maybe that's when we should have called the doctor."

Second, family members learn that certain behaviors they previously attributed to "laziness" or "your hyperactive nature" are really symptoms of depression or mania that may not be controllable by the patient (FFT Goal 4: separating personality from the disorder). Third, learning that the patient has had many symptoms consistent with the diagnostic criteria for bipolar disorder helps family members and patients to begin to resolve their doubts about whether or not the illness is a reality. This is particularly helpful for patients and families coping with a first or second episode. In introducing the symptom list, proceed as follows:

Symptoms of Bipolar Disorder

Symptoms of mania

- High (euphoric or elated) mood or irritable mood
- Decreased need for sleep
- Increased activity level
- Increased sexuality
- Pressured, fast speech
- Racing thoughts
- Appetite disturbance
- "Grandiose" or unrealistic beliefs
- Distractibility
- Loss of self-control and judgment

Symptoms of depression

- Low mood or sadness
- Increased or decreased appetite and weight changes
- Sleeping too much or too little
- Loss of energy: excessive fatigue or tiredness
- Loss of interest or pleasure in activities
- Changes in activity level
- Suicidal thoughts or actions
- Decreased ability to think or concentrate
- Feelings of worthlessness or excessive guilt
- Decreased sex drive
- Tearfulness

Symptoms of psychosis

- Unusual or unrealistic beliefs
- Hallucinations
- Speech that is difficult to understand
- Impulsive, dangerous, or irrational behaviors
- Slowness, apathy, lack of emotional responsiveness

HANDOUT 2.

"One of the ways we want to help you is to look at the symptoms of bipolar disorder and show you how a diagnosis is made. We want to identify which of these symptoms you had so we can know what you went through during your episode, as well as when you were becoming ill. Some people find it easy to talk about their symptoms, and others find it hard—they feel embarrassed or ashamed, or sometimes they just can't remember. But let's give it a try."

Briefly review the definitions of each of these symptoms, and explain that they tend to occur in clusters that compose a *syndrome.* Explain, for example, that "tearfulness" is not synonymous with "major depression"; "irritability" is not the same as mania. Several symptoms must occur together before the diagnosis of bipolar disorder (manic or depressed) is made.

Next, the patient is given the floor and is asked, "Which of these symptoms do you remember having during your last manic (depressive) episode?" Each parent or spouse is separately asked to recount the symptoms he or she observed (e.g., "Which of these symptoms were you aware of William having?" "Did this cause any difficulty in the family?"). Table 6.2 lists some useful probing questions to elicit discussions of specific symptoms.

Discussing the patient's symptoms often generates uncomfortable feelings within the family, whether or not these are voiced. Within the patient, the discussions may bring up feelings about being labeled mentally ill (see Chapter 8). Thus, offer much encouragement, support, and empathy for all participants as they review the patient's symptoms (e.g., to the patient: "It must have been hard for you, coping with these symptoms and trying to make sense of it all"). As discussed further in Chapter 8, "spreading the affliction"—asking each of the patient's relatives to recount his or her own experiences with depression or other symptom states—helps to keep the patient from feeling that he or she is being unfairly labeled, singled out, or scapegoated by the psychoeducation process.

The Symptoms Leading Up to the Acute Episode

In reviewing the symptom list, you can help the patient and family identify the prodromal signs of the most recent episode. This is an important component of the "relapse drill" (Chapter 7).

CLINICIAN: So you couldn't sleep?

WILLIAM: Yeah, I was staying up later and later. It didn't happen all at once, kind of gradually.

TABLE 6.2. Examples of Questions to Elicit the Experience of Manic and Depressive Symptoms

	Question/probe
Manic symptoms	
Elated mood	Did you feel high, on top of the world, like you could conquer anything?
Irritable mood	Were you feeling very angry, whether you showed it or not? How did you show it? Yell at people? Break things?
Decreased sleep	Did you have trouble falling asleep or staying asleep? Did you feel like you didn't need to sleep, and weren't even tired the next day?
Increased activity	Did you get involved in lots of extra projects? Did you feel like you were going a mile a minute? Talking to lots of people on the phone?
Racing thoughts	Were your thoughts going very fast? Was your mind racing along almost like you were watching a DVD in fast-forward?
Depressive symptoms	
Depressed mood	Were you feeling low, down in the dumps, sad, hopeless?
Loss of interests	Was nothing any fun? Did everything seem like it was too much effort?
Suicidality	Did it feel like life wasn't worth living? Did you want to hurt or kill yourself? Did you have a plan as to how you would do it? Did you act on any of this?
Decreased concentration	Did your mind seem like it was going slower than usual? Were you able to read or watch television and know what was going on? Did you have trouble making decisions?

STAN: And I spoke to him on the phone and he was coherent, but talking too fast for me to follow. Something about cell biology.

WILLIAM: I started reading all the time. I couldn't put down my biology book, which is weird 'cause I had thought before that biology was super boring.

CLINICIAN: So sleep disturbance and this sudden interest in biology were your first signs?

WILLIAM: Yeah.

CLINICIAN: And then you started having more energy for work?

WILLIAM: Yeah, but I also had this sense that I had gained a few IQ points. I felt I understood things like never before.

In the above vignette, the clinician helps the patient identify four different prodromal symptoms (decreased need for sleep, increased interests, increased energy, grandiose or rapid thinking) that may in the future herald the development of new manic episodes. Consider the following case vignette from a different family including an 18-year-old:

CLINICIAN: Sam, do you remember what your experience was like when you were first getting manic?

SAM: Yeah. I remember basically, pretty much, noises . . . and voices.

CLINICIAN: Yeah?

SAM: I was really sore all over my body, and I kept going off on tangents. I was yelling and screaming. I did some pretty funny things. I read in books now of people who've had similar experiences and stuff.

CLINICIAN: Certainly, sure.

SAM: Racing thoughts, superintelligence, and mental communication with objects and flowers. Colors were really bright. It was a really interesting LSD trip . . . (*Pause*) . . . whatever an LSD trip is like.

CLINICIAN: I'm glad you added that for your mom. (*All laugh.*)

These same questions about the development of the patient's episode are then directed to family members:

CLINICIAN: Mrs. Clancey, what do you remember about how Sam's episode developed?

MRS. CLANCEY: Well, I had known he'd been racing for weeks, and we had talked about him seeing a psychiatrist, but I thought he was, you know, calming down. . . . But then we made the mistake of going into a restaurant . . . and then he went into the kitchen and started screaming at the chefs. . . . Then I had to talk to the owners, and I had to borrow their phone to call Jeff [one of her other sons] to see if he could come help.

CLINICIAN: So he was racing and acting impulsively. Jeff, do you remember that?

JEFF: Yeah, that's where I came in. I got a call. I was at my desk working, and Mom said she was having trouble controlling Sam. So I said, "I'll come down and see what I can do."

MRS. CLANCEY: Uh-huh. It seemed like forever. 'Cause, see, that's when he was ready to jump up on the chandeliers. . . . Oh, God, it was a traumatic experience. And luckily they didn't hurt him.

JEFF: Yeah, and then there was that convertible, a car—I think it was an MG—wide open. (*to Sam*) And you said, "Here we are, Jeff! How do you like my new car? Let's go for a ride!" You had opened the door and you were getting in the car. . . . So I pulled him out of that. But it was at that point that I said, "No, we're not gonna be able to take this guy peacefully."

SAM: (*Giggles.*) I don't know why I was screaming at the time. I was like, "Aah! I'm being attacked!"

MRS. CLANCEY: "They're kidnapping me!" he was hollering. And here I am.

SAM: We can laugh about it now, but that was horrible.

In discussing the events and the prodromal symptoms leading up to the full episode, it is healthy for the family and patient to laugh about the events that occurred. However, make sure to reflect empathically upon the disturbed, often frightened emotions each family member probably experienced during the escalation of the episode.

Summarizing the Symptoms Associated with the Episode

Before moving on to the discussion of the life events precipitating the episode, summarize what has been learned so far about the patient's symptom profile:

> "It sounds like you've had a number of symptoms of mania, and they were quite disorganizing to you and your family members. We understand better now what you've gone through—you felt quite euphoric, you weren't sleeping, you had more energy, and you felt like you could do almost anything. Your mom and brother noticed you were acting dangerously and impulsively. These are common attributes of manic episodes. There was also a period of time when these symptoms were accelerating but they hadn't gotten out of control yet—your prodromal period, when you began to feel ultraintelligent, where colors seemed brighter, and your thoughts raced and you were going off on tangents. Soon, we'll talk about how we can use this information in preventing these episodes from escalating in the future."

It was helpful to this family to realize that the patient's initial "racing" behaviors (e.g., his feeling of superintelligence) constituted the initial prodromal symptoms, whereas the symptoms described by his mother and brother (euphoria, irritability, impulsivity, reckless and dangerous behavior) reflected manic symptoms that had spiralled out of control. Thus, the presence of racing behavior and grandiose thinking could be identified in the future as triggers for the need of early medical and psychosocial intervention.

Events Leading Up to the Episode: The Life Events Survey

The discussion of the symptoms associated with the index episode, although providing an extremely important addition to the family's knowledge base, tends to raise the tension level. In contrast, discussing the environmental precipitants of the episode tends to bring participants together. Often, a life event has affected all members of the family, as well as playing a role in the patient's episode. Thus, discussing important life events that occurred prior to the episode allows the patient and family to unite against a common enemy (life stress).

Identifying precipitating events may also help the patient and family to anticipate and plan for periods in the future when similar events occur. These may be especially high-risk intervals for the patient. Finally, discussing precipitating life events sets the stage for presentation of the vulnerability–stress model, presented in full after the review of the index episode (see Chapter 7).

Surveying Life Events

Begin the discussion of precipitating events with the following:

> "As we mentioned earlier, episodes of bipolar disorder seem to be brought on by a person's stress level in combination with his or her biological predispositions. Let's talk for a minute about the events that occurred in the last 3 months, some of which probably created stress in your family."

In our experience, simply asking, "Was there something unusual that happened in the months just before your episode?" usually generates null responses. Instead, give each participant a copy of the Recent Life Events survey (Handout 3), which lists a number of events—some minor, some major—that may have occurred prior to the patient's episode.

The patient and his or her family members are each asked to review the list and report on which events occurred in the preillness period. Some of the events reported by relatives will have directly involved the patient (e.g., marital separations in a couple, financial problems), whereas others may have occurred quite independent of him or her (e.g., death of a spouse's parent). In reviewing these events, the patient usually feels less in the "hot seat," as he or she begins to realize that family members have been dealing with problems of their own.

When discussing the events that affected the participants, it is important to assess their *appraisals of* and *emotional reactions to* each event. For

Recent Life Events

Please read this list of events and circle those that you have experienced in the *last 3 months*.

1. Change in residence.
2. New person moved into household.
3. Person moved out of household.
4. Made a major purchase.
5. Contracted for a loan or mortgage.
6. Started new school or training program.
7. Started a new job.
8. Promoted to a new job.
9. Received a substantial increase in salary.
10. Changed school or job.
11. Finished school or training program.
12. Vacationed.
13. Started dating someone new.
14. Fell in love.
15. Became engaged.
16. Married.
17. You/spouse became pregnant.
18. Birth or adoption of child.
19. Significant gain or loss of weight.
20. Stopped an addictive habit (e.g., smoking).
21. Problem with parent(s).
22. Problem with romantic partner.
23. Problem with spouse.
24. Problem with child.
25. Problem with in-laws.
26. Problem with close friend.
27. Problem with neighbors.
28. Problem in school or training program.
29. Trouble with boss.
30. Excessive workload.
31. Discriminated against or overlooked at work.
32. Problem with associates at work.
33. Did not receive expected promotion.
34. Demotion or reduction in salary.
35. Loss of job.
36. Charge in spouse's school or job status.
37. Financial problems.
38. Personal illness or injury.
39. Serious illness or injury of parent(s).
40. Serious illness or injury of spouse.
41. Serious illness or injury of child.
42. Serious illness or injury of other family member.
43. Serious illness or injury of close friend.
44. Death of parent.
45. Death of spouse.
46. Death of child.
47. Death of other close family member.
48. Death of close friend.
49. You/spouse had abortion.
50. You/spouse had miscarriage or stillbirth.
51. Learned you/spouse cannot have children.
52. Breakup of a close friendship.
53. Separation or divorce of parents.
54. Your infidelity discovered by partner.
55. Partner's Infidelity discovered by you.
56. Breakup of a romantic relationship.
57. Separation or divorce from spouse.
58. Victim of sexual harassment.
59. Victim of theft or burglary.
60. Victim of assault.
61. Arrested.
62. Other: ______________________

    ____
    ____
    ____
    ____

HANDOUT 3. *Source*: Adapted by permission from Dohrenwend, Krasnoff, Askenasy, and Dohrenwend (1978).

example, say, "It sounds like there were some real important things going on that were difficult to handle and may have contributed to ___________'s episode. Which of these do you think were the hardest to deal with, and why?" Useful probing questions include "Was this event expected or unexpected?" "How did you react to it?" "What did you do immediately after *X* happened?" "Why do you think this event was particularly difficult for you?"

The Patient's Emotional Vulnerabilities

A core justification for identifying precipitating life events is to gain a sense of what kinds of events are likely to precipitate the patient's episodes in the future. Patients may be more affected by certain kinds of life events than others. For example, some patients with mood disorder become depressed after achievement-related events (e.g., failing a school course), whereas others are more affected by events in interpersonal relationships (e.g., relationship terminations; Hammen, Marks, Mayol, & deMayo, 1985).

It may be useful to help the patient categorize recent events as reflecting losses, role transitions, or interpersonal disputes (Frank, 2005; Weissman, Markowitz, & Klerman, 2000). Where possible, the patient is asked to generate examples of previous events in his or her life that (1) are in the same conceptual category as the precipitating event and (2) provoked similar, although perhaps less intense, emotional reactions. In this manner, the patient learns to identify areas of emotional vulnerability for him or her, vulnerabilities that, when activated by life stressors, decrease his or her threshold for new mood disorder episodes.

Connecting the Event with the Episode

Ask the family to rank two or three life events that occurred in the 3 months prior to the episode, in order of severity (e.g., [1] grandmother died, [2] the family moved to a new house, and [3] patient had trouble with boss). Then, explore with the family the possible connection between the occurrence of these stressors and the onset of the episode. You can facilitate this process by probing with questions like "Was this period a more stressful time than usual? When did event *X* occur in relation to when you [the patient] started having your symptoms?" If the patient and family are able to see these connections, summarize the discussion of the precipitating events:

> "I think this gives us at least a partial answer as to why this manic episode happened to you at this time. This was a high-stress time for you—you had several important life events within a short space of

time. Most of us get more vulnerable to illnesses when we get overwhelmed with stress. So, at least in this way, it makes sense that your episode happened at this time."

Notice that the clinician does not say that the stressful event caused the patient's episode. A patient whose manic symptoms have been building will be more prone to experiencing certain stressful events, such as conflicts with an employer or being kicked out of school. Likewise, a depressed patient may withdraw from others or become overly needy, in a way that fosters rejection from others. Nonetheless, events caused by the patient's behavior still have an impact on his or her mood states, which can then lead to a vicious circle of more dysfunctional behavior and more stress.

Resistances to Accepting the Role of Life Stress

Occasionally, patients or family members will deny the importance of stress in precipitating mood disorder episodes, arguing that the disorder is fully biological and that episodes are simply "time bombs" that go off at random intervals. Sometimes these discussions make clear the different beliefs family members hold about the origins of the disorder, beliefs that may precipitate family conflicts (see the discussion of these conflicts in Chapter 8). Consider the following vignette, in which the clinician addresses this perspective:

STAN: I think we're grabbing at straws here. OK, so we moved to a new house. Why should that make him get manic?

CLINICIAN: You're making a good point, and I agree that it's easy to fall into the trap of thinking one event caused this disorder. I hope we haven't communicated that it's that simple. [Validates father's question.]

STAN: But this disorder is mostly biological, isn't it?

WILLIAM: To you, maybe.

CLINICIAN: [*Ignores conflict brewing.*] Well, I can see why you might view it that way. It is biological, but nothing is *only* biological. As you'll see when we talk more about how we understand the causes of this disorder, both biological predispositions and stress must be present before episodes occur.

STAN: So are we never supposed to move again?

CLINICIAN: It's not moving per se that's important here, but rather the overall level of stress you as a family experienced before William became ill. If William were not already biologically predisposed to having these episodes, I'm sure moving would have had little or no effect. [Sets the foundation for the vulnerability–stress model.]

STAN: So, I guess if he was predisposed we shouldn't have moved at that time. Now I'm starting to feel guilty.

CLINICIAN: I want to make clear that I'm not trying to blame anybody here, or imply that the family shouldn't have done certain things. I also want to make clear that William is not the only one in the family who has experienced stress and tension from the events you've listed. The value of discussing these issues is that in the future you may know what kinds of stress are important in William's disorder and affect the family as well, and how to avoid those stressors or better manage them once they've occurred. [Addresses father's guilty feelings, and emphasizes that learning about life stress empowers the patient and family.]

Family members may also raise the very reasonable question of whether the event caused the episode or the episode caused the event. You can point out that such distinctions are indeed difficult to make, and that a certain event can be one of many causes *and* one of many effects of a developing episode. The point needs to be clear that no one event caused the disorder, but rather collections of events create cumulative levels of stress that would be upsetting to anybody.

Planning for the Future

Toward the end of this exercise, offer a summary statement that gives the patient and family hope for the future:

> "I appreciate how much each of you has offered to this discussion. One of the things we'll do in this treatment is keep this list of events in our pocket, so that as the year goes on, when things happen that we suspect you're vulnerable to—for example, loss or change experiences—we'll know this is a high-risk time and that you need to work extra hard to manage these events and your mood states.
>
> "Soon, we'll be discussing with you some skills you may be able to use to keep stress from getting to you. For example, if you're beginning to get into conflicts with your boss, we'll teach you some new ways to communicate with her so that you can keep your stress level from getting too high."

The clinician concretizes for the family the prevention concept by offering an example of how one might use skills learned in FFT to mitigate the effects of stress. In so doing, he encourages the participants to feel they have a certain degree of control over their mutual fate. In addition, he praises each family member for his or her input.

Discussing the Hospitalization Experience

Not all acutely ill bipolar patients end up in the hospital. In fact, hospitalization is getting to be a rarer alternative because of the financial limitations imposed by managed care companies. However, when hospitalization is a part of the acute episode, a unique set of issues is raised for the family.

The Trauma of the Hospitalization

For virtually every patient and family member, the process of hospitalization and the hospitalization itself are quite traumatic experiences, even independent of the symptomatic behaviors of the patient. Their reactions—anger, frustration, confusion, sadness, guilt, and anxiety—are most acute if they are dealing with the patient's first or second hospitalization. However, in our experience, even families who have dealt with multiple hospitalizations can have these reactions.

Consistent with the goal of helping the family to make sense of the most recent episode, encourage a discussion of the hospitalization experience. Begin with a question to the patient: "How did your hospitalization come about?" If the patient is able, encourage him or her to discuss the process of admission, the inpatient treatment, the other patients whom he or she encountered on the ward, and reactions to the inpatient physician. Express empathy for the trauma associated with the hospitalization:

> "I know this is something you've been struggling with. I don't know anybody who's liked being in the hospital or the process of being hospitalized, or of seeing their relative on an inpatient ward. Also, people sometimes learn afterward what they did while in the hospital, and this can be a source of shame and guilt. I bet each of you sometimes feels that the whole event was a big injustice to you."

In this passage, the clinician communicates that the patient and family are not alone in their experiences of these events. The following is a vignette from a family in which two brothers, Jim and Todd, have had hospitalized manic episodes, one of them (Todd) quite recently.

CLINICIAN: Jim, what do you remember about Todd's episode? What do you remember having to deal with at the time? Did you recognize the signs from your own experiences?

JIM: Immediately. Yeah. It was torture for me because I knew what he was going through, and I just wanted to get him to the hospital as soon as possible. He was, like, in la-la land.

CLINICIAN: Do you remember that, Todd?

TODD: I remember I was in the hospital. I think I just called you guys up, and all of a sudden, next thing I know, there's more doctors piling up . . . eight or nine of them after me and start tearing me up and lifting me and putting me in some room. (*Chuckles.*)

JIM: I wonder if there really were eight or nine doctors, or if it just seemed that way. Maybe there were really two doctors. (*Laughs.*)

TODD: There was a lot of 'em. They were all lifting me. Like, herds of 'em.

MRS. RODRIGUEZ: I'm sure it was scary, though, having eight people drag you into a room.

CLINICIAN: Good point, Mrs. Rodriguez. I think it is scary to be dragged into a hospital, even if you can laugh about it later.

TODD: (*Brightens.*) Yeah! And then I . . . I was gone after that. . . . I don't know how many days went by till I woke up and had . . . a beard and everything. I went in and out, thinking all these thoughts.

CLINICIAN: I appreciate how frank you're being about your experiences, Todd. I'm sure it was a very frightening thing for all of you. I'm glad that you're able to talk about it so openly.

In this vignette, the patient is "given the floor" to discuss his hospitalization experiences. The clinician highlights the patient's fearful reactions accompanying his otherwise jovial recollections of the hospital.

The family's experiences should also be drawn out (e.g., "Mrs. Rodriguez, how did Todd's hospitalization come about? What happened during that time that you'd like to discuss?"). Many relatives—whether they voice it or not—have been deeply humiliated by the hospitalization experience, particularly if the police were involved or if they were embarrassed in front of their neighbors. Alternatively, they may have been treated with disrespect by hospital staff members. Clarify with them their anger, hurt, fears, or avoidance reactions, always maintaining a nonblaming stance:

"I think many family members feel the way you did. Here you brought your son in for care, and the reaction you had was that your feelings weren't important. I think there are cases when inpatient staff members are insensitive to family members, not because of malice but sometimes because they have so many demands on them or they simply don't know what to say. But I'm sure those interactions with the nursing staff made you wonder whether the hospitalization would be helpful to your son." [Empathizes with family but also indicates that the family has probably not been "singled out" for this kind of treatment.]

The Patient's Feelings of Betrayal

Prepare yourself for the possibility that the patient feels betrayed by his or her family's involvement in the hospitalization. For example, one patient of ours said to his wife, "You didn't take care of me. Instead, you just stuck me in that snake pit." Another patient said, "When you visited, I felt worse. You looked at me like I was an animal in the zoo."

This issue should be addressed with much empathy and sensitivity. If possible, the fact that the parents or spouse hospitalized the patient should be framed as evidence of their caring for the patient's well-being. Avoid implying that you agree with the patient, that the hospitalization should not have occurred.

In the case below, the patient had bitterly complained about his parents having called the police, who had quickly and rather aggressively taken him to the hospital.

PATIENT: You didn't have to call the cops. I'm not some goddamn criminal.

FATHER: But what else were we supposed to do?

CLINICIAN: When someone in your family is showing behavior that is so radically different from what he's usually like, it's understandable to take the stance that he needs treatment, even if it does involve a hospitalization. Family members often have to call the police because they're afraid that if they don't, the person may hurt himself or someone else. [Validates the wisdom of the family's decision to take action.]

PATIENT: So you think they're right?

CLINICIAN: I don't think the issue is whether it was right or wrong. I think what you're saying is that you felt quite betrayed—perhaps you felt as if your family abandoned you. Although it's understandable to feel this way, I think it's important to keep in mind that this was the only thing your family members felt they could do at the time, because they were very concerned about you. And although the experience may have been frightening, embarrassing, and ugly, I think you must realize that your family was doing this out of a sense of caring for you, not as a punishment.

A related issue is the quality of the inpatient care the patient received while in the hospital, a frequent source of anger and dismay. Nowadays, patients feel that they are quickly checked in and out, overmedicated, and shown little personal respect during their hospital stays. Although these perceptions are often quite realistic, make clear that the patient's family should not be held accountable for the quality of the inpatient care:

> "It sounds like those experiences on the unit were not exactly beneficial to your recovery. On the other hand, your family wasn't there all the time and really had no control over this. And although they may have chosen the hospital you went to, they really didn't have much of a say in what treatments you got."

There may be other aspects of the hospitalization experience that the patient or family members wish to discuss. In particular, family members may want to explain to the patient why they felt it necessary to call the police, arrange the hospitalization, or perhaps, visit him or her on the ward infrequently. These discussions cap the exploration of the development and course of the patient's recent episode and allow you to transition to the topic of the long-term prognosis of the disorder.

The Expected Course of Bipolar Disorder

The course of bipolar disorder is often of great concern to family members. Their core question is usually "What does the future hold?" or "Will he (or she) keep having these episodes?" Alternatively, they may ask, "Will he (or she) be able to hold down a job . . . or have a family?" Patients may have similar questions about their own futures.

Presenting the Facts

Avoid becoming overly academic when discussing these issues. That is, family members are not usually interested in the fine distinctions between different course patterns (see the discussion of these in Chapter 2). Instead, offer some basic statistics about recovery and relapse. For example, over a 1-year period, the chances of remaining well without a recurrence—if the patient is adequately maintained on lithium or other mood-regulating drugs (i.e., divalproex sodium, atypical antipsychotics)—is about 50–70%, and about 40% over 2–3 years; the amount of time needed to recover from a manic episode averages about 2 months, and about 3–4 months for a depressive episode; and, although many patients recover fully from their episodes, some (25–50% in some studies) show significant residual symptoms and/or continuous periods of illness (dysthymia, hypomania, rapid cycling) following episodes (Perlis et al., 2006; Judd et al., 2002; Gitlin et al., 1995; Keller, Lavori, Coryell, Endicott, & Mueller, 1993).

A key notion to communicate to the family is the importance of minimizing expectations for the patient's immediate functioning during the recovery period. Even patients who are symptomatically recovered need time to regain their previous level of social and occupational adaptation, and some do not ever recover to this level. However, point out the many individual differences in patients' abilities to handle work, go to school, or socialize following an episode. This issue is discussed in more detail in Chapter 7.

First Episode versus Chronic Patients

In giving information about the course of the illness, make a distinction between a multiple-episode patient versus one who has had only one or two episodes. With first-onset patients, assess the degree to which the patient and family appear ready to accept the notion of vulnerability to future episodes (FFT Goal 2). In most cases, it is best to paint a cautious but optimistic view of the future:

> "Bipolar disorder is usually a recurrent illness, and episodes tend to come and go over time. But you've only had one episode, so in reality we don't know what the future holds. We know most people who have a manic or a depressive episode do go on to have another one, so our basic position is 'Assume you're at risk but hope for the best.' If you're able to follow a regular medication plan and get some psychotherapy—at least for this first year—we think your prognosis over the long run is going to be much better."

Although one might assume that multiple-episode patients and their families are more ready to accept the inevitability of recurrences, this is not always true. Many recurrent patients and their family members continue to believe that the most recent episode will be the last one:

> "I think you've seen that whenever you go off your medications or stress gets too high, you have another episode. I think this is a reality you and your family have had to deal with for quite some time. But learning the facts about what sets you off puts you in a much stronger position. For example, perhaps you'll be able to identify when you're in a high-risk period. Then, you can get the help you need sooner rather than later."

Concluding Comments

This chapter has addressed several issues pertinent to the beginning phases of psychoeducation. In the initial sessions, the clinician develops a therapeutic alliance with the family and reviews the most recent episode and/or hospitalization, which have often been quite traumatic for the patient and family. In discussing these issues, he or she imparts didactic information about the disorder: its prodromal signs, acute symptoms, psychosocial precipitants, and expected course.

If well delivered, family members and patients should walk away from these initial sessions with several benefits. First, they will feel that you understand them and care about each of them as a person. Second, the treatment will feel less intimidating to them, and the potential benefits clearer. Third, they will feel that their experiences and emotional reactions during the episode are within the normal range. Fourth, they will have a beginning sense of the syndrome of bipolar disorder, including its signs and symptoms and how to recognize when episodes are recurring. As a result, their anxieties about the future will be tempered.

chapter 7

Family Psychoeducation

Etiology, Treatment, and Self-Management

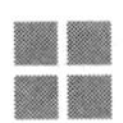

When the family clinicians raised the issue of the etiology (causes) of William's bipolar disorder, it became clear that each family member had a different explanation. William was convinced that the LSD he had taken about 1 year before his hospitalization was the primary cause of his disorder. His father argued that "he's really always been like this. This is just an exaggeration of his personality." His mother explained that "Stan [her husband] has several mentally ill people in his family. I'm sure William has inherited those genes." Stan expressed a great deal of annoyance at this explanation. Referring to his wife's own history of depression, he argued, "Well, Alyssia, if we're going to place blame, we could also say your unavailability while he was growing up could have contributed, too, couldn't we?"

Chapter Overview

This chapter describes the psychoeducational information pertinent to the causes and treatment of bipolar disorder. It reviews the practical suggestions given to patients and their family members about how to manage the disorder (e.g., keeping family stress and performance expectations to a minimum). The goals of providing this information include (1) empowering patients and family members through acquainting them with available medical and psychosocial treatments, (2) alleviating the guilt of family members who believe they may have caused the disorder, and (3) encouraging family members to think of the disorder's symptoms as signifying an illness syndrome rather than a set of willfully produced behaviors.

The Etiology of Bipolar Disorder

There is a series of questions on the minds of family members when one of their relatives has had an episode of psychiatric disorder. These questions can be summarized as "Why this member of our family?" "Why now?" and "What will happen in the future?" These are very loaded questions, because family members may experience more or less guilt, depending on the way you, as the clinician, address these questions. Keep in mind that behind these questions are often other questions of the form "Am I at fault?" or "Did I hurt him (or her) somehow?" Table 7.1 presents general guidelines for imparting etiological information.

In transitioning to the discussions of etiological factors, the following is a useful opening:

> "Bipolar disorder is caused by many factors that all interact with each other. No one person, event, or experience makes this disorder occur. In this session and the next one, we're going to present to you a theory, called the vulnerability–stress model, for understanding the interplay of these factors. And although we may not know what caused William's particular symptoms, we do know, in the more gen-

TABLE 7.1. Guidelines for the Delivery of Etiological Information

- Take a nonblaming, accepting stance.
- Show interest in the patient as a person; look beyond the illness.
- Talk about multiple etiological pathways involving genetic, biological, and psychosocial factors.
- Avoid overly technical, impersonal explanations of genetic transmission or neuronal communication.
- Do not accept the argument that any one event, factor, or person caused the disorder.
- Emphasize the roles of protective as well as risk factors.
- Discuss elements of treatment that are likely to bring about change.
- Do not assume genetic or biological explanations produce less guilt in family members than psychological ones.
- Instill optimism about the future course of the illness.
- Address the patient's and relatives' emotional reactions to the material.

eral sense, some of the things that make people get these symptoms. We hope this information will be helpful to you."

In this opening, the clinician already communicates that family members are not to be blamed and sets the stage for introducing a multipathway etiological model. He also points to the limitations of our knowledge about the origins of the disorder.

The Vulnerability–Stress Model

From the beginning, make clear your stance that episodes of the disorder, including the disorder's first onset, are a product of a complex interaction between a person's (1) genetic vulnerabilities (i.e., the number of first- or second-degree relatives who have had the disorder or a variant of it), (2) biological vulnerabilities (sometimes better understood by family members as "predispositions," or biochemical imbalances of the central nervous system), (3) his or her levels of and styles of coping with socioenvironmental stress, and (4) the protective effects of close relationships. Handout 4—a graphic display of the vulnerability–stress model—provides a useful schematic for families in their attempts to understand these notions. Handout 5 is supplemental to Handout 4, because it offers specific information about some of the presumed causes of the disorder. Plan on referring to these handouts throughout the discussions of etiological mechanisms. However, these handouts are not simply passed around and explained in a mechanical way, nor are they an end in themselves. Rather, they serve as stimuli to guide family-wide discussions of the various pathways to the disorder. They also often elicit emotional reactions from the participants, which you should take time to explore.

Socioenvironmental Stress

Perhaps most accessible to families learning the vulnerability–stress model is the environmental component, which is introduced first. Because you will have already explored with the family the role of stress in the onset of the most recent episode (see "Surveying Life Events" in Chapter 6), it is not necessary to spend a great deal of time reiterating these notions. However, underlining the importance of environmental stress in the etiology and course of the disorder is crucial to justifying the skill-training tasks that come later in the treatment.

A good entry is to elicit from each participant examples of what he or she considers stressful. Consider the following interchange:

CLINICIAN: Let's take a look at Handout 4 depicting the vulnerability–stress model. First, a major cause of episodes of mania and depres-

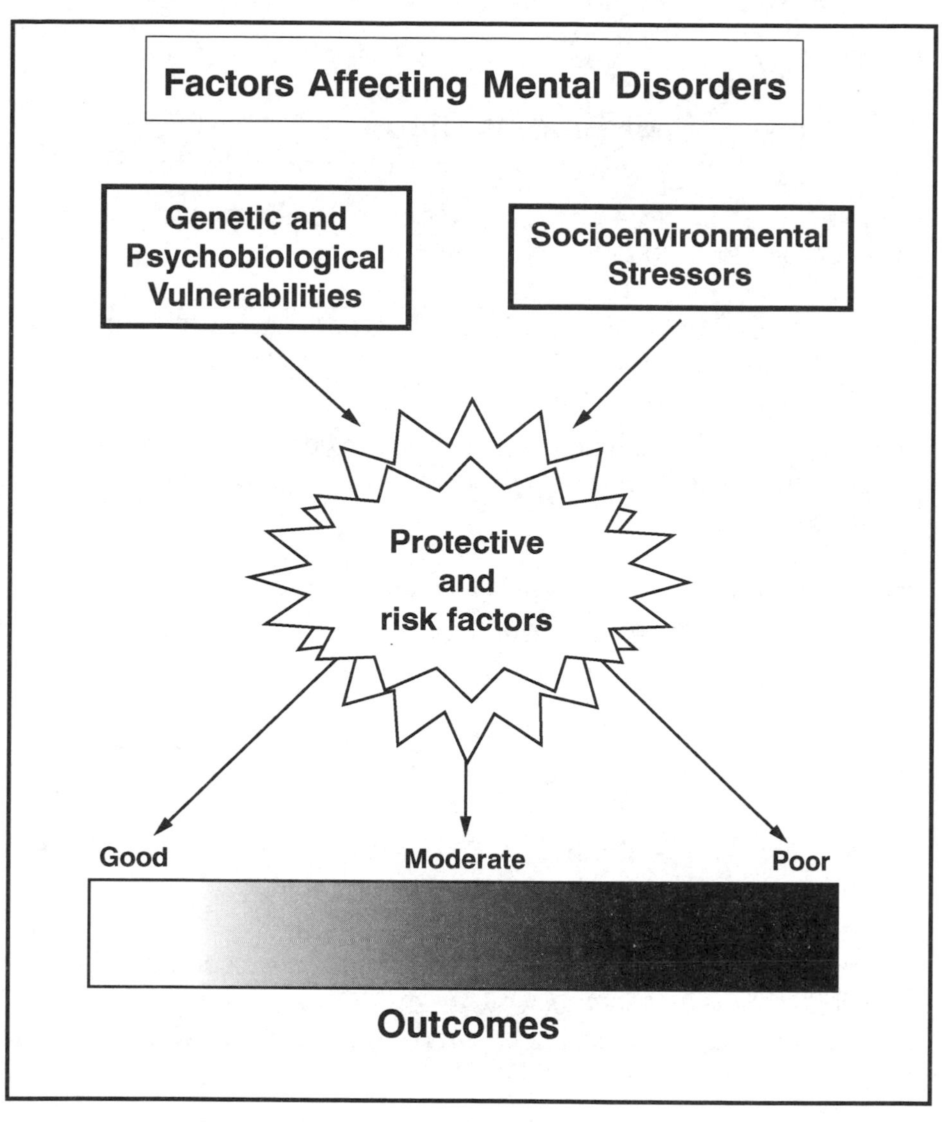

HANDOUT 4. *Source:* Adapted from Anthony and Liberman (1986) (public domain).

How Do People Get the Symptoms of Bipolar Disorder?

People are born with a genetic or biological predisposition to develop bipolar disorder.

- The rate of bipolar disorder in first-degree relatives of people with bipolar disorder is about 9% and the rate of major depression is about 14%.
- People have a "biological vulnerability" to develop it (i.e., a tendency for the nervous system to become overactive under stress).

The environment may become more stressful (e.g., increases in social or job demands, life events). A stressful environment may interact with a genetic or biological vulnerability.

Coping skills (e.g., communicating well with others) may be inadequate for dealing with environmental stress.

Drug abuse (e.g., PCP, alcohol, amphetamine, LSD, cocaine) can set off an existing biological vulnerability.

Sleep deprivation and changes in daily schedules can set off an existing biological vulnerability.

sion is stress, or events in your environment that make life more difficult and require you to use certain coping skills. We talked about those events that occurred in the last 3 months and how they may have contributed to William's episode, as well as how they affected the family during that period. Now, I'd like to get an idea of what role stress generally plays in your lives, both during periods of illness and at other times. [Makes clear that stress disrupts everyone's life, not just the lives of persons with bipolar disorder.] Stan, can you give me an example of what stressors you face in your own life?

STAN: Well, when the bills come due. That's when I get really stressed! (*Laughs.*)

CLINICIAN: Good example. How about for you, William?

WILLIAM: (*sullen*) When my mom and I get into an argument, and she starts ranting and raving.

ALYSSIA: (*defensively*) Or, when he does things that make me rant and rave!

CLINICIAN: Those are all good examples. Stress can be due to events like financial demands, or to conflicts in the family, or even to positive events, like starting a new relationship or getting a job promotion. All of these stressors increase the demands on us to perform and can lead to some difficult emotional states.

If you're predisposed to having bipolar disorder—which we'll be discussing in a minute—then one or more stressful events or a great amount of family conflict can be enough to "overwhelm the system" and bring about the symptoms of a manic or depressive episode. For some people, especially those with strong predispositions, even a small amount of stress can be influential. William, your examples of getting the flu, having finals, and then losing all that sleep were good examples of how stress can contribute to an episode.

In this passage, the clinician explains that stress does not operate in a vacuum but instead interacts with a person's constitutional vulnerabilities. Note that the clinician does not, in this case, choose to follow up on the conflict this discussion generated between the patient and his mother. Arguments of this kind are usually best dealt with in the context of CET (Chapters 9 and 10).

Illness Episodes as Discrete Life Events

A point that can be easily forgotten is that illness episodes are in themselves stressful life events for the patient and family. The patient often experiences shame and guilt over the bizarre behaviors he or she performed while manic, or the dependency and demandingness shown while depressed. For the family, the episode can mean financial strain from debts incurred while the patient was ill, public embarrassment or humiliation, or the encumbrance of having the patient return to the family home. Close relatives often have to increase their work hours or child care responsibilities during the postepisode period.

The various ways that illness episodes can serve as stressors should be incorporated into these discussions. The most recent episode may serve as an example. However, be careful not to imply that the patient's illness has irrevocably damaged the lives of his or her relatives, an implication that can only increase the patient's often considerable feelings of guilt:

> "William, I guess one thing you're now experiencing is the stress and disappointment of having to quit school and move back home. I know you felt like you 'graduated' from your family's home and this community a long time ago. Likewise, your parents are experiencing stress and are having to make their own adjustments. I think some of the conflict you're having as a family can be attributed to these transitions, this readjustment period. I think these are temporary stressors that will eventually return to normal. [Empathizes with the loss of role status experienced by the patient, and attributes family conflict to the stress of the postepisode period.]
>
> "However, I want to underline that I'm very optimistic about your abilities to handle the stress associated with this period. I think you're all working very hard to adjust, and with the communication and problem-solving skills we'll be teaching you later on, you should have some additional ammunition against these kinds of stressors."

In this passage, the clinician engenders hope and expresses optimism about the future. He encourages the patient and family to unite against the mutually disruptive effects of life stress brought about by illness episodes and their aftermath.

Genetic and Psychobiological Vulnerability

It is quite important for the patient and family to understand the notions of genetic and biological vulnerability, concepts central to justifying the importance of taking medications (FFT Goal 3) and learning to mitigate stress (FFT Goal 5). With reference to Handout 4, the clinician explains this concept:

> "As you can see in the handout, we believe stress interacts with a person's genetic and biological vulnerabilities or predispositions. Pre-

dispositions mean that some people are susceptible to having manic or depressive episodes because of a factor within themselves, like the genes they inherit or the particular chemistry of their brains. For example, many people are predisposed to being overweight because they inherited this predisposition—being overweight runs in their families. As a result, their bodies may not metabolize food or fat in the same way as other people's do.

"We know that bipolar disorder runs in families. We also know that people can have certain biochemical imbalances in the brain that make them predisposed to mood disorder episodes. Does all of this make sense to you?"

To concretize these issues for the family, explore the possible role of genetic factors in the onset of this particular patient's disorder. This is done by examining the patient's family tree to see if anyone had bipolar disorder or some variant of it. If it seems appropriate to do so, review with family members what they disclosed about their family histories during the functional assessment interviews. Patients and family members sometimes have an "aha experience" when discussing other relatives in their family trees who may have had similar symptoms that, at the time, seemed mysterious to everyone in the family.

If family members cannot identify anyone in the family who had the disorder, explain that the genetic basis of bipolar disorder does not follow simple rules. For example, a first- or second-degree relative carrying the genetic predisposition may have had a subsyndromal disorder that went undetected. Alternatively, the affected individual may have been several generations back. However, make clear that there are cases of bipolar disorder with no clear genetic basis. Further, explain that "genetic predisposition" is not the same as "genetic inevitability":

"I want to make clear that 'genetic predisposition' does not mean that if you've got the genes, you'll get the illness. These predispositions interact with the kinds of stress a person experiences and how a person lives his or her life. For example, some people are predisposed to hypertension, but they may not get it unless they don't eat right, don't exercise enough, smoke, or are constantly under stress. Likewise, we think that a person only gets bipolar disorder if the genetic vulnerability and certain stressors are both operating."

It also helps to give more general facts about the genetics of bipolar disorder: that rates of affective disorder in first-degree relatives of bipolar persons average 20–25% (about 9% with bipolar disorder, 14% with unipolar depression), and that identical twins have higher concordance rates for bipolar disorder than fraternal twins (Smoller and Finn, 2003). In discussing these figures, point out their dual meaning: Although the disorder has a genetic basis, it clearly has causes that are not explained by genes alone. It is crucial to make this point to buttress the key arguments about the roles of family and life events stress in the onset of episodes.

Gene Guilt

Some relatives will be relieved to hear that the disorder has a genetic basis. This is particularly true for a parent who previously believed the illness was due to poor parenting or to "the time I dropped him." However, parents can also feel worse after hearing the genetic evidence. Some will feel "biologically defective" and guilty about having passed on these defects to their son or daughter. Alternatively, a parent may blame his or her spouse for contributing the gene, sometimes leading to arguments about who came from the crazier family (see the example of William's family at the beginning of this chapter).

You may begin to wonder, "Why raise the issue of genetic predisposition if it's going to upset people?" In our opinion, the family and patient must understand that the patient may have inherited the disorder in order to accept that he or she (1) is vulnerable to future episodes, (2) cannot fully control his or her behavior, and (3) needs to take medication on an ongoing basis. In parallel, understanding that hypertension is in part heritable is critical to accepting the lifestyle adaptations one must make to reduce the risk of future heart disease. Patients and family members who are not exposed to the vulnerability concept may mistakenly believe that the most recent episode was a one-time occurrence brought about by stress or hard living, and will be correspondingly unlikely to accept the necessity of a medication regimen. Thus, on balance, discussing the genetic underpinnings of the illness is of value to the patient and family even if it generates difficult emotions.

Empathize with the guilt and associated anger of relatives being acquainted with the genetic etiological model. Take steps to alleviate this guilt:

> "I can understand why you might feel bad after hearing this, but let's face it—none of us can control the genes we come into this world with. This is not a question of fault. Also, as we've said, genes are not the only cause of this disorder.
>
> "On the whole, I don't think the debate you're having about whose family contributed the genes will help in getting clarity on all of this. We don't know if William inherited genes from one side of the family, the other side, or both. And although I understand your desire to know the truth, I think this discussion can only make things more painful."

Arguments between parents over who contributed the genes are probably masking other emotional issues, such as long-standing marital problems or resentments held by a spouse about his or her mate's family of origin or parenting styles. It is best to save discussion of these underlying issues for the subsequent phases of treatment (e.g., the communication enhancement module), when they can be dealt with in the context of skill-building exercises.

Fears about Heritability

An issue that often arises in couples is the risk of bipolar disorder to their existing or planned children. They may ask whether they should have children at all. Likewise, parents of a diagnosed bipolar patient may wonder whether their other children—particularly those who are not yet through the age risk period (broadly defined as ages 15–39, with a peak frequency of onset in the 15–19 age range)—will develop the disorder.

Although it may be helpful to remind them of the actual risk to children of bipolar parents (about a 1 in 10 chance of developing bipolar disorder and a one in seven chance of developing major depression), do not take a directive stance on the issue of whether the couple should have children. The decision to have children is a complicated one that should be based on many factors other than one's genetic loading for affective disorder. Consider the following session segment:

WIFE: (*Jokes.*) So, if we have 10 kids, one will be depressed? If we have 5, will one of them have half a depression?

CLINICIAN: (*Laughs.*) It may not work quite that way, but those are the odds, kind of like betting on a horse.

HUSBAND: Well, maybe we shouldn't have kids at all.

CLINICIAN: I think the decision to have children is a very personal one, and one that should be influenced by many things, including the quality of your marriage, your careers, your values and religious beliefs, and, of course, your mutual desire to have children. My feeling is, if you're wanting to have children, and you think all the other arguments are in favor of having them, I wouldn't let these statistics deter you. We all have illnesses that run in our families. If the disorder were deadly and the odds were more like 50%, then I think you might want to reconsider.

In this interchange, the clinician broadens the issue of childbearing beyond the question of the heritability risk. You can also suggest that the issue be put on the agenda for the later communication enhancement and problem-solving exercises.

Biochemical Imbalances

Understanding that there are chemical imbalances operating in this disorder helps patients and family members comprehend the role of medication in preventing episodes. However, it is not essential that the family grasp all of the complexities underlying biological dysregulations. In fact, if the patient and family members learn that the patient has "a chemical imbalance over which he or she has little control," the task of acquainting the family with this vulnerability factor has been largely accomplished.

If you do not feel you have the expertise to explain neurophysiological imbalances adequately, dispense with this section or encourage the treating psychiatrist (if he or she is not also the family clinician) to explain these phenomena to the patient and family. If you prefer to acquaint yourself with the literature on the neurobiology of bipolar disorder, we recommend a review article by Manji et al. (2003).

If you do decide to explain the role of biological imbalances in the brain, proceed as follows:

> "We know from much research that people with bipolar disorder have certain imbalances in neurotransmitters, or chemical messengers in the brain. These neurotransmitters have names like norepinephrine, dopamine, and serotonin. Neurotransmitters are important in how cells communicate with each other. Nerve cells are connected to each other and have a little space between them called the synapse. Whenever a message is sent from one part of the brain or the body to another—for example, when we have a new idea, play a musical instrument, or decide to make a sandwich—each one of these cells ignites the next one, kind of like a string of firecrackers going off. These neurotransmitters jump across the synapse and ignite the next cell.
>
> "In bipolar disorder, we think that sometimes the cells have too much neurotransmitter activity and communicate messages too quickly. When this happens, a person may get manic. During depression, the messages are not coming through fast enough. These 'chemical imbalances' are not something you can consciously control. In fact, that's what the medications you take are designed to do—they maintain a balance in your nervous system and regulate the level of chemical activity in your brain."

Be careful when explaining these notions to observe the nonverbal reactions of the patient and family members. These reactions may vary from disinterest, to quizzical looks indicating lack of comprehension, to doubt about the applicability of these concepts to the patient. When observing these reactions, stop and address questions the family may have, and pursue an open-ended discussion of the meaning of this information to the family (see also Chapter 8).

Addressing Questions about Psychobiological Vulnerability

Family members may raise quite sophisticated questions about the concept of biological vulnerability. For example, some family members ask about the availability of a blood test or brain scan to determine who is "at risk" or carries the vulnerability to the disorder (there are none currently). Others may question the stability of the vulnerability over time. Consider the following segment:

ALYSSIA: Do you mean the vulnerability is always there? Or is it there only when he gets sick?

CLINICIAN: That's an excellent question. We think that the vulnerability is a constant, meaning that a person with bipolar disorder, even when he's well, is susceptible to getting ill again, given certain factors like stress, drug abuse, or not being protected by medication. [Reiterates vulnerability–stress notion.]

ALYSSIA: So, even though he looks well, he's really sick now?

CLINICIAN: No, not exactly. The vulnerability is more severe during the time a person is ill and immediately after. This is why we keep emphasizing the importance of William's staying on his medications during the recovery period, because this is when a person is most susceptible to getting ill again. But the predisposition is always there, even though the potential for these imbalances to cause trouble may wax and wane. For example, when a predisposed person is feeling well it may take more of an outside "push"—like an important life event—before that person gets any symptoms.

In explaining these notions, it may help once again to make analogies to medical disorders like hypertension. For example, point out that a hypertensive person's blood pressure may be highest when that person is under stress, but may still be abnormal even when the person is relaxing.

Risk and Protective Factors

The vulnerability–stress explanations are rounded out by introducing the family to the notions of risk and protective factors. Risk factors can be defined for the family as "those things that increase the chances of getting ill in someone who is already susceptible." Risk factors include but are not limited to external stressors. They can include abusing drugs or alcohol or leading a chaotic life and not getting regular sleep. Protective factors can be defined as "those things that keep you from getting ill when you're predisposed." Although protective factors are often equated with supportive relationships, they can also include illness management behaviors such as keeping regular daily and nightly routines or keeping a mood chart (see below).

Point out that "when risk factors outweigh protective factors, outcomes are worse, and a person can end up having symptoms. When protective factors outweigh risk factors, outcomes are better, and a person can show a remission of his or her symptoms and begin to live and work independently." Handout 6 is a useful starting point for discussing risk and protective factors.

The notions of risk and protection will not come alive for the family members until they have generated their own examples of each. Begin with a question posed to the family: "When each of you has been under a lot of stress, what has been helpful in keeping you from getting depressed or upset in other ways?" Patients often mention having their medications adjusted; having good working relationships with their physicians or therapists; or the presence of external social supports, such as having someone to talk to. Other members of the family may cite "being able to turn to my work," "going to church," "working out," or "feeling like I'm doing well in other areas of my life." Emphasize the protective roles of these medical and social factors and underline the importance of utilizing them when risk factors are present. From these examples, you can begin to set the stage for the upcoming communication training:

> "I think what you're all saying is that being supported by others, and feeling like you have the skills to function well in various domains, can be protective factors that help you through some tough times. Actually, that's going to be a core issue in our later sessions: What ways of communicating with other people, and what ways of solving problems, are most useful when one is under a lot of stress?"

You should also point to the risk factors that often overwhelm protective factors. For example, in the case of William above, the clinician reminds the family of the stressful life events that may have precipitated his manic episode (the flu and his school finals). He also points to other potentially relevant risk factors (i.e., his drug abuse, family conflict, irregular routines, and sleep deprivation). From these discussions, the patient and family become acquainted with what stressors or high-risk behaviors place William at risk for future episodes.

Risk and Protective Factors in Bipolar Disorder

Risk factors

- Alcohol/drug abuse
- Sleep deprivation
- Stressful life events
- Family conflict or distress
- Provocative interpersonal situations

Protective factors

- Taking appropriate medications
- Using social/family/community supports
- Using communication or problem-solving skills
- Getting regular therapy
- Keeping regular daily routines
- Keeping a mood chart

HANDOUT 6. From *Bipolar Disorder: A Family-Focused Treatment Approach, Second Edition,* by David J. Miklowitz.

Use of a Mood Chart

This is often a good time to introduce the use of a mood chart. Mood charts help patients to track the cycling of the disorder from day to day and to identify triggers (and often, protective factors) that influence cycling patterns. Ask the patient to keep track of his or her daily moods, medications, sleep cycles, and stressors using a chart such as the one provided at *www.manicdepressive.org* (click on "Resource Center," "Tools for All," and then "Blank Mood Chart"). Have some sample blank charts available and explain the rationale as follows:

> "One of the best things you can do to manage your disorder is simply to keep track of your moods. This is one of the few concrete things you can do for yourself other than just taking medications. If you make a daily rating of whether you feel up, down, or stable, you will start to see your mood patterns from day to day and then from week to week. If you also keep track of your sleep, whether you take all of your medications, and any stressors you experience, it will give a more complete picture of what is affecting you and how. Here's an example of a mood chart (*hands copy to patient and family members*), but you can, of course, devise your own."

If you get reactions like "I hate doing that" or "I'll never remember to do it," simply nod and ask, "Would you be willing to try it this week?" If the patient refuses, drop the issue for now but revisit it later when the family is ready to transition from the psychoeducation to the CET module (approximately Session 7 or 8).

Summarizing the Vulnerability–Stress Model

The family has been given a great deal of information at this point, and it is a good idea to step back and review what has been learned. Handout 5, How Do People Get the Symptoms of Bipolar Disorder?, reviews the didactic information imparted. Address some of the emotions that may have been generated by these discussions:

> "There are a couple of things I'd like to emphasize. First, I think it should be clear that this disorder has multiple pathways, and that no one factor or person is responsible for why someone gets ill. [Addresses the possible guilt of family members and tries to deter family members from "linear thinking."] I also want to point out that this information should make you feel hopeful about the future (*to the patient*). In fact, the next time you think you're at risk for getting ill, you'll know what things to avoid and what things to get more of,

like support from other people, a more effective medication regimen, or talks with your therapist. (*To the parents or spouse*) This helps put you in the driver's seat. I also think you are now armed with a knowledge of the disorder and how to recognize its signs and symptoms, so I think you're also in a more powerful position than you were before."

Treatment of the Disorder within the Vulnerability–Stress Model

The thorough discussions of the etiology of the disorder set the stage for reviewing effective treatments. Treatment information should focus on two major issues: what the patient can do to help him- or herself (i.e., take medications, monitor these medications, and develop skills for self-managing the disorder) and what the family can do to help (i.e., participate in and facilitate the patient's treatment, keep the environment low in stress, and keep performance expectations to a minimum).

Medications as a Way of Treating a Biological Vulnerability

Paralleling the vulnerability–stress model, the treatment of bipolar disorder consists of two primary components: a medication management approach for correcting underlying biological vulnerabilities associated with the disorder, and a psychosocial management approach to mitigate the effects of stress triggers. It is important to support both components of the overall treatment program. In fact, a patient protected by medication is more likely to benefit from psychosocial/stress-management strategies than one not so protected, and vice versa.

Drug nonadherence is sometimes driven by a lack of knowledge about medications or what they do. For this reason, we think it quite important for patients and family members to become fully educated about the pharmacological treatments available to them. Here we present the didactic approach to encouraging medication usage and adherence. In many cases, however, a patient's nonadherence is indicative of his or her denial about having the disorder, as discussed in Chapter 8.

We assume the patient's psychiatrist (who, of course, may also be the family clinician) will do most of the education of the patient concerning medication dosages, monitoring strategies, side effects, and blood tests. If this is the case, a collaborating family clinician should not step into this role. If, however, the psychiatrist does not routinely conduct this education, or if the family has many unanswered questions about medication usage, you can offer general information to participants about the classes of medications available, their purposes, and the linkage between pharmacotherapy and the vulnerability–stress model.

Classes of Medications

First, make an assessment of how much the patient and family already know about psychiatric medications. Depending on the outcome of this assessment, you may begin by offering the family Handout 7. This list is not exhaustive, but helps to give the patient and family members an idea of the various classes of drugs used to treat bipolar disorder and the pharmacological alternatives to the patient's current regimen. Review with the family the patient's medications and give a general explanation of the function of each (e.g., "You're on Depakote, which helps regulate your mood; Seroquel, which helps control agitation and should help control the voices you've been hearing; and Lamictal, which is to help you with depression.")

Many times, simply knowing the general purpose of a given medication is a relief to the patient and family members. For example, many patients believe that taking two medications means they are twice as ill as patients taking one, not realizing that one of these medications may be controlling the side effects of the other.

How Medications Work

We recommend avoiding complicated explanations of the biological actions of psychiatric medications, such as reuptake inhibition, receptor sensitivities, or down regulation. However, consider the following interchange:

MOTHER: So why does he have to take lithium?

CLINICIAN: Lithium is used to correct biological imbalances in the brain. For example, if the brain is producing too much of the neurotransmitters—which are the chemical messengers we talked about—lithium can act to slow down their production so that the brain operates at normal speed. Likewise, when a person is depressed, lithium can help "jump start" the system and get it to operate at a more productive and energetic level.

PATIENT: Is that just when you're ill? Why do you have to take it when you're well?

CLINICIAN: That's a very good question. The reason is that lithium prevents future episodes *and* controls symptoms that you already have. We think it actually alters the underlying predispositions we've been talking about, although it doesn't erase them. It helps regulate chem-

Medications Used to Treat Bipolar Disorder: Mood Stabilizers, Antipsychotics, and Antidepressants

Generic name (alphabetical)	*Brand name*	*Class of drug*	*Use*
Aripiprazole	Abilify	Atypical antipsychotic	Mania, prophylaxis
Bupropion	Wellbutrin	Antidepressant	Depression
Carbamazepine	Tegretol, Carbatrol	Mood stabilizer	Mania, prophylaxis
Duloxetine	Cymbalta	Antidepressant	Depression
Fluoxetine	Prozac	Antidepressant	Depression
Fluvoxamine	Luvox	Antidepressant	Depression
Lithium	Eskalith	Mood stabilizer	Mania, depression, prophylaxis
Lamotrigine	Lamictal	Mood stabilizer	Depression, prophylaxis
Mirtazapine	Remeron	Antidepressant	Depression
Olanzapine	Zyprexa	Atypical antipsychotic	Mania, prophylaxis
Olanzapine/ fluoxetine	Symbyax	Combination atypical antipsychotic/ antidepressant	Depression
Paroxetine	Paxil	Antidepressant	Depression
Phenelzine	Nardil	Antidepressant (MAOI)	Depression
Pramipexole	Mirapex	Novel antidepressant	Depression
Quetiapine	Seroquel	Atypical antipsychotic	Mania, depression, psychosis
Risperidone	Risperdal	Atypical antipsychotic	Mania, prophylaxis
Selegiline	Emsam patch	Antidepressant	Depression
Sertraline	Zoloft	Antidepressant	Depression
Tranylcypromine	Parnate	Antidepressant (MAOI)	Depression
Trazodone	Desyrel	Antidepressant	Depression
Valproic acid	Depakote, Depakene	Mood stabilizer	Mania, prophylaxis
Venlafaxine	Effexor	Antidepressant	Depression
Ziprasidone	Geodon	Mood stabilizer	Mania, depression, prophylaxis

HANDOUT 7.

ical activity in the brain, which makes you less vulnerable to having other episodes. That's why going off your medication when you're feeling well is generally not a good idea—it means you won't have this protective effect.

As illustrated here, the clinician repeatedly links the use of medications to the vulnerability concept, a linkage that is not always obvious to the participants. He also makes clear that mood-regulating medications serve the purpose of preventing future episodes as well as controlling current ones.

The Importance of Psychosocial Treatment

At this stage, it may not be necessary to build additional arguments for the role of FFT or other forms of psychosocial treatment, beyond simply restating their value in helping participants to cope with environmental stress. However, there will still be cases in which you must address the participants' ongoing misgivings about and resistances to FFT. First, a minority of families believe they have no problems that need to be addressed. These families often have fundamental misunderstandings about the nature of the psychosocial treatment being offered. Second, some families state that they have a history of very severe, long-standing family problems (e.g., histories of incest; physical abuse; or severe, unresolved conflicts) that are distressing to one or more family members and need resolution, independent of your psychoeducational agenda.

The Family That Denies Problems

Some relatives will argue that they have no need to come in as a family, because "he's the one with the problem!" These relatives may argue that theirs is a well-functioning, healthy family, and that the problem is entirely the patient's disobedient behavior. This is particularly true of families that include a teenage bipolar patient.

You will likely have encountered this thinking when first introducing the program to the family. Consider the following interchange, which occurred in a family in which members had been fighting daily since the patient's hospital discharge:

FATHER: I'm glad we're talking about this therapy stuff, because, to be honest, I don't think we need family therapy.

CLINICIAN: Can you say more?

FATHER: Well, I'm not trying to be difficult, but it seems to me, he's got to take his medications, and other than that we're doing just fine.

CLINICIAN: I'm glad you're telling me this, and I certainly don't perceive you as being uncooperative. I want to make it clear that we're offering you this program not because we think you have severe family problems. Rather, this is a time of great stress, and anybody going through this recovery period is going to need some support and guidance. Does this make sense?

FATHER: Yeah . . . but we're usually pretty good at dealing with things that happen to us, at communicating and stuff.

CLINICIAN: That may very well be true, and you may find as we go along that this treatment is not for you. But we've found that a hospitalization for bipolar disorder, as well as its aftermath, tends to disrupt a family's communication and its abilities to solve day-to-day problems. These are normal reactions, not just those of families who've had problems before. Families need to be superefficient in their communication and tap into abilities they've never had to use before. Our purpose is to help you, through learning about the disorder and through the communication tasks we've described, to cope better with what would otherwise be a very difficult time.

The clinician here does several things. First, she does not challenge the notion that the family has no problems, even though she may very well believe they do. Second, she frames the disorganization and conflict experienced by the family during the recovery period as a normative reaction to a stressful event—the recent mood disorder episode. Thus, she makes a distinction between psychosocial treatment for long-standing family problems and treatment for time-limited problems that could exceed the coping capacities of even the most healthy people.

A related issue is misunderstandings about or mistrust of the psychotherapy process itself. That is, FFT can become merged in the family's mind with any of a number of other therapies that promise the world or carry assumptions that the family may not agree with. Consider this interchange:

ALYSSIA: There's still one thing I don't understand. If he's inherited this disorder and has a biochemical imbalance, why should he spend a lot of time and money talking to someone and digging up things from his childhood? Won't that make things worse?

CLINICIAN: Those are good points, but I want to put our therapy back into the context of the vulnerability–stress model we talked about before. The goal of psychosocial treatments like the one you're in with us is not to discuss childhood, but to help a person with bipolar disorder, and family members, to learn some ways to cope with their day-to-day stress. [Reconnects FFT to the vulnerability–stress model.]

ALYSSIA: (*Interrupts.*) But how is coming up with memories from his childhood going to help him do that?

WILLIAM: (*Defensively.*) He just said how!

CLINICIAN: Hold a second. Alyssia, I think you're asking a good question, and maybe I didn't make things all that clear. The kind of psychotherapy you're describing can be of help to some people, but what we're offering is quite different. The kind of counseling we recommend for bipolar disorder focuses on the present: It's educational and oriented around teaching skills. Some people do need to discuss their childhoods. Other people rely on a therapist to help them deal with their day-to-day lives, like how to handle the boss at work, how to communicate with one's family members, or how to handle a problem with moods. Have I answered your question? [Provides education about types of psychotherapy, and explains how FFT is different from more traditional psychotherapies.]

ALYSSIA: Sort of.

CLINICIAN: Can you say more?

ALYSSIA: Well, I guess I'm just not convinced therapy helps anybody. (*chuckles nervously*) At least not the kinds I've had.

CLINICIAN: I know you've had some negative experiences with therapy before, and I can certainly understand your skepticism. I think it's healthy to enter any new treatment with a degree of skepticism. But, as far as our work is concerned, I think we have to be fair and give it a chance. I wouldn't be recommending this for you if I didn't think it had a chance to be helpful to you, Stan, and William.

In this vignette, the clinician relabels the mother's resistances as healthy and understandable. She also, without promising the world, expresses optimism about the potential helpfulness of the treatment.

In cases in which participants continue to be very resistant to family treatment, it may be helpful to schedule individual sessions with these participants to determine whether there are other issues—perhaps conflicts they do not wish to discuss in front of other family members—operating in the background (see Chapter 8).

The Family with Severe, Long-Standing Problems

On the other side of the coin, some family members argue that a psychoeducational treatment will be unhelpful unless their rather severe, long-standing problems are addressed first. Some of these problems may be current and, in fact, should be addressed before proceeding with the FFT agenda (e.g., one family member is abusing, victimizing, and/or endangering the life of another member). In these cases you may wish to conduct a family or individual therapy not specifically targeted toward bipolar disorder (e.g., a treatment focused on abuse or PTSD), and proceed with FFT once these problems have been effectively addressed. Alternatively, refer the family to clinicians with greater specialization in these problem areas.

In other cases, family members bring up historical issues that are of a quite dramatic nature. For example, they may reveal that an adult patient has been a victim of childhood incest; that there were highly traumatic events in the history of the family or couple that have never been addressed; or that there are long-standing, severe marital problems between parents. Although the family must eventually address these issues, the postepisode recovery period is usually not the best time to do so. In particular, addressing these issues when the patient has just been discharged from the hospital may very well interfere with his or her recovery.

In these cases, encourage the family to delay discussion of these problems until the FFT protocol is completed. At that point, the family may wish to address them in a different venue with you or another consultant. Alternatively, you may deem it best to refer the patient or various family members to adjunctive individual therapy during the FFT treatment (see a discussion of the termination process in Chapter 13).

The following interchange occurred with a couple in which the patient had been a victim of sexual abuse in early childhood. She was still quite symptomatic following her recent depressive episode (note that early sexual abuse is a predictor of more serious episodes of bipolar disorder; Post & Leverich, 2006). The clinician had just given information about the roles of pharmacological and psychosocial treatments in the postepisode recovery phase.

PATIENT: (*talking rapidly*) I think this program sounds very good, and I've been wanting to deal with the things I told you about before, like having been abused. Maybe now's the time to do it.

CLINICIAN: I can certainly see why you'd want to deal with that, because it's an extremely important issue. But we've found that when people are coming off an episode, they and their family members aren't really able to deal with these very loaded issues. During the recovery period people really need to get stabilized on their medications, and they and their family members need help dealing with day-to-day, practical problems.

PATIENT: But how will I get better if I don't deal with these things? They eat away at me.

CLINICIAN: I'm sure they do, and I certainly don't want to play down how important those issues are. On the other hand, it will be hard to really deal with them until you've been stable and free from your depression for a while. Once you're fully recovered and we've finished our program, then we may very well want to get into these things in our work with you, or you may prefer to get into them with someone else. But to do so now would probably be counterproductive.

The clinician validates the importance of these long-standing issues. In no way does he imply that these problems are not real or do not impact on the patient's and family's emotional life. However, he also encourages the patient and husband to delay addressing these problems until they are acquainted with the facts about the disorder and have learned coping strategies for dealing with daily life.

How the Family Can Help

A question often on the minds of spouses, parents, and other relatives is "How can we help?" Spouses and parents are particularly interested in how they can encourage their bipolar relative to maintain emotional stability and get back on his or her feet, and thereby keep their own caretaking burden to a minimum. Offer family members much reinforcement and praise for asking this question. It may imply a willingness to work toward a lower stress (low-EE) environment, one that may be associated with a reduced risk of relapse for the patient.

Role of the Family in Treatment

Handout 8, How Can the Family Help?, is a useful starting point for these discussions. Begin by encouraging family members to support the recommended treatment regimen:

> "Stan and Alyssia, one thing I think you can do is help William to get the kind of treatment he needs, by encouraging him to see his physician often enough, get the right blood tests, and support his use of medication. For example, Alyssia, when you called the hospital last time and arranged for him to see Dr. Jones, that was quite helpful. If you felt William was having a hard time with our treatment sessions,

How Can the Family Help?

- Help your son/daughter (or husband/wife/partner) to obtain treatment and keep all appointments.
- Help him or her to be consistent about taking medications.
- Help him or her to maintain regular daily routines and sleep cycles.
- Get help for yourself or other members of the family who are having a difficult time.
- Learn as much as you can about bipolar illness so that you can recognize early warning signs of relapse.
- Develop a plan as a family for controlling the escalation of mood swings.
- Maintain a tolerant and low-key home atmosphere.
- Reduce expectations of what your son/daughter/spouse should be able to accomplish during recovery; recognize that for most medical illnesses, recovery is a gradual process.
- Try to continue on with normal family life as much as possible; attend to the needs of other kids in the family.
- Use good communication skills:
- Praise good behaviors and positive changes.
- Listen actively.
- Express anger as constructively as possible.
- Use problem solving.
- Exit interactions that are becoming unproductive.

HANDOUT 8. *Sources*: Falloon et al. (1984); Liberman (1988).

or if you suspected he was not taking his medication, it would be helpful to have a heart-to-heart talk with him, and let him know why you think these treatments are important. William, can you think of how your mom might address these issues with you if they came up and she were concerned?"

The clinician communicates that *family members are allies in the treatment process.* This is quite different from the message given to families in the 1950s and 1960s, when family members were told simply to leave the patient alone. We now know that parents or spouses often play quite instrumental roles in encouraging the patient to obtain the appropriate treatments.

It is important to obtain feedback from the patient as to what the family members might do to support his or her adherence to medication or other psychosocial treatments. For example, the clinician in the above vignette later introduces the triad to a structured role play and has them practice with each other ways to discuss the patient's reluctance to take medication or attend psychosocial treatment sessions. In so doing, the patient gives his mother feedback about her style of relating to him and makes suggestions as to how she could approach him differently. Likewise, his mother articulates the "no-win" situation she experiences when she tries to help and how he could help her get out of this bind.

Increasing Tolerance and Acceptance

The issues of maintaining a tolerant and low-key home atmosphere and reducing performance expectations are complicated and emotionally loaded. In fact, difficulties with these issues are often at the core of the family's conflicts.

The rule in discussing tolerance and acceptance within the family is to present both sides of the issue. That is, never imply that the family caused the patient to become ill; that relatives are reacting in a vacuum, unprovoked by the patient's behavior; or that the patient's illness or aversive behavior is entirely responsible for his or her parents' or spouse's reactions. In the following vignette, the clinician addresses the high-conflict situation that has developed in William's family, centering on the issue of when he will return to work and school.

CLINICIAN: If you remember the handout on vulnerability and stress factors, you'll note that people with this disorder do best when stress is kept to a minimum. That includes family stress. For example, when relatives get overcritical with a bipolar person, or do not allow him or her enough independence, this creates stress for that person. Likewise, we know that bipolar people in low-stress family environments seem to do much better over time. So, a low-stress home can be a protective factor. [Introduces family to the EE construct.]

ALYSSIA: (*laughs*) So mothers *do* make their kids crazy!

CLINICIAN: No, and while I can appreciate why you might hear it that way, that's not what I have in mind. I think parents get angry or protective for very good reasons. For example, when a son or daughter does something annoying—whether or not he or she is bipolar—most parents will try to get him or her to stop. Likewise, if a son or daughter seems not able to take care of him- or herself fully, it's natural and understandable to become protective. [Reframes critical and overprotective behavior as natural reactions to disturbing, confusing circumstances.]

On the other hand, I think it's important to keep in mind that although you clearly care about him or her, it's also possible to care too much. There are certain battles that are worth going to the mat over, and others that are better left untouched, especially during this period when William is still getting over the episode. So, you may have to bite your tongue from time to time. These issues that cause problems for you may be able to be addressed later when he's in a better state, and certainly, these sessions will be one venue for addressing them.

The clinician encourages the family to maintain a low-EE home atmosphere during the recovery period. Recognizing the volatility of the situation for both the patient and the relative, he encourages family members to walk away from battles rather than engage in destructive conflicts.

Pay careful attention during such discussions to the emotional reactions of the patient. The patient may object to the notion that he or she performs behaviors that are annoying to others, or may conclude that you doubt his or her ability to take care of him- or herself. So, be sure to supplement such discussions with questions such as "How are you receiving this, ___________? Do you agree with what we're saying?" Further clarification of your central position may then be in order.

Reducing Performance Expectations

It is almost always best for the patient and family to reduce their expectations for the patient's social and occupational performance during the immediate postepisode period. If the patient is still hypomanic, he or she may try to resume the work habits of the preillness period, but may be cognitively and/or emotionally unable to handle the demands of these tasks. Likewise, if the patient is depressed, he or she may not have the motivation, energy, or mental stamina for these renewed responsibilities.

As discussed further in Chapter 8, sometimes it is the patient who holds high standards for his or her performance during the recovery period, and sometimes it is the family members. In either case, family members may aid the recovery process by encouraging the patient to slow down and focus his or her energies on low-stress activities.

The following interchange occurred between a family clinician; a recently manic, recovering female patient, Liz, who had been a tournament tennis player; and her husband, Bob, who has been "egging her on" to return to her rather demanding work and athletic life. Conflict between the spouses had resulted.

HUSBAND: (*proudly*) Well, right now she's rarin' to go. She wants to get right back to her job and her tournaments. That's my girl!

CLINICIAN: (*to Liz*) It's certainly understandable and healthy to want to get back into your work and your old life, but is it possible you're rushing it a bit? [Underscores the notion of a gradual reentry into society following an episode.]

LIZ: (*defensively*) Well, he says I'm all better. And I'm taking these medications. Why shouldn't I?

CLINICIAN: We've talked about these months as being a recovery period. I know you're feeling a lot better right now, and I'm very glad about that. But one thing we've noticed about people with this disorder is that after they've been manic, they often want to jump back into things too quickly. Then, when things don't work out as well as they used to, they're left feeling cheated and depressed. Bob, I know you've said you've seen some things in Liz that worry you and make you think she's not ready to jump right back in. [Enlists husband's help in clarifying that the patient is not fully recovered.]

BOB: Well, yeah. She's still not sleeping soundly, and she's certainly irritable.

CLINICIAN: Liz, I think it's important for you and Bob to keep your expectations for yourself to a minimum, at least until you're fully recovered. Maybe we should talk about what's realistic and what's not realistic right now. For example, you may not be able to go back to your job full-time just yet; maybe part-time is more realistic. [Encourages the setting of reasonable, achievable goals.]

LIZ: Tell that to him.

CLINICIAN: I will. One way you can help, Bob, is to make it clear to Liz that you find it acceptable for her to spend some time recovering, and that you don't necessarily expect her to jump back into doing everything— her work, her tennis, her social life—like she used to do. That's, of course, assuming you do find this acceptable, which you may not. But keep in mind that this is probably the way things will be just for now.

In this vignette, the clinician gently encourages the patient and husband to accept the recovery period as a temporary setback. The patient in this couple needed to hear from her husband that it was acceptable for her to take a hiatus from her fast-paced lifestyle: She had feared that he would find her unattractive if she "put the brakes on."

Conclusion

As listed in Handout 8, there are some concrete things family members can do to aid in the patient's recovery. However, keep in mind that patients and family members often need skill training to implement these recommendations effectively. Thus, introducing your recommendations during the education phase helps you achieve more focused goals (e.g., how a spouse can communicate acceptance of his or her partner's limitations) during the later, skill-oriented modules of FFT.

The Self-Management of Bipolar Disorder

A frequently overlooked issue in the outpatient care of bipolar disorder is the degree to which the patient can take responsibility for his or her own care. Patients often wish to learn the concrete things they can do to manage the disorder, beyond simply taking medications. Self-management strategies help them gain a sense of control over the disorder.

We have already mentioned two of the ways that patients can self-manage: through becoming educated about and cooperating with a recommended treatment regimen, and by keeping a regular mood chart. Other ways include (1) eliminating or at least limiting one's intake of alcohol or street drugs, (2) maintaining regular daily routines and sleep–wake cycles, and (3) avoiding provocative interpersonal situations (see Handout 6).

Avoiding Alcohol and Drugs

Make absolutely clear to the participants that alcohol and drug abuse are particularly hazardous to the bipolar patient, because of the effects of these substances on the biochemical dysregulations outlined earlier. The following excerpt was taken from a session involving a bipolar patient who had been using cocaine prior to his most recent episode.

CLINICIAN: One thing to remember about drugs is that they can make both your manic and your depressive symptoms worse, depending on which ones you take. Cocaine can make you feel better temporarily, but then . . .

PATIENT: (*Interrupts.*) In the end you're more depressed.

CLINICIAN: Right. What happens after you come down from the cocaine high? You go through a crash period, right? And that's because you keep building up your neurotransmitters and the cells suddenly say, "We've produced enough. Let's stop producing it." And then you feel depressed. [Links the action of street drugs to the biological vulnerabilities outlined earlier.]

PATIENT: What about booze?

CLINICIAN: Booze can make depression much worse. It's strange that people drink to feel better, because in fact, over time, it makes them feel worse even if they feel temporarily better. In fact, sometimes the way to help someone to become less depressed is to get him or her off the bottle.

Needless to say, providing educational information is not sufficient to treat a severe substance or alcohol abuse or dependence problem, but it is a beginning. Consider supplementing FFT with referrals to outpatient drug or alcohol rehabilitation programs. Chapter 12 addresses further the use of FFT in treating substance abuse.

Standardizing Daily Rhythms and Maintaining "Sleep Hygiene"

The patient can also obtain a degree of mood stability from having predictable "social rhythms" (i.e., when he or she eats, socializes, exercises, etc.) and "circadian rhythms" (sleep–wake cycles; Ehlers et al., 1988, 1993). The patient can be encouraged to track his or her daily routines with a self-monitoring schedule, the Social Rhythm Metric (Monk, Kupfer, Frank, & Ritenour, 1991; Frank, 2005), or even with the mood chart discussed earlier. This schedule acquaints the patient with the interrelations between changes in his or her daily rhythms, sleep, and mood, and the beneficial impact of one's mood on standardizing social rhythms.

If you are treating a patient who appears to have irregular routines, ask him or her to keep track of them and to experiment with keeping them regular (i.e., going to bed and waking up at the same times, even during weekends; exercising at similar times of the day). He or she may quickly realize a benefit to his or her mood state from this form of self-management (Frank, 2005).

Avoiding Provocative Interpersonal Situations

Beyond what has already been discussed about keeping family stress to a minimum, make clear that, during the postepisode phase, the patient should also avoid excessive interpersonal stress outside the family (see Handout 6):

> "One point I want to emphasize is the degree to which you can control your mood by controlling the level of social stress you encounter. This is a good time to keep your work and social stress to a minimum. For example, you may want to avoid situations with your boss in which you'd be tempted to tell him off. Can you think of some ways to do this?"

Some bipolar patients will object to the notion that they should alter their lives to minimize stress, arguing that this would interfere with their natural spontaneity. Explain that these kinds of changes are particularly important during the recovery period, and that the patient may be able to introduce more spontaneity later:

> "I can understand why you'd object to keeping stress to a minimum. After all, you're a person who has thrived on spontaneity—it's part of who you are. On the other hand, keeping stress down doesn't mean life has to be boring, nor does it mean you have to follow this rule forever. Right now, you're in a high-risk period, during which time family arguments, conflicts with friends or lovers, or high-demand jobs should be avoided."

The Relapse Drill

The relapse drill (Marlatt & Gordon, 1985; Miklowitz & Goldstein, 1990) caps these discussions. In this drill, the patient and his or her family members do a "dress rehearsal" for the actions they will perform when the patient shows the incipient signs of a manic or depressive recurrence.

The drill drives home the point that the patient is vulnerable to subsequent episodes of mood disorder (FFT Goal 2). As discussed at length in Chapter 8, patients, particularly those with a recent onset of the disorder, can be quite resistant to this notion, and you may wish to delay the relapse drill if you feel the issue of relapse proneness has not been adequately addressed.

If done well, the relapse drill can be the family's first exposure to problem solving. That is, the family or couple will at some point in the future be faced with a specific problem (the patient shows signs of relapsing) and will have to consider the steps necessary to solve this problem (getting him or her the appropriate treatment). There are several steps to the drill. First, review with the family the patient's prodromal signs. Second, ask each participant (including the patient) what he or she might do if these signs became evident, without simultaneously evaluating the pros and cons of these alternatives. Third, consult the patient and family members as to which of these alternatives would be most helpful (and least threatening) when manic or depressive symptoms recur. Fourth, encourage the patient and family members to choose one or a combination of these alternatives for future implementation. Finally, discuss with them the practicalities of implementing these solutions:

> "Later in this treatment we'll be introducing you to problem solving, which is basically a framework for defining a problem, generating solutions, and picking the appropriate solutions. Today I'd like to introduce you to this technique around a specific problem, namely, what would you do if William seemed to be getting ill [manic, depressed] again? This is what we call a 'relapse drill.' "

At this point, of course, the patient may object to the notion that he or she will have a subsequent episode. If so, depart from the relapse drill to examine the patient's resistances to the illness notion (see Chapter 8). If you decide to proceed, you can make the drill more palatable by analogizing to other types of emergency drills with which the patient and family members are probably familiar:

> "The relapse drill is a bit like the fire drills you probably went through in school. In a fire drill, you try to find the best way to behave, treat other people, and get out of the building so no one gets burned. A fire drill is preparation for something that may never happen, but *could* happen. Likewise, we're not saying a new episode will happen, only that you need to be prepared in case it does."

The fire drill analogy often brings smiles of recollection to the faces of patients or family members and makes the relapse drill seem less onerous. Further, you have communicated via this analogy that taking part in the drill does not mean admitting that the patient is likely to have a recurrence.

The following is an example of a relapse drill as applied to the prevention of manic recurrences. A similar process can be undertaken in discussing depressive recurrences. Notice the way the clinician addresses but does not get immersed in the patient's resistances:

CLINICIAN: William, let's again review the signs that you were getting manic. Do you remember what they were? [Reviews prodromal symptoms.]

WILLIAM: Well, like I already said, not sleepin', my thoughts goin' fast, and stuff. Everything racing.

CLINICIAN: Alyssia, what do you remember?

ALYSSIA: Well, as you know, I wasn't there at the dorm, but when we came to see him, right before the hospital, he looked disheveled—he didn't look like he'd showered in a while—and he was very angry.

CLINICIAN: Stan?

STAN: Don't remember much, just a lot of yelling and being frantic-like.

CLINICIAN: So would it be fair to say that when you start getting manic, William, the first signs are that you lose sleep, start looking disheveled, get irritable, and your thoughts start going fast?

WILLIAM: Probably.

CLINICIAN: OK. Now let's picture this scenario. William starts showing these signs again. William, what do you think your parents should do? [Begins problem-solving portion of the relapse drill.]

WILLIAM: Have me locked up.

CLINICIAN: Well, I know that's a concern of yours, that your parents will just lock you up. But that's really why we're having this discussion, William, to see what could be done to keep you from having to go back into the hospital if you have these symptoms again. [Casts relapse planning as a way for the patient and family to gain some control over the disorder.]

ALYSSIA: You see, the attitude he's showing now gets exaggerated when he's manic. He gets oppositional.

WILLIAM: I'm not being oppositional. I'm just being realistic.

CLINICIAN: I want to emphasize that it's not always clear what you should do when someone's getting manic. Yes, you can call the police and try to get a person locked up. But what are the other alternatives? [Gets family back on task.] William, how could your parents calm you down if you felt that way?

WILLIAM: Like I always say, get off my case, and don't be buzzin' around my head.

CLINICIAN: OK, you've told them what not to do. What can they do that's positive?

WILLIAM: (*reluctantly*) Just talk to me, find out what's wrong.

CLINICIAN: Nice idea. Alyssia, what else could you imagine doing?

ALYSSIA: Well, obviously, call the doctor.

CLINICIAN: OK. What would you imagine the doctor doing?

ALYSSIA: Probably change his medication or take a blood level. And then bill us, of course.

CLINICIAN: I'm sure you're right on all counts. William, do you think you'd be amenable to seeing a doctor when you're feeling like that?

WILLIAM: I don't know. When you're getting manic everything seems awesome, like you can do whatever you want. The last thing you want to do is go see a doctor.

The clinician continues to examine with the family the ways they can communicate with each other, and who will perform what behaviors, when the patient is in need of immediate care. Patients who remain sentient during the height of an acute episode can be encouraged to take primary responsibility during these crises for making the call to the doctor. Of course, other patients become too psychotic during an acute episode to perform such functions effectively. These patients should be encouraged to make a contract agreeing that, at such times, the parent or spouse will take control of the situation.

You should also convey the importance of knowing what hospital resources are available to the family:

CLINICIAN: Let's imagine the symptoms were bad enough that all of you agreed William needed to be in the hospital. What would you do then? William?

WILLIAM: Probably call you.

CLINICIAN: Well, you could certainly do that. But what if you couldn't reach me? Stan?

STAN: Probably call the doctor and get him admitted?

CLINICIAN: Good choice. What hospitals do you imagine him going to?

ALYSSIA: Well, City Hospital didn't have a bed last time, but it was around Christmas.

CLINICIAN: So, that may be one alternative but maybe not the only one. What are the others?

Conclude the relapse drill by summarizing—or, if possible, asking the family members to summarize—their list of acceptable solutions. To increase the chances of the successful implementation of this plan, encourage the family to keep appropriate phone numbers handy, and come to final (albeit revisitable) agreements on who will do what. It's usually best to ask the patient and/or family members to summarize the agreements.

CLINICIAN: So, William, if you were showing signs of not sleeping, or if you got disheveled and became unusually irritable, what did we agree you and your family should do?

WILLIAM: Just to talk to me and calm me down.

ALYSSIA: At least keep things low-key.

CLINICIAN: And if that didn't work?

ALYSSIA: Call you and his psychiatrist . . . or do we call the hospital then?

CLINICIAN: Possibly, but it might be that things could be handled on an outpatient basis with changes in the medications. If not, Stan, what would you do?

STAN: I'm supposed to call City Hospital and see if he can get in there.

It is helpful to end the drill by praising each participant for his or her willingness to discuss this difficult topic. Be optimistic about their future:

"I appreciate how seriously each of you took this exercise. I think it will feel better to you in the long run to have a plan of action that you can use at times of distress. However, I want to make clear that I'm not saying a relapse is just around the corner. In fact, William looks good right now. I just don't want to see the same traumatic things happen all over again, particularly things that could be avoided. I suspect you all feel the same."

Addressing Unanswered Questions

Family members often wait until the end of the psychoeducation module to ask important questions. For example, they may once again ask, "What does the future hold?" Others will ask whether medication will always be necessary, or whether the patient will be able to achieve his or her life goals. You may not be able to give fully satisfactory answers to these questions, and if so, acknowledge this. Nonetheless, offer a general sense of what the future may hold:

"These are, of course, excellent questions, and I wouldn't want to pretend to have a crystal ball. In reality, William, the fact that you've had a few episodes makes it likely that you'll have others. That's the bad news. Now here's the good news. For now, I think if you're willing to commit to taking medication and learning to manage the disorder in some of the ways we've talked about, and if your family can continue to serve the supportive function it has already served, then I think the future looks quite bright. As we've talked about, lots of people have this disorder and lead quite productive and happy lives, so you're in good company."

As illustrated here, the clinician avoids painting a rosy view of the future, but also offers hope, in light of the patient's and family's decision to partake in medical and psychosocial treatments.

Concluding Comments

The seven or more sessions of psychoeducation should help patients and family members to feel that they have a certain degree of control over, or at least can to some degree predict, what will happen in the future. The sessions should also lead to the understanding that mood disorder symptoms are the result of an illness, and are not willfully produced by the patient. Equally, it should be clear that parents or spouses are not to be blamed for the disorder's onset or recurrences. Accomplishing these goals will go a long way toward reducing tension and enhancing coping in the postepisode family environment.

In this and the prior chapter I have focused on the nuts and bolts of imparting didactic information. However, there are frequently resistances to accepting the illness notions that are at the core of the psychoeducational approach. In the following chapter, I describe specific methods for dealing with denial of the disorder (on the part of patients, relatives, or both), the participants' concerns about the stigma associated with mental illness, and the patient's unwillingness to take medications.

chapter 8

Family Psychoeducation

Dealing with Resistances

Arturro was a 19-year-old Latino man who had been a drama major at college. His parents were quite proud of him; he was the first member of the family to go to college. They described him as a high-energy, bubbly type of person who had always been "a mover and a shaker." After auditioning for a number of acting roles, he was chosen for the lead in a college production of *A Streetcar Named Desire.* His excitement about his acting career—and his accompanying energy level—started to mount. However, shortly after he landed the role, his grandmother died.

Arturro had been very close to his grandmother. Her death hit him hard, and he sank into a deep depression. He lost interest in his acting career, missed rehearsals, and, when he did attend them, "blew his lines" frequently, complaining that the scenes were too confusing and fast paced. Eventually, the director dropped him from the play. His depression grew considerably worse, and he was hospitalized.

Shortly after his discharge, Arturro decided, against his physician's advice, to discontinue his medications. He soon cycled into mania: His speech became rapid and disorganized, and his mood, euphoric and irritable. Returning to school, he attempted to make his way back into the drama production, but was quickly dismissed. One night he appeared on his parents' doorstep, "high as a kite" and "screaming lines from Shakespeare." When they refused to let him in, he tore off his clothes and ran down the street shouting, "Stella! Stella!" He was hospitalized again.

At the end of this hospitalization, Arturro agreed not to immediately return to school and was discharged to his parents' home. When he and his parents began the family psychoeducational program, he was still quite symptomatic. Moreover, learning that there was a name for his condition gave Arturro little relief. He refused to believe his manic symptoms were anything more than his natural, energetic personality. He intoned, "You guys just want to stamp a label on my forehead and put me in some corner."

In contrast, upon receiving the psychoeducational materials, Arturro's parents became quite entranced—and perhaps obsessed—with his syndrome. They began to rethink his whole history: Their descriptions of him during his teen years changed from "energetic and popular" to "hyper and excitable." Arturro was angered by the notion that his personality strengths were now being labeled by his parents as signs of an illness. He continued to deny that he had been ill or would have future episodes. Although he took his lithium and Depakote tablets, his parents feared he would again discontinue them.

Arturro's parents began pressuring him to quit his acting career, arguing that this was the root of his problems. He became sullen and uncooperative in the psychoeducation sessions. When the clinician explored these reactions, he said, "You always just side with them. All your theories and handouts are just giving them reason to destroy who I am and keep me under their thumb."

Chapter Overview

It is important to keep in mind the real meaning of "psychoeducation": It means, literally, "psychological education." By this, we mean that the family clinician must go well beyond the delivery of facts and theories about bipolar disorder to address the emotional reactions—both those expressed and those unexpressed—that are often stirred up by these materials. More specifically, there is a core resistance among patients and family members to accepting the reality of the disorder, a resistance that is normal and expectable. However, denying the reality of the disorder is usually a recipe for disaster, as it often leads the patient to terminate his or her medications or psychosocial treatments, engage in high-risk behaviors, and, finally, become ill again.

Patients and family members in FFT may express this core resistance to the illness notion by refusing to discuss the symptoms, course, prognosis, or etiology of the disorder; discounting the family- or self-management strategies that may improve the long-term prognosis; or other behaviors indicative of resistance (see below). However, the underlying issues frequently center on anger about the events that have occurred, sadness over lost dreams and hopes, anxieties over the social stigma attached to the illness, and fears about the future.

Addressing these underlying themes is often the core of the FFT treatment, and can make the difference between a successful and an unsuccessful treatment outcome. However, a great deal of clinical skill is necessary to explore and resolve these issues successfully. In this chapter I present numerous clinical examples describing the specific therapeutic interventions pertinent to confronting and exploring these resistances. You will probably want to mold these suggested interventions to fit your particular style.

I first describe the various manifestations of denial and resistance. Second, I present a method for preempting resistance before it has been expressed. Third, I address the core issue of lack of acceptance of the disorder among patients and family members, including its various "deep structure" (preconscious or unconscious) manifestations. Finally, I describe the interventions recommended for the most common manifestation of resistance to the illness notion: medication nonadherence.

Manifestations of Denial and Resistance

Inputs and Outputs

In understanding denial and resistance, it is useful to think in terms of emotional inputs and behavioral outputs. As you will see, these inputs and outputs are conceptually linked to, and in many ways form the basis of, the six FFT objectives (Chapter 1).

The inputs are the underlying fears and belief systems in patients or family members that motivate their resistances to accepting the reality of the disorder. These include (1) the anxieties evoked by trying to make sense of what happened during the episode (FFT Goal 1); (2) a fear of the negative, stigmatizing effects of being labeled mentally ill, as manifested by the patient feeling singled out within the family or by the family feeling alienated from or rejected by society; and (3) among patients, the fear that all one's feelings, behaviors, or reactions—even those attributes that are core to the patient's personality—will from now on be interpreted by others as signs of an illness (FFT Goal 4). With this fear may come a hopeless feeling—often shared by family members—that the patient will never achieve his or her dreams or aspirations.

The "outputs" refer to the concrete, behavioral manifestations of this denial or resistance. The patient may *underidentify* with the illness by refusing to acknowledge his or her vulnerability to future episodes (Goal

2), the need for psychotropic medications (Goal 3), or the role that socioenvironmental stressors have played (Goal 5). He or she may act out by abusing alcohol or drugs or by performing high-risk behaviors (e.g., sexual indiscretions) to prove to his or her family, or to the clinician, that he or she "can handle it" and is not ill.

Rather than denying the reality of the disorder, other patients or family members *overidentify* with the illness. For example, the patient may give up and commence "living the life of a mental patient." He or she may believe that, from now on, all he or she does, thinks, or feels should be construed as manifestations of bipolar disorder. Likewise, family members may overidentify with the disorder and interpret the patient's ordinary, understandable reactions to environmental challenges as signs that he or she is once again becoming ill.

Over- or underidentifying with the disorder can become the source of intense family conflict. This is particularly the case when one member of the family (often, but not invariably, the patient) underidentifies with the disorder while others in the family overidentify with it. During psychoeducation the clinician must address these variable reactions to the illness notion, as one means of helping to restore healthy family relationships after the episode (Goal 6).

Resistance as Manifested in Family Sessions

These underlying themes are often behaviorally expressed by participants through resistance to the family psychoeducational sessions. For example, patients or family members may refuse to accept or may ridicule the psychoeducational materials, complain that the sessions are unhelpful, act sullenly or with overt hostility, or simply refuse to attend. Patients may express their resistance through grandiose stances (e.g., "I can control my problems without any help from anyone"). Alternatively, participants may express resistance to only certain of the educational information. For example, patients or family members who overidentify with the disorder often "overbiologize" it as well, dismissing any role for social stressors or family relationships.

These overt manifestations of resistance are to be distinguished from signs of tension, which may or may not be related to feelings about the disorder. For example, during FFT sessions the patient or family members may fidget, become restless, or get up and pace frequently. These behaviors may be due to unresolved symptoms, medication side effects, fatigue, boredom, anxiety about other matters, or, simply, feelings about being in treatment with one's relatives. You should plan on exploring the nature of these reactions to determine whether they indicate uncomfortable feelings stirred up by the psychoeducational materials versus other important matters.

Anticipating and Preempting Denial and Resistance

We have identified three therapeutic maneuvers that are effective in preventing or at least minimizing the negative effects of denial and resistance. In some cases, these interventions bring to the surface the family's underlying conflicts or fears about the disorder. Thus, these interventions are helpful even in cases in which the patient or family has not yet shown signs of denial or resistance.

Predicting and Reframing Denial and Resistance

Recall that most forms of resistance are expectable reactions to the slow, painful process of accepting the disorder. The reactions will be most salient among young first- or second-episode patients, but they can occur in highly recurrent patients as well. You can head off these reactions at the pass by anticipating and predicting their occurrence. The following intervention can be a prelude to introducing the symptom list and reviewing the most recent episode:

> "Although you are now expressing feeling comfortable with what you were told in the hospital—that you've had a mood disorder episode and that it's necessary to take medication—I'm going to guess you're not always going to feel that way. In fact, you may have some important questions about how much this diagnosis applies to you. Coming to terms with having a mood disorder is a very painful process, and many people find it difficult to accept. This struggle is a normal and healthy struggle—people shouldn't accept an identity as someone with a psychiatric disorder too easily. So, if these issues come up for you, let's talk about them."

The clinician does three things in this passage: He predicts the occurrence of resistance and noncompliance, reframes this expectable resistance as healthy and understandable, and asks for an agreement that such resistance become a focus of discussion should it arise.

In the example below, Arturro and his family have expressed some initial discomfort about discussing the symptoms of bipolar disorder.

MRS. YBARRA [mother]: He's really only had the one episode, and it seems like jumping the gun to go through these symptoms and assume he's got this terrible illness.

CLINICIAN: That's a very good point. After a family has gone through something like this, I think it's completely understandable for family members to be confused and to feel that what happened did not really happen. If you're a parent, it's understandable to feel that this was a product of circumstances that won't ever occur again. [Validates the question, and normalizes denial and puts it in the context of the larger problem of accepting a chronic illness.]

ARTURRO: Are you saying it will happen again? Because I sure don't want to go through this again. And I know I won't have to.

CLINICIAN: I can appreciate why you wouldn't want to go through it again, and I think your reactions are quite understandable. If you're the person who's actually gone through the hospitalization, it's hard to believe that you've really been ill, and you may feel like you've been mistreated and misunderstood. We can't predict what the future will bring, but we do know one thing: No one likes to think that he or one of his close relatives has a chronic illness. [Avoids challenging the patient's or the parent's denial, and labels it as healthy and expectable.]

In the example above, no one in the family is fully convinced that the patient is ill. However, the clinician does not get into a debate with the patient or family about whether the patient really has the disorder. Instead, she focuses on the emotional underpinnings of this belief: that accepting a chronic illness is a difficult and painful process.

Spreading the Affliction

As discussed below, being labeled mentally ill puts the patient in a one-down position in the family, a position that can make him or her feel increasingly annoyed by the psychoeducational materials. When reviewing the symptoms or expected course of bipolar disorder, you can help prevent or minimize these reactions by "spreading the affliction," or eliciting from other members of the family their own experiences of depression, anxiety, or other symptoms. The goal of this intervention is not to identify these other family members as psychiatric patients, but to normalize and destigmatize within the family context the patient's experiences of a mood disorder.

In the example below, the clinician has noticed the patient's anxious behavior as the symptoms of depression are being discussed. The patient, 17-year-old Kevin, seems avoidant, uncomfortable, and nervous, although he has not expressed any direct opposition to discussing the symptoms.

CLINICIAN: Kevin, what is your mood like when you get depressed? Can you describe it to us?

KEVIN: (*defensively*) Well, just the things people get when they get depressed. I'm probably just like everyone else.

CLINICIAN: Good point. I think you'd be hard pressed to find anybody who hasn't at some point in his or her life experienced depression. How about you, Mrs. Williams [mother]? Have you ever had a depression? [Spreads the affliction.]

MRS. WILLIAMS: (*Pauses, somewhat surprised.*) Well, I would imagine that I have, although I didn't link it with depression. I have had what I would call "blue days" and I think that's really depression, now that I'm finding out more about it. I don't feel like talking. I've never labeled it depression; I would just say, "Oh, I've got the blues today."

CLINICIAN: I think getting the blues is a good description. What happens when you get the blues? [Does not challenge mother's label, as calling it "major depression" may be perceived by her as threatening.]

MRS. WILLIAMS: I would rather just stay in bed and sleep all day, you know, to keep from being confronted with anything. But I've never felt suicidal.

CLINICIAN: (*Points to symptom list.*) You've just mentioned three symptoms of depression or the blues: sad feelings, not wanting to get out of bed, and suicidal thoughts.

KEVIN: (*Brightens.*) I never knew you had depressions. I thought it was just me.

CLINICIAN: I think it's a matter of degree. I think we all get depressed or blue sometimes, but some people get it more severely than others. [Normalizes depression and casts patient's disorder as an extreme variant of everyday sadness.] How about you, Mr. Williams? Do you ever get blue or depressed periods?

Try to avoid lumping together great differences in people's experiences of mood swings. That is, don't imply that a father who reports periods of high energy (without other manic symptoms) is himself bipolar, or that a mother with the blues has major depressive disorder. Instead, normalize the experiences of mood variations in different members of the family and cast the patient's mood swings as extreme variants of these experiences.

Using Analogies to Chronic Medical Disorders

As explicated later, a key difficulty in accepting the diagnosis of bipolar disorder is the stigma associated with mental illness. It is much easier for the patient or family to accept the diagnosis if it is described in the same terms as one might describe a traditional medical disorder that requires medication, long-term care, and family support. Thus, one way to pre-empt resistance to the illness notion is to make analogies between bipolar disorder and medical disorders:

> "I think bipolar disorder is a lot like a chronic medical illness such as diabetes. People with diabetes also have a biochemical imbalance, only it's in their body's ability to use sugar. Without a drug called insulin, diabetic people can go into insulin shock and die. As a result, they need to learn to manage their disorder over time—become educated about it and its treatment and gradually come to accept it. Their families also have to come to terms with the fact that their loved one has a chronic illness that requires ongoing care. This can create a lot of tension and conflict in the family. Perhaps what they experience is a little bit like what you're experiencing."

Some patients or family members will disagree with this medical analogy, arguing, for example, that diabetic patients are likely to receive sympathy from others, whereas patients with bipolar disorder elicit fear or rejection. The stigma of mental illness in society—a problem that also fuels resistance to accepting the disorder—is discussed later. Nonetheless, it is generally helpful to place bipolar disorder in the context of other medical disorders.

The Meaning of Bipolar Disorder within the Family Context

Denial of, or alternatively, overidentification with bipolar illness often leads directly to family systems conflicts. In fact, the psychoeducational process can precipitate a crisis within the family, as members attach different meanings to the didactic material and draw different conclusions about its implications for their respective futures. You can feel quickly drawn into being asked to side with relatives or with the patient around issues pertaining to the reality of the disorder (as illustrated in the case study of Arturro, above and below).

In this and the following section, I address the core issue raised for many patients and family members in their struggle to accept the illness: the new role the patient may have to accept in the family and in the larger society. I first discuss the underlying emotional issues in the patient's, and separately, the relatives' struggles. I then describe interventions designed to address the splits that occur when patients and relatives are in different places in terms of their readiness to accept the disorder.

Accepting the Disorder: The Patient's Conflicts

> "I feel like everything I do is now somehow connected to me being sick. If I'm happy it's because I'm manic; if I'm sad it's because I'm depressed. I don't want to think that every time I have an emotion, every time I get angry at somebody, it's because I'm ill . . . some of my feelings are justified. People say I'm a different person every day, but that's me! I've never been a stable person."—*A 25-year-old woman with bipolar disorder*

The experience of bipolar disorder, including the altered experiences of reality, the heightened or decreased activity levels, the bizarre behavior, and the alienation of other people, can precipitate a crisis in an affected person as to who he or she really is. The experience of a manic or depressive episode is very difficult to integrate or place into a proper context. Moreover, when a patient is not fully recovered from an episode, he or she is likely to experience a host of residual affective and cognitive symptoms (e.g., loss of memory and attention, inability to "track" or concentrate), which may further cloud the patient's ability to make sense of the episode, or even remember what he or she used to be like.

A patient in this state, particularly one who has had only one or two episodes, is asking him- or herself many uncomfortable questions. These questions are often brought to the surface by the psychoeducational materials but may never be voiced directly. Some of these questions are listed in Table 8.1.

The threat valence of these questions is heightened by the new role the patient perceives him- or herself to have in the family. Patients may feel labeled and scapegoated by their parents or other members of the family, and that their previous accomplishments and developmental

TABLE 8.1. Questions Considered by Patients Following Manic or Depressive Episodes

- Am I "only bipolar" now, or do I still have a separate identity? Where do I stop and where does the disorder begin?
- Do my prior accomplishments mean nothing? Were my prior periods of high energy and productivity just signs of mental illness?
- How much mood variation am I "allowed" before everyone thinks I'm getting ill again?
- How much responsibility do I have for my own behavior?
- Will I ever have a normal life? Will I achieve my goals? Will my mental abilities ever come back?

advances are now being discounted. The married patient may feel that he or she has let down the spouse, that the spouse now thinks he or she is inadequate, or that the future of the relationship is in jeopardy.

The questions in the table can be summarized as "Why me? Why this? Why now?" When faced with these difficult questions and conflicts, an *attributional process* occurs in which the patient fights to make internal sense of what has happened. As discussed above, the patient frequently responds by underidentifying with (denying) or overidentifying with (merging one's self-concept with) the disorder. Optimally, the patient should come to a place where he or she can accept the disorder and its necessary treatments, while at the same time pursue his or her life goals to the degree possible. Thus, a major objective of FFT is to bring about a realistic balance in the patient's understanding of the disorder and its relevance to his or her future.

Underidentification: Distinguishing Personality from the Disorder

Underidentification or denial can often be linked to the patient's difficulty in discriminating his or her premorbid character attributes from the symptoms of the illness. This is a very real issue, because many bipolar patients have premorbid and intermorbid (between-episode) personality styles that are characterized by wide mood swings and heightened experiences of emotion (Akiskal et al., 2000). In fact, trained clinicians have a great deal of difficulty in distinguishing the personality of the bipolar patient from the residual or prodromal symptoms of the disorder. However, often the real conflict for the patient is one of wanting to find some continuity in the self. Understandably, he or she does not want to feel fully identified with the disorder. Instead, the patient struggles with how to carry forward those personality traits that he or she has found in the past to be valuable and attractive to others.

Patients experiencing this core conflict often attribute all of their symptoms to "my usual self or "the fact that my family (or spouse) has never really accepted who I am." Such patients rebel against the illness notion and refuse to maintain themselves on medications. The hypomanic, grandiose patient is particularly prone to this way of thinking. Naturally, this stance is quite upsetting to relatives, who fear that the patient's denial will set in motion events that will precipitate another episode.

Because the family psychoeducation sessions tend to bring these questions to the surface, you must be prepared to identify, validate, and normalize them. As a beginning example, when patients raise the question of personality versus disorder (or, alternatively, when family members raise this question), a useful approach is as follows:

"I can see why you would struggle with this question. In fact, just coming off the episode, it's hard to tell what's personality and what's illness. During the recovery period a person's personality can be quite different. As you recover, we'll be in a better position to answer this question.

"But in a way, the question is too abstract. I think the real question you're asking is, 'How do I want to deal with life? Are there ways I used to deal with things before I got ill that I'd like to continue to do now, and are there ways I'd like to deal differently?' I suspect that as you begin to recover you may remember ways you've dealt with stress in the past, some of which may have been healthy and some not so healthy. These are some things I'd like to see us focus on."

In the above example, the clinician attempts to get the patient off the rather academic issue of distinguishing personality from disorder and onto the harder issue of how he or she will cope with life stress, and what features of his or her premorbid personality can be carried forward to cope with current environmental challenges.

Overidentification with the Illness

On the opposite side, the patient may deal with fears and anxieties about the future by merging his or her identity with the disorder. Some patients come to believe that they have been bipolar all of their lives, that they have been continuously manic or depressed since early childhood, and that they can expect to accomplish little or nothing in their lives. A patient may say or imply, "All I am is bipolar, and I can't change. It's all biochemical, and I can't take responsibility for myself." Like underidentification, overidentification is quite troubling to parents, spouses, and other family members, who see the patient as giving up, fearing adult responsibility, refusing to work, and taking the family's goodwill and caretaking for granted.

A question to consider is whether the patient is being more realistic than the family or the treatment team in evaluating his or her capabilities. That is, he or she may be experiencing cognitive deficits or residual affective or psychotic symptoms that may be unobservable to others. Ongoing assessments of the patient's symptomatic state, and in some cases neuropsychological testing, can help you to determine whether the patient is indeed ready to take on renewed responsibilities.

A beginning approach to the problem of overidentification is as follows:

"Yes, you have bipolar disorder, but you're also a person, a person with many qualities. It would be unfortunate if you narrowed your definition of yourself to only somebody who has a mental illness. It may be comforting in some ways, but in other ways it limits you terribly as to what you can do. What are some of your qualities or abilities that are not the same as your illness? What positive things did you accomplish before you became ill, and what qualities in yourself do you value? Let's see where you can go with these, because there are obviously some great parts of you that are not your illness."

This kind of intervention is an icebreaker. It puts on the table for discussion the patient's overidentification with the disorder and communicates that the patient has a self separate from his or her illness. However, as discussed below, family members often chime in with their own attributions about the patient's illness or tendency to overidentify, resulting in systems conflicts that must be addressed.

Accepting the Disorder: The Family's Conflicts

The experiences of the acute episode, the hospitalization (if one occurred), and the patient's postepisode recovery period, combined with the discussion of these experiences in the psychoeducation sessions, raise in family members a similar set of uncomfortable questions. Once again, these questions may not be voiced directly. Table 8.2 lists a subset of the questions raised for family members, and these are usually accompanied by much affect. As was the case for patients, family members engage in an attributional process in which they ask, "Why did this happen? Why to him (or her)? Why now?" In answering these questions, family members may also under- or overidentify with the disorder as an explanation.

Family members who underidentify with the disorder imply or make explicit that they do not believe the illness is real. Like the patient, a parent or a spouse may blame the episode on the patient's premorbid personality (e.g., "He's always been hyper"; "She's always been too much of a party girl"—or, as we often hear among parents of teens, a "drama

TABLE 8.2. Questions Considered by Relatives after a Manic or Depressive Episode in a Family Member

- Will he or she ever get better?
- Will he or she be able to work and be productive, and live independently? Are my hopes and dreams for him or her gone?
- Will I always have to take care of him or her? What will happen to him or her if I die?
- (For spouses) Should I leave this relationship? Did I marry the wrong person?

queen") or on specific unstable circumstances (e.g., "It was the medications they gave him in the hospital that made him sick"; "She was hanging with the wrong crowd").

In contrast, family members who overidentify with the illness are usually quite worried that the disorder will recur at any moment. Often, one sees an overidentifying family member paired with a patient who is quite ill, and the family member's overidentification—which may take the form of emotional overinvolvement or overprotectiveness—can reflect adaptive responses to the patient's symptomatic state. However, overprotective home environments can be associated with high relapse risk (Fredman, Baucom, Miklowitz, & Stanton, in press; Butzlaff & Hooley, 1998), so it is important to encourage the same kind of balance in family members that one encourages in patients: a balance between accepting the disorder and the necessity of treatment, and holding realistic expectations for the patient's life functioning:

> "I know this is something you've been struggling with. You care a great deal about him, and you want to make sure he'll get well. On the other hand, I don't think that means you can't expect ___________ to take care of himself in some basic ways. I think it can be very unclear to family members how much to take over versus give a person more autonomy—at what point are you pushing too hard and at what point not hard enough? As we go along, we're going to rely on you, ___________, with the support of your family, to figure out what you're able to do for yourself versus what is too much at this time."

In this example, the clinician normalizes the family's tendency to be overprotective, while gently suggesting that the patient is not as incapable as the relatives may think.

Differing Perceptions of the Disorder as a Source of Family Conflict

Understanding the internal attributional processes of the patient and relatives is central to understanding the family dynamic issues roused by the psychoeducational process. That is, the didactic material often upsets the balance of forces within the family, resulting in harsh disagreements about perceptions of the disorder and its implications for the future. Examples of these conflicts are given in Table 8.3.

In each of these conflicts, the clinician can feel caught in the middle. For example, in the second case, if you insist that the patient has bipolar disorder but do not explore the meaning attributed to this diagnosis by the patient, he or she is likely to become alienated. If you support the patient's belief that his or her behaviors were simply a product of personality attributes, you can confuse and alienate the family.

Your job in these cases is essentially one of mediation. Mediation requires validating each person's point of view, labeling each as understandable, and encouraging resolution of the conflict through negotiation and compromise. However, in performing this mediational role, do not back off from the central point that the patient has had an illness episode requiring medication treatment, family support, and self-management.

The "Patient Accepts/Family Rejects" Conflict

Sometimes family members do not acknowledge the seriousness of the illness, whereas the patient may be very aware of his or her moods and functional impairment (first example, Table 8.3). This is most common when the patient has recently experienced a depressive episode. The relatives' lack of acceptance of the disorder may be accompanied by pressure on the patient to immediately, and prematurely, resume his or her former functional roles.

Convalescence

In these cases, the notion of "convalescence" may be quite useful to the family. This term suggests that the patient is in a temporary and

TABLE 8.3. Examples of Family Conflict Related to Different Understandings of the Disorder

<u>Example 1</u>

Patient embraces illness notion, or overidentifies
("I'm depressed and unable to work")
+
Family denies or underidentifies with illness
("No, you're just being lazy and afraid")
= Family conflict

<u>Example 2</u>

Patient denies or underidentifies with illness
("I'm not irritable; I'm just an assertive person")
+
Family embraces illness notion, or overidentifies
("No, you're getting sick again")
= Family conflict

expectable period of recovery. The following is a case of a married woman, Christine, who had been discharged from the hospital after an episode of bipolar depression with psychosis. Although she appeared well physically, she was still quite dysthymic and low in functioning. Her husband, Ralph, was supportive at first, but became unsympathetic when she proved unable to return to her former job and when most of the child care fell on his shoulders. Although he had been rather quiet during the presentation of the symptom list, he began to voice his displeasure during the discussions of the vulnerability–stress model.

RALPH: I don't understand this stuff. If she has all this vulnerability and biological springs gone loose, how come she looks so good? How do I know she's not just taking an unpaid vacation?

CLINICIAN: I can appreciate why you're asking this, Ralph. Christine may look good to you right now, and Christine, you seem much healthier to us now than you did when you were in the hospital. But, Christine, you may not *feel* very good right now, and you may not be ready to do all those things you did before. [Points to discrepancies between wife's observable mental status and her actual level of functioning.]

CHRISTINE: That's very true.

CLINICIAN: This is a tough time for both of you, and it's understandable that you, as her husband, want to see her get back on track. But, Christine, you may need to convalesce for a while, in the same way that someone who's had a bad flu needs to spend a few more days in bed after the worst symptoms have gone away. [Validates husband's concerns, and normalizes the period of recovery.]

Next, the clinician examines with the couple their changed dynamics, brought about by these differing perceptions of the disorder.

CHRISTINE: You know, he was so supportive to me before, and now it's all just criticism.

RALPH: No, it's just that I think you aren't trying hard enough.

CLINICIAN: (*to Christine*) You know, when someone gets depressed, and is showing all the signs of depression we've reviewed, family members are usually sympathetic at first, but then they get angry and frustrated. This is partly because they want to help and don't know how, and sometimes they feel that their efforts go unrewarded. [Reviews interpersonal processes that surround a depressive episode, and reframes frustration of family member as coming out of a desire to help.]

RALPH: You're telling me!

CLINICIAN: But it's also because family members often assume that the depressed person can control it, even though he or she often can't. Most people don't want to stay in bed and be dysfunctional, but it's really hard to mobilize yourself when you're in an episode of depression. [Makes it clear that the dysfunctional behavior is not willfully produced.]

Offering Hope

Next, offer the family some sense of what to expect in terms of improvement. Emphasize that the depression will not last forever, but steer away from making predictions as to when the person's prior functioning will resume.

RALPH: So, is she always going to be like this? Am I both mother and bread earner from now on?

CLINICIAN: Ralph, all the evidence we have suggests that Christine will recover from this depression, especially if you, Christine, keep taking medication and learning to cope with stress. But sometimes this takes a while, even just for the medications to take effect. Again, I think you have to consider this a temporary period of convalescence, even though I know that means you [Ralph] have to carry the ball for a time. [Supports treatment regimen and empathizes with the difficulties associated with husband's increased stress level.]

The clinician encourages the husband to "back off" for a period of time, but instills the realistic hope that the patient will eventually regain, at least to an extent, her premorbid level of functioning.

The "Patient Rejects/Family Accepts" Conflict

Family conflict also occurs when a patient disagrees that he or she has an illness, whereas family members accept or overidentify with the disorder. Although the following example pertains to a first-episode male patient living with his parents (Arturro, in the case study introduced earlier), we have observed this same type of family disagreement in chronic, multiple-episode patients, as well as patients living with spouses.

The clinician had just presented the list of symptoms of bipolar disorder to the family. Arturro's parents showed keen interest in the list, but Arturro sneered, fidgeted, and cast angry looks at his parents.

MRS. YBARRA: Why are you looking at me that way?

ARTURRO: Because, as usual, you're not saying what really happened. I couldn't sleep because I had a roommate who partied till all hours, not because I was getting "manic."

MRS. YBARRA: But there you go again, denying what happened! You're forgetting how sick you were! (*to clinician*) Is this a sign of the illness, forgetting what really happened to you?

ARTURRO: Let's take a break. I need to go to the bathroom.

Dealing with "the Process"

In this interchange, the introduction of the symptom list serves as a stressor, aggravating the patient's irritability and encouraging his withdrawal. However, rather than backing off from the importance of this didactic material, the clinician focuses on the process in the room. The following series of interventions opens up the issue of the family's differing perceptions of the disorder and labels these as important topics for discussion and negotiation.

CLINICIAN: (*Takes symptom handouts off the table.*) I'm noticing that this topic is upsetting everyone. I wonder why this is happening? Arturro, why did you get so upset? [Communicates that the agenda is not immutable, and that emotional reactions to the material are just as important as are the facts about the disorder.]

ARTURRO: Because they seem to want to cram this stuff down my throat.

CLINICIAN: Mrs. Ybarra, I doubt that's what you wanted to do. But I'm wondering why it was so important to you that he admit to this illness right now? What was going on for you just then?

MRS. YBARRA: I don't know. Just worried, I guess. Maybe I'm just being insensitive.

CLINICIAN: No, I don't think this is about being insensitive. Actually, I suspect you feel a need to get him to admit to these symptoms at this instant because, understandably, you're worried that if he doesn't admit to them, he'll not take medication, not work with you, and get sick again. [Interprets mother's reactions as due to underlying fears and concerns over her son's health, and normalizes her reactions.]

ARTURRO: I don't see why I should have to admit to anything, especially when I don't even agree with the diagnosis.

CLINICIAN: Maybe you don't have to just yet, Arturro. I suspect you feel like we're all pointing to you and your symptoms and losing sight of who you are. [Begins to address patient's feelings of alienation.]

ARTURRO: (*Mumbles.*) Whatever.

CLINICIAN: Mrs. Ybarra, maybe his admitting to an illness doesn't have to come today. Maybe we should just be satisfied that he's willing to join us and try this treatment, which I imagine, Arturro, is rather hard at times.

The clinician clarifies the differences in perceptions of the disorder held by the patient and his parents. In addition to validating the mother's viewpoint, he reframes the patient's willingness to attend treatment sessions as a sign of cooperativeness with the family.

Exploring Feelings of Alienation

Exploratory interventions such as the above have the effect of lowering tension in the room and making it safe to explore the patient's underlying feelings of alienation.

CLINICIAN: Arturro, tell us more about your views on what happened.

ARTURRO: (*Sullen*) It's just weird talking about this with my parents here. I just don't like being singled out like this, as "Mr. Bipolar."

CLINICIAN: I can understand how you'd be uncomfortable with that, almost as if you were an outsider to the family. Maybe you're also feeling like we're treating you as an "object of discussion" or just "an illness" rather than recognizing you as a person. Maybe sometimes you even feel like you're being labeled the "bad child" in the family.

ARTURRO: "Bad child" is exactly right. I feel like I've accomplished a lot in the last 2 years, and sometimes it seems like they just want to throw it all away, and now I'm back to being a little kid again.

CLINICIAN: I hope that I haven't communicated that that's what I think. The purpose of these discussions is certainly not to make you feel uncomfortable, but rather to understand what you went through, what symptoms you had, and what brought about these symptoms. [Empathizes with patient's feeling of being stigmatized and clarifies the purpose of discussing these events at all.]

ARTURRO: (*Softening*) It's not that I don't think it was a serious event. It's just that some of what happened was awful, and some of it was great. I don't like the idea that it's all being summed up in this little term "bipolar." I don't think that does it justice.

MR. YBARRA: But what you're forgetting is that, for us, it was all pretty awful. There wasn't much good about it.

CLINICIAN: You know, not everyone has the same experience of a manic or a depressive episode. In fact, I suspect, Arturro, you feel very much like you were never really ill. I think this is a very understandable belief. You may feel that you can explain the things that happened to you and why you did what you did without including any discussion of illness. But looked at from the outside, this was a very disturbing and frightening event to your family. [Further validates and normalizes patient's experiences, but shifts attention toward the family's viewpoint.]

MRS. YBARRA: Yes, it was. And I don't think it's over yet.

Validating the Family's Point of View

Next, the clinician emphasizes that the differing perceptions among family members are not due to family pathology but, rather, to differences in the subjective experience of the disorder.

MR. YBARRA: I just find it hard to believe that, after all that happened, he still thinks he wasn't sick. That just strikes me as very odd.

CLINICIAN: (*to Mr. Ybarra*) You witnessed what went on before and during Arturro's hospitalization. It may be quite frustrating to you to not have his cooperation now or have common goals.

MR. YBARRA: I can't imagine we'll ever agree on what happened.

CLINICIAN: You may be right—the three of you may not be able to come to a full agreement about this, because the person living with the disorder has a very different experience and perspective than a family member who's observing it. [Validates father's point of view, but maintains that the experience of bipolar disorder will differ depending on the perspective one takes.]

ARTURRO: Dad, you weren't there. You didn't go through these things. I was gaining insight into what acting is all about. I began to see how one becomes an Orson Welles or a Laurence Olivier, and it was all coming together (*pause*) . . . I don't think anybody in this room knows what that was like. [Implies that clinician is siding with his parents.]

CLINICIAN: Arturro, I think you're right that the experience of mania can be a very profound one, and someone who hasn't gone through it won't ever fully get it. You and your relatives are in very different places with this stuff. As we go through our information about bipolar disorder you may feel that it fits their experiences better than yours, and in fact some of it may. This may make you feel that I'm more on their side than on yours, which I'm not. Nor am I on your side against them. [Addresses split clinician has found himself in, maintains neutrality, and does not confront the patient's grandiose beliefs.]

Examining Underlying Feelings of Shame and Guilt

In exploring the "patient rejects/family accepts" conflict, you are often addressing the underlying motives, beliefs, and fears fueling this conflict. Therefore, you can expect certain strong emotions (e.g., shame, guilt, anger) to rise to the surface, particularly within the patient.

In the final segment, Arturro expresses shame, accompanied by the fear that he has forever lost his life goals. The clinician reframes his struggle as part of a developmental step in learning to accept the disorder, and therefore a healthy struggle.

MR. YBARRA: (*angry*) And when you were thinking that way, that you were the next Laurence Olivier, you were up all night screaming lines from Shakespeare and running down the street naked.

ARTURRO: (*Eyes tear up.*) Why do you have to remind me of all this stuff?

MR. YBARRA: So you won't do it again.

ARTURRO: (*angry*) So, all that stuff I discovered about acting, that was just craziness, is that what you're saying? You think I'm never going to be able to act again, because it gets me crazy? Because *that's* what's crazy.

MR. YBARRA: (*solemn*) Maybe not.

CLINICIAN: (*Hands Arturro a tissue.*) I would guess it's pretty hard when people tell you what you did when you were ill, and it's perfectly normal to want to fight it. A lot of people feel shame later on, and want to believe these things didn't happen. You may have been a quite different person when you were ill.

ARTURRO: Maybe those things *were* crazy. But that doesn't mean there weren't some good things to learn along the way.

CLINICIAN: You're absolutely right, Arturro. I'm sure you did learn some important things, and we certainly want to hear about them. But I think the issue is whether or not you think you had an episode of bipolar disorder, not what we make of specific events. I think it's very normal not to want to see yourself as ill.

I think, rather than wishing the disorder would go away, it's better to get all the evidence about it, which is one of the things I'm encouraging you to do here. If you work your way toward understanding the disorder and, eventually, learning what you can to control it, I think you'll feel much more like you're in the driver's seat. [Offers hope by pointing to the control the patient gains by accepting and learning to manage his disorder.]

Throughout these discussions, the clinician does not take sides with members of the family but consistently maintains that the disorder is real.

He normalizes but does not overindulge the patient's denial and resistance to the illness concept.

The Grieving over the Lost Healthy Self

Once you have explored and worked through some of these family conflicts, you may notice a sadness settling on the patient and, perhaps, the family members. This sadness may signal a beginning acceptance of the reality of the disorder, the realization that one must adjust to changed life circumstances, and the associated feelings of loss generated by these realizations. As discussed earlier, the patient may begin grieving over the lost hopes, aspirations, and dreams he or she once had, and may begin thinking about his or her life as if it were bifurcated into those periods before versus after the illness (Frank, 2005). This grieving process can be a motivating factor in the patient's denial of the disorder. Thus, try to address these underlying issues during psychoeducation.

Distinguishing Short-Term versus Long-Term Goals

In the short term, take a fairly authoritative stance and recommend that the patient and family set low expectations for the patient's performance during the recovery period (see also Chapter 7). However, support those long-term goals or aspirations that appear realistic. The patient and family may especially benefit from understanding three notions: (1) that having bipolar disorder, although forcing certain setbacks, does not fundamentally change who a person is; (2) that having a psychiatric illness does not mean one cannot have a happy, productive life, nor does it mean one cannot pursue one's muse; and (3) that many quite creative individuals (musical composers, writers, artists) have had bipolar illness, suggesting it may have its positive sides (Jamison, 1993). In the following vignette, the clinician addresses Arturro's sadness over his lost hopes.

ARTURRO: I'm crying because I feel like you're saying, "All is lost"! There are a lot of things I wanted to do and now it seems like I have to give all these things up and be this sedate, calm person who "keeps stress to a minimum" and all that.

CLINICIAN: Well, are we really saying you have to give up everything? Can we make a distinction here between what you do now, for the next 3 months or so, and what you do later?

ARTURRO: But I want to get back to school full-time, and get back on stage. Otherwise, everyone else will pass me up. You're not young as an actor for very long.

CLINICIAN: Well, I can understand why you'd want to do that, but I think it's a mistake to assume that because you've been discharged from the hospital, you're all better, and you should be ready to take on the world. [Revisits notion of residual impairments.]

MRS. YBARRA: If he's not better, why did they let him go?

CLINICIAN: Well, of course, that's really a question about the health care system, but given our short hospitalizations, people are often very fragile when they get out. (*to Arturro*) So this may not be the best time to jump back in full-bore; I'd rather see you reenter gradually, maybe take a half course load or only one course.

The clinician has not yet taken a stand on the longer-term issues raised by the patient, but instead emphasizes that the patient should set goals that are more in line with his current level of functioning. Next, the clinician transitions to discussing longer-term goals.

MR. YBARRA: I think you'd better give up the acting, too. I think that's part of your problem.

ARTURRO: (*to clinician*) Do you agree with that, that I can't be an actor?

CLINICIAN: No, not necessarily, but I don't think your dad's saying this to be mean. I think this is a time when your family is confused and trying to figure out what they think about all this. But let me suggest that you're really asking a different question, namely, "Can I still think of myself as a person with wishes, needs, and goals? Can I still do those things I wanted to do?" Certainly you can think of yourself that way, and you should. Actually, many very creative and successful people, including artists, writers, and actors, have had bipolar disorder.

MRS. YBARRA: I read about that.

CLINICIAN: Yes. But I think it's important to remember that whatever decisions you make now may not be the same ones you make over the long term. For now, Arturro, I'd like to see you focus on the next 3 months, the next 6 months, and so on, until you're fully recovered and stable on your medications. Then I think you'll be more in a position to decide for yourself whether acting is the right career for you.

In this interchange, the clinician validates the patient's desire to see himself as a person separate from the disorder. He encourages the patient and family to distinguish long- from short-term goals. Finally, he gives the patient a greater sense of control over his long-term career decisions and frames the patient's participation in treatment as an avenue for achieving his goals.

Challenging the Health of the Former Self

Akiskal (Akiskal et al., 2000) has discussed the various "core temperamental disturbances" that often presage the development of bipolar disorder: mild to moderate swings in mood and behavior (cyclothymia, dysthymia, and hyperthymia) that are often associated with high productivity but also disturbances in interpersonal relations. In FFT, patients and family members are often recalling and idealizing a preillness self that was hypomanic, antisocial, or at minimum, immature and irresponsible.

You have to walk a fine line between challenging the health of this former self and at the same time (1) appreciating the attractiveness of the patient's personality characteristics and (2) allowing the patient to experience continuities between his or her former and current self. This challenge can be made more acceptable to the participants by predicting that the patient has matured and advanced in his or her self-understanding from the difficult experience of having gone through an episode and hospitalization. However, you should actively discourage the patient from testing the waters (i.e., by discontinuing medications) to determine if his or her former lifestyle, strengths, or abilities are still retrievable.

In the following vignette, Arturro has made reference to the life he led in San Diego prior to college, before the onset of his manic episode. This period was characterized by many exciting adventures, friendships, girlfriends, nights of drunken rowdiness, and daredevil activities. His parents laughed with him in appreciation of this period.

ARTURRO: That was when I was happiest. I wasn't in college yet, I didn't have all these responsibilities, and people just couldn't get enough of me.

MRS. YBARRA: (*admiringly*) Every time he came home the phone never stopped ringing. He was so popular!

MR. YBARRA: (*Smiles.*) Our phone bills were ridiculous.

CLINICIAN: That sounds like it was a pretty exciting period. I think we can all point to times in our lives when we didn't have many responsibilities, and we often wish those periods would happen all over again. I think you'd be missing this period even if you hadn't become ill. [Joins with patient and family in appreciating the patient's premorbid self.]

ARTURRO: But then you grow up and get boring. And in my case, you get mentally ill.

CLINICIAN: Well, I think you're not giving your adult experiences much credit. In some ways, it sounds like you were just a kid then. I think you've grown up a lot since then. You've had more life experiences, you've gone to college, and now you've gone through this difficult period of having been hospitalized, and you're handling it in a mature way. In some ways, you're way ahead of where you were then. [Reframes current self as a more mature version of the prior self.]

ARTURRO: Well, sometimes think I should just move back there. Some of the people I knew still live there.

CLINICIAN: I think what you're saying is that, if you went back to San Diego, you'd find who you used to be waiting for you.

ARTURRO: (*Pauses*) Maybe so.

CLINICIAN: What makes you so sure you aren't still that same person? How do you know that after you recover from this episode you won't still be an energetic, popular person, only with some more life experience under your belt? [Emphasizes continuities between prior and current personality attributes, and instills hope.]

The Relatives' Grieving Process

Although we have discussed only the patient's grieving process so far, family members often undergo a grieving process of their own. This is especially true if the patient has had more than one episode, and the reality of the illness now seems unavoidable. To close relatives, the person they used to know, who may have been talented, popular, energetic, and seemingly destined for success, is now dull, sedate, and unmotivated, or, alternatively, grandiose and unrealistic. For parents of children with bipolar disorder, this has been called "grieving over the lost healthy child" (Miklowitz & George, 2008).

Be prepared to explore these themes with relatives. However, be simultaneously aware that such discussions may become quite painful for the patient. Once again, keep the focus on the distinction between long- and short-term goals, and on what continuities in the patient's premorbid self can be drawn upon in his or her, or the family's, attempts to cope with the recovery period.

Special Issues with Child and Adolescent Patients

Most preadolescent and adolescent patients—and sometimes their parents—disagree with the bipolar diagnosis. Their resistance is not unfounded. Our field does not fully agree on the diagnostic criteria for childhood-onset bipolar disorder, and few studies have examined the course of its early presentations. Thus, we are on shaky ground in telling family members that their child will grow up to have adult bipolar disorder with classic manic or depressive features. In many cases, it will even be premature to make predictions about recurrences or rehospitalizations. Consider the following two cases:

Caitlin, age 14, had sudden outbursts of rage that alternated with despair, suicidal ruminations, and self-destructive behavior. When rageful, she would become severely agitated, break things, cut herself with glass, scream, curse, and run away from home, sometimes overnight. At other times, she would become "filled with passion" and seek a sexual liaison with one of several boys she knew at school. She went through periods of sleeping very little, but usually caught up the next day or on weekends. In between these episodes, she had periods of mild depression and often spoke of empty and hopeless feelings, but did not report extreme fatigue, lethargy, or sleep disturbance. Her functioning at school deteriorated when her mood was cycling, and she had been hospitalized twice for suicidal behavior.

Josh, age 17, had been hospitalized four times since he was 10. His episodes were invariably precipitated by going off his lithium and atypical antipsychotic medications. Most of his episodes included a significant psychotic component, such as his belief that he was being followed by CIA agents who were "trying to steal my inner self." He would shake his head when he heard voices. He was both elated and extraordinarily irritable when his delusions or hallucinations emerged, and would go for days without sleeping. His behavior became erratic and bizarre. His "crash" periods usually began as soon as his mania stabilized, and consisted of weeks of deep sadness, loss of interest, feelings of worthlessness, insomnia, inertia, and suicidality.

Can we be sure that both of these patients will develop adult bipolar disorder? The path seems relatively clear for Josh—he has classic manic, depressive, and psychotic (possibly schizoaffective) symptoms precipitated by medication nonadherence. But what about Caitlin? Do we know that she will develop an adult form of bipolar I or II disorder? Are any of her problems related to the hormonal changes associated with puberty? Does she have conduct disorder, or the beginnings of a borderline personality disorder? Or are her rage periods simply extremes of teenage behavior?

The question of long-term outcome is often posed by parents during FFT sessions. With younger patients, it is usually best to admit to your uncertainty about the long term and to focus instead on the immediate episode stabilization period. For example, you can say:

"Although Caitlin meets the diagnostic criteria for bipolar disorder now, we really don't know for sure whether she'll have major episodes when she's an adult. The studies that would answer that question haven't been done. But maybe that's not the most important question right now. Caitlin, I'd like us to focus instead on how you're going to get stabilized so that you can go on with your life. How do we get you back to school and doing those things you're best at? How do we keep you stable over the next 3 months so that you can complete the semester?"

In the absence of information to the contrary, parents often assume the worst about their child's future. Discourage them from assuming that their child is lost, that he or she will have a life of diminished potential, or that the child won't be able to go to college, get married, have a career, or have his or her own children. Provide an optimistic but realistic view of the future, much as you do with parents or spouses of adults, but targeted toward the younger age group:

"I know that this last episode was very disappointing for you, and that you're really worried about Caitlin's finishing high school. But we really don't know enough about this disorder to make predictions of that kind. We know that some people have very difficult courses of illness as adults, but many others straighten out as they age; they become more stable, more responsible, and get a better handle on what factors contribute to their mood cycling. You are getting good treatment for Caitlin and educating yourself about the disorder. Kids in families whose parents do these things have a much better outcome."

The Stigma of Bipolar Disorder within the Larger Society

"We can talk about it [the illness] in front of certain people, but, you know, people at work, or some friends come up to you and say, 'Hey, where were you those couple of months?' Or, 'What happened to you, and why are your hands trembling?' You can say, 'Hey, well, I'm a manic–depressive, and I've been in a mental hospital.' You know, it's a burden you have to carry."—*A 22-year-old male bipolar patient*

Accepting a psychiatric diagnosis means accepting being different. This is a very real issue for many patients, who usually feel uncomfortable telling friends, lovers, bosses, or coworkers about their symptoms or hospitalization. They believe, often realistically, that others will reject or avoid them and no longer desire their companionship. They fear they will be fired or demoted from their jobs. For these reasons, patients or family members often want to believe that the illness is not real or was simply a one- or a two-time occurrence.

In our experience, this problem is best discussed around a specific interpersonal problem, such as the patient's relationships with friends or employers. You can help the family to break this issue down into several smaller questions: (1) Whom do you tell about the disorder? (2) How much do you tell them? (3) What is the likelihood that these persons will actually respond with rejection? (4) How can you destigmatize the disorder for these persons so they will not be afraid? While empathizing with the difficulties the patient may have in making such self-disclosures, point out that friends or employers who are informed of the illness may not be as insensitive or rejecting as he or she fears.

In the vignette below, Ralph had raised the question of whether his currently depressed wife, Christine, should tell her employer about the recent hospitalization.

CLINICIAN: This is indeed a difficult and a touchy issue, and I certainly appreciate why you're raising it. Everyone has to come up with his or her own way of handling disclosures of this kind. Christine, how do you feel about disclosing your bipolar disorder to people? Is there someone you want to discuss this with now? [Concretizes the issue.]

CHRISTINE: My boss. I've been out for almost 2 months now. At first he asked me if I was pregnant, and I said no. But now I feel I have to tell him something.

CLINICIAN: How is he likely to react? Is he a very judgmental person?

CHRISTINE: (*pauses*) I hadn't really thought about that. He's stern, but he's not really that judgmental.

CLINICIAN: Has anyone else in your office been out sick for a period of time?

CHRISTINE: Yes, Clarissa was. She had breast cancer. Actually, he was very understanding.

CLINICIAN: So he may not be as judgmental as you fear. [Challenges the assumption that others will be rejecting.]

CHRISTINE: I just don't know how he'd react to a *mental* illness, and that I was locked up, in restraints, and all that.

CLINICIAN: I understand why it would be difficult to tell him those things. In fact, I'm not sure you need to tell him all the gory details, but maybe you can do some basic education with him so that it won't seem so awful, kind of like what we're doing with you here. I think you may have to "destigmatize" the disorder for your boss so that he's not afraid of it.

Practical manifestations of this stigmatization issue, such as described in this vignette, are often good introductions to communication enhancement training (see Chapter 9). You can pose as the patient's boss and role-play with the patient different ways she might disclose her illness, while coaching her as to how much to disclose, how to frame the hospitalization experience, and how to address the difficult question of the impact of her disorder on her work performance. You can also coach her on ways to ask for special accommodations at work, such as later work hours, taking more breaks, or taking leave time for medical appointments (see also Miklowitz, 2002).

Similar issues come up for children and adolescents regarding how much to tell teachers or guidance counselors at school. Usually, schools need to know the nature and extent of the disability in order to develop an Individualized Educational Program or make other special accommodations. How to coach families on communicating with school officials is discussed in Miklowitz and George's (2008) *The Bipolar Teen*.

Medication Nonadherence: Its Management within the Family Context

> Accusing me of mania, my elder sister's voice has an odd manic quality. "Are you taking your medicine?" A low controlled mania, the kind of control in furious questions addressed to children, such as "Will you get down from there?" . . .
>
> As if by going off lithium I could erase the past, could prove it had never happened, could triumph over and contradict my diagnoses; this way I would be right and they would be wrong. It had always been the other way; they were right and I was wrong. Of course I had only to take the lithium in order to be accepted back . . . on lithium I would be "all right." . . . But I am never all right, just in remission. If I could win this gamble. . . . (Millett, 1990, p. 32)

Perhaps in no other domain is denial and resistance to the illness notion, and to the psychoeducational process, more evident than in the patient's approach to taking medications. You will often be in the position of treating a patient who does not want to take medication, or who is so inconsistent about tablet taking that the medications are unlikely to be effective.

FFT is conceptualized as a treatment within a larger community program, and one of its goals is to support and reinforce the patient's medication treatment. There are two reasons behind this objective. First, because of the significant biological dysregulations associated with the disorder, FFT is unlikely to be effective unless the patient is also being managed pharmacologically. Second, issues around medication nonadherence can be the product of family dynamics during the recovery period. For example, nonadherence may reflect the patient's battle for autonomy with parents or a spouse.

The Role of the Family Clinician versus the Role of the Psychiatrist

If you are not the patient's psychiatrist or general practitioner, avoid stepping into the physician's role when discussing medication adherence with the family. It is primarily the physician's job to monitor medications, assess side effects, obtain blood serum levels, avoid toxic reactions, and educate the patient about the importance of medications; these are all basic components of good clinical management (see, e.g., Yatham et al., 2005).

When nonadherence occurs, regular communication should occur between you and the psychiatrist or general practitioner. Otherwise, "splitting" may occur. For example, you may become aware of a patient's nonadherence, but the patient may refuse to allow you to disclose this information to the psychiatrist. As discussed in Chapter 4, release-of-information permitting this communication should be obtained from the patient very early on and made a condition of the patient's continued participation in FFT.

Identifying the Reasons for Nonadherence

The first step in addressing nonadherence is to assess the reasons underlying it. Pose several questions to the patient and family: Why is the patient being nonadherent now? Did some event precipitate the decision to discontinue? To what degree is he or she nonadherent—completely or only partially (e.g., missing the evening dose only, missing the second medication in a two medication regimen)? What are his or her (or the family members') thoughts and feelings about it?

The reasons for nonadherence are quite varied (Colom, Vieta, Tacchi, Sanchez-Moreno, & Scott, 2005). They include, but are not limited to, the following:

- A lack of understanding about the purposes of medication
- The complexity of the regimen
- Side effects
- Residual manic or depressive symptoms
- Discomfort with blood tests
- Negative feelings about having one's mood controlled
- Missing high periods
- The stigma associated with psychiatric medications
- The loss of creativity
- Disbelief in the diagnosis/lack of acceptance of the disorder
- Desire to rebel against parents or spouses

- Comorbid personality disorders
- Simple forgetting

In understanding these diverse causes, one can make a distinction between nonadherence based on (1) specific beliefs about the medication, its side effects, or its associated management strategies (cognitive–informational factors) versus (2) feelings about what the medication symbolizes (affective factors).

The sections that follow describe various intervention strategies for dealing with nonadherence, each of which is consistent with the goals of the larger psychoeducational program. We have developed three primary strategies for addressing nonadherence: a preventative, a cognitive–informational, and an exploratory approach.

Addressing Nonadherence: The Preventative Approach

As in the case of addressing resistance to the illness concept, one can use a preventative approach to nonadherence by *predicting* that it will occur at some point during the treatment. The approach opens the door for discussions of the patient's feelings about medications. This approach is particularly useful for (1) patients who are young, living with parents, and experiencing their first or second episode of illness (a high-risk group for nonadherence; Miklowitz et al., 1988); and (2) patients who deny having bipolar disorder but nonetheless agree to take medications.

This approach can be implemented as follows:

> "Although you're taking your medications now, at some point during our treatment I'm guessing you'll want to stop taking them—you'll reach a point where you're feeling better and you'll feel like you don't need them. Most people don't like to take medications, perhaps because of the side effects, or perhaps because of not wanting to feel dependent on them. It's very understandable to feel this way. But we'd like you to agree that if you start having these feelings, you will bring them up here and with your psychiatrist so we can discuss them *before* you actually decide to do anything."

Some clinicians feel uncomfortable about predicting nonadherence in a patient who is adherent. However, most patients who have been diagnosed recently, and virtually all patients who deny the validity of the diagnosis, have considered discontinuing their medications at some point. Making this prediction is unlikely to precipitate nonadherence, in the same way that asking about suicidal ideation is unlikely to precipitate the corresponding behaviors.

Addressing Nonadherence: The Cognitive–Informational Approach

With certain patients, you may believe that nonadherence is due to lack of information, and that the patient would continue medications if he or she were able to place medication taking into a proper informational perspective. In fact, lack of information is a major cause of nonadherence (Aagaard & Vestergaard, 1990). Specifically, you may see value in exploring and discussing with the patient (1) the relapse risks associated with nonadherence, (2) ways to handle (and communicate with one's psychiatrist about) side effects, and (3) the patient's feelings about having regular blood tests.

Relapse Risk

Some patients benefit simply from knowing the risks they face by not taking medications. In most of these cases, the patient or family has not understood the meaning of "prevention" and sees the medication as a "one-shot deal," like an inoculation or an antibiotic. These patients or family members need to have the concept of preventative maintenance explained again (see Chapter 7), and they need information about relapse risk. For example, we tell patients that one's chances of having a recurrence in a 1-year period are cut in half by taking medications (i.e., from about 80 to 40%). You can also tell them that the risk of hospitalization is cut by 82% by taking lithium (Tondo et al., 2001).

Some patients will say, "I'll just take it if I start getting sick again." There are two counterarguments to this position: (1) Most mood-stabilizing agents take several weeks to become fully therapeutic, and symptoms may escalate before the medications take effect, and (2) when one is becoming manic, one feels good and judgment becomes impaired. People in this state do not want to "spoil the party" by taking medication.

Side Effects

Many patients want to discontinue their medications because of legitimate complaints about side effects. For example, patients on lithium or Depakote (divalproex sodium) may experience weight gain, nausea, trembling, sedation, or abdominal pain. People on olanzapine (Zyprexa) may experience weight gain and daytime sleepiness. The patient will experience you as empathic and validating if you encourage him or her to discuss the unpleasantness of side effects. Side effects may be a major issue for the patient, but perhaps not one given much credence by family members. Point out that any medication's benefits go along with certain costs, but that there are ways to lessen these costs:

ARTURRO: I'll tell you why you don't have any more episodes on lithium. Because you're spending all your time in the bathroom, peeing.

CLINICIAN: You've raised the point I was going to get to next. All of these medications have certain side effects that make them difficult and annoying to take. With lithium, the side effects include having to pee a lot, as you mentioned, as well as thirst, weight gain, and nausea.

ARTURRO: So you just have to live with them?

CLINICIAN: Actually, what many people don't know is that side effects are sometimes controllable—you don't have to quit taking your medications to make them go away. For example, you can have frequent blood tests to make sure you're getting the right dosage, and if not, your physician can adjust your dosage or switch you to another medication so that the side effects are less severe. Alternatively, you may get adjunctive medications that control these side effects. If the side effects are bad enough, your doctor may want to try you on a different medication.

To coordinate further the goals of FFT with those of medication management, you should separately discuss with the physician the patient's side effects and their potential to precipitate nonadherence. You can also conduct a role play exercise with the patient focusing on how he or she might discuss these issues directly with the psychiatrist.

Blood Tests

Clinicians are often surprised at the extent to which having blood drawn is an emotional issue for the patient. In addition to the unpleasantness of being pricked by a needle, blood tests can remind the patient that he or she has a chronic illness, or that society deems him or her "still sick" even though the patient may feel well. Many patients skip their blood tests (usually recommended once a month for lithium, and somewhat less frequently for Depakote, at least during the stabilization phase) and as a result do not know whether they are getting too high or too low a dose of a medication.

Children are often needle phobic and will refuse taking the medicines for no other reason than that they require blood tests. For younger patients, doctors often recommend medications that stabilize mood but don't require blood monitoring (examples: Lamictal and Seroquel).

Open up this issue by asking, "Do you mind having your blood drawn?" or "What are your feelings about this whole issue of blood samples?" Taking a didactic stance, review the advantages to the patient of getting blood tests, including that blood work (1) verifies therapeutic dosages and may be one way of controlling side effects and (2) helps minimize the likelihood of toxic reactions (for lithium: drowsiness, severe nausea, slurred speech, muscle twitching, and disorientation; for Depakote: severe dizziness, drowsiness, irregular breathing, severe trembling, or coma). However, explore and, where appropriate, normalize the patient's resistance to having his or her blood monitored:

> "I think having your blood drawn is a stressful experience. I certainly don't like having my blood drawn when I go in for a checkup. I guess it's also upsetting because it can remind you of having an illness. That's entirely understandable—after all, who likes having a blood sample taken to see if he (or she) is healthy?"

Interventions of this type often lead into more general discussions of the patient's feelings about having an illness, as discussed in other parts of this chapter.

Addressing Nonadherence: The Exploratory Approach

Often of greatest impact are interventions that explore the psychological significance of taking medications. Medication nonadherence can frequently be tied to feelings about the disorder and its stigma either inside or outside the family. As one patient of ours stated, "You've been healthy all of your life, and then to be subjected to taking these pills and stuff, it's kind of like, 'This isn't me . . . it can't be happening.' "

In this section we describe several interventions designed to explore the psychological factors underlying nonadherence. These include (1) clarifying the symbolic significance of taking medications, (2) interpreting nonadherence as a battle within the family for autonomy, and (3) using supportive analogies to other medical disorders. In evaluating these interventions, remember a single caveat: Taking medication is often interpreted by bipolar patients as the giving up of independence or control. Therefore, your core task is often one of encouraging the patient to view medication as a way to gain—rather than give up—independence and control.

Note the similarity here between FFT and motivational enhancement therapy, a therapeutic strategy for substance abuse (Miller & Rollnick, 1992). People tend to be more motivated to give up substances when they seem them as potentially interfering with their individual life goals. Likewise, accepting medications is easier for the bipolar patient if tied to the achievement of his or her aspirations.

Clarifying the Symbolic Significance of Medications

Encourage the patient to discuss what taking medications means to him or her. For many patients, taking each pill is tantamount to admitting that he or she is sick, disturbed, lacking in independence, or defective. The patient may express a great deal of anger and frustration over experiences such as having been "spied on" by other family members, having lovers terminate relationships because of side effects of the medications (for example, sexual side effects with SSRIs; weight gain with atypical antipsychotics), or being humiliated in sports or other activities due to side effects such as trembling hands.

Prior to the interchange below, Arturro announced that he had discontinued his medication 2 days prior:

ARTURRO: (*angry*) Taking medication makes me feel like I'm a kid all over again. And then when you add the fact that Mom follows me around the house, trying to see if I've taken it . . .

MRS. YBARRA: I do not follow you around the house!

CLINICIAN: I realize, Arturro, that taking lithium is a decision you make every day. Every day, you have to think in terms of what it means to you and what its significance is. Of course, you know my position, that you'd be much better off staying with it, but that doesn't mean I don't understand how uncomfortable these daily reminders must be.

ARTURRO: It feels like each little pill digs me in deeper.

CLINICIAN: In other words, it reminds you of not having the independence and control you feel you used to have.

In the vignette above, the clinician (1) clarifies the connection between medication taking and Arturro's perceived lack of independence within the family and (2) restates that the medications are essential to Arturro's recovery. In the next section, the clinician goes further with this theme and frames Arturro's nonadherence as a way of rebelling against his parents.

Nonadherence as a Battle for Autonomy

Nonadherence can be a way of saying, "I am feeling one-down in this family [or marriage], and I will stop my medications as a way of proving that I'm independent, healthy, and normal." Of course, this stance backfires when the nonadherent patient relapses and, in the aftermath of the episode, becomes even more dependent on family members than ever before.

Evidence that a patient's nonadherence is a way of rebelling against the family includes (1) his or her angry criticisms of parents or spouses for their actions relevant to medication taking (see the vignette above), (2) "clues" left for family members suggesting that he or she is not taking medications on schedule (e.g., leaving pills around the house), or (3) frequent arguments with family members about whether or not the disorder is real. These behaviors tend to elicit overcontrolling, domineering, or overprotective behaviors among parents or spouses. To the chagrin of all family members, parent–child dynamics that were salient in the patient's childhood begin to reemerge.

In the following segment, the clinician opens up the issue of Arturro's rebellion against his family.

CLINICIAN: I think that when you refuse to take your medication, it's not so much the medication that concerns you, but rather you're communicating that you want to be treated more like an adult and to be able to do things on your own. You're wanting your family to recognize your individuality, and in the same way you want to make it your decision to take or not take medication. [Reframes nonadherence as signifying a battle for autonomy.]

ARTURRO: (*sarcastically*) They're forgetting that I used to eat, sleep, and take showers, and even go to the bathroom by myself. They're acting like I'm some sort of incompetent, that I can't even remember to take a pill every morning and evening. I just couldn't deal with it anymore, so I stopped.

CLINICIAN: I think taking medication *can* make someone feel like he or she is being treated like a child. Sometimes, when people feel this way, it's easy for them to fall back into a child-like role. In fact, not taking medication can be a way of rebelling against your family, almost like you were a kid again. [Reframes the behavior as a reenactment of earlier parent–child dynamics.]

MRS. YBARRA: That's what it feels like. Like he's refusing to eat his string beans.

CLINICIAN: If you do take your medication, do you think you're really giving up that independence?

ARTURRO: If I take my medicine, it's like saying, "You've won, Mom and Dad. I really am crazy, and you were right."

CLINICIAN: I think that's very insightful, Arturro. Sometimes a person's family may really want him to take medication, and the person may even want to take medication himself, but to do so means somehow admitting to his family that he's sick or different in some way. So the problem can become, "How do I take this medicine without feeling like I'm giving in to my family?"

The clinician attempts to ally with the adult side of the patient. He frames nonadherence as a childish solution to a real problem of adult independence. But at this juncture, the clinician wonders whether nonadherence signifies the latest in a series of adolescent autonomy battles that Arturro has been fighting with his parents for years. We have also observed this dynamic in couples, where nonadherence becomes a way of wresting control from a domineering spouse with whom the patient has long battled for independence.

ARTURRO: I'm 19 years old. That's too old to be under your parents' thumb.

CLINICIAN: That's true, no one at your age likes to be told by his family what to do. But I'm beginning to think this autonomy thing has been a battle between you and your parents for quite some time. In fact, maybe we have to separate this issue of medication from your battles with your family because, really, this is a bad way to express your individuality. Once you go off your medication, you can easily get sick again. When people get sick they have no ability to stand up and say, "I'm independent." [Points out that the patient is self-sabotaging.]

ARTURRO: (*Pauses.*) So, what am I supposed to do? Just give in and be their little pet?

CLINICIAN: Well, let me put it back in your court. If you go off your medication, what does this get you?

ARTURRO: A chance to prove I'm really OK—which, as you've said, can backfire.

CLINICIAN: Yes, of course it can. Does it get you anything else?

ARTURRO: Not really. But I just don't see what taking medication buys me either.

CLINICIAN: Well, actually, what I'm thinking is that taking your medication, in the longer term, may actually give you *more* independence from your family, and more control over your own fate. If you take it regularly, get a therapeutic dose and all that, you'll be likely to recover more quickly, and then you'll be more in a position to move out, go back to school, or acting, or whatever it is *you* decide you want to do. [Frames adherence as an avenue for achieving independence.]

A useful next step is to steer the family toward problem solving (see Chapter 11). Specifically, the family may be able to solve the following conceptualization of the problem: How can the patient feel like an adult even when taking medication, and at the same time relieve some of the anxieties of his parents? For example, one of our patients agreed to take his medications independently but to report to his parents at the end of each week as to any missed dosages or side effects. Family members are often relieved by such solutions, because reminding the patient on a regular basis is stressful and places them in an old role they no longer wish to play.

Supportive Analogies to Other Medical Disorders

Patients often find taking a psychiatric medication more acceptable if it is compared to medications used in the treatment of medical disorders. This is particularly true among patients whose feelings about medication are inextricably tied to the stigma of the illness within the larger society. Consider the following interchange, which occurred in the treatment of the above-described marital couple, Christine and Ralph. In this vignette, the clinician had been coaching the patient as to how to discuss her illness-based absence with her boss.

CHRISTINE: I wish I weren't taking these damn medications. That's part of the shame of the whole thing. He'll probably see me taking them, or see my hand shaking, or something.

CLINICIAN: Maybe when you discuss the illness with him, you can describe the medication in terms of the analogies we made earlier to high blood pressure or diabetes. Both of these medical problems require long-term medications to correct chemical imbalances.

CHRISTINE: Actually, I think *he* takes a high blood pressure medicine.

CLINICIAN: Well, I'm not sure Depakote, Risperdal, and Lexapro are really all that different. Of course, bipolar disorder carries a social stigma that medical illnesses like high blood pressure don't have, but, in fact, both illness are brought about by biological vulnerabilities and stress, and they're both treated with daily medications.

A goal of this interchange, of course, is to make the patient more comfortable with the idea that she must take medications on an ongoing basis. Once a patient understands and agrees with the rationale for his or her regimen, it will be much easier for that person to discuss it with others.

Addressing Nonadherence: When Does One Stop the Family Treatment?

Despite the clinician's, the family's, and the psychiatrist's best efforts, the patient may nonetheless decide to discontinue his or her medications during FFT. This places you in a dilemma: Should you continue family treatment despite the patient's nonadherence? If so, aren't you implicitly sanctioning the patient's behavior? If not, are you removing the patient's only lifeboat?

Setting Limits

In many cases, the patient will simply discontinue medications and family treatment sessions simultaneously. In these cases, you may wish to continue seeing the parents or spouse for a limited number of sessions, with the rather circumscribed goal of familiarizing them with the prodromal signs of mood disorder recurrences and the steps necessary to intervene in such circumstances (see "The Relapse Drill" in Chapter 7).

In other cases, the patient may state that he or she wishes to continue in the FFT program (with the parents or spouse) as a substitute for taking medications. He or she may try to win you over with statements like "You're so much more understanding than my psychiatrist." In general, I do not recommend continuing the family program with an unmedicated patient. Instead, contract with the patient for one or two more family sessions to work through his or her resistance to taking medications, with the stated expectation that he or she will resume a similar (or perhaps modified) regimen once these issues have been explored.

Patients can be intimidated by the notion that agreeing to medication means agreeing forever. Therefore, ask the patient to commit to a time-limited trial of medication (i.e., 3 or 6 months), especially while he or she is in FFT:

> "Of course, no one can force you to take medications, but I want to make it clear that I cannot continue seeing you under these circumstances. It would be irresponsible of me to provide counseling sessions if I didn't think they'd be effective. If you're off medication, you're at a greater risk for having another episode, and I don't want to convey the message that you can get along with these family sessions alone.
>
> "On the other hand, perhaps you'd be amenable to a few more sessions where we just discuss your feelings about your medications and try to get you back on it for some agreed-upon period of time, let's say, 3 months. Would this be useful?"

Engaging the Help of the Psychiatrist

If the patient is amenable to a time-limited contract, the next step may be to have a meeting involving the attending psychiatrist, the family clinician, and the patient, with no family members present. In this session, the various treatment options can be considered, such as switching from one medication to another (e.g., from Depakote to Lamictal), adjusting dosages, arranging a more comfortable blood-monitoring plan, or introducing side effect medications (e.g., propanolol). This session is likely to give the patient a greater feeling of control. The meeting with the physician should be followed up by a family session in which the agreements reached are shared with the patient's relatives.

Medication as a Cost–Benefit Decision

If all attempts to get the patient back on a medication have failed, leave the patient with the notion that he or she (1) has made an important "cost–benefit" decision and (2) retains the ability to rescind this decision should he or she weigh the costs and benefits differently:

> "I think in discontinuing your medications you've made a cost–benefit decision. I view things in one particular way from what I've learned from other patients. For me, the benefits of being able to stay out of the hospital and not go through again what you've gone through, as well as being able to continue in the family program, would outweigh the costs of the side effects, the blood tests, and the uncomfortable feelings about taking medications. But, clearly, as the one who has to take them, you weigh the costs and benefits differently and have made a different decision than I would.
>
> "Let's keep the door open. Should you decide to go back on your medications in the near future, we may be able to resume our sessions then. In the meantime, you can call me if you want to discuss this further. Keep my number in case there are any emergencies like your symptoms getting worse or if you want another referral."

Concluding Comments

In this chapter, I have discussed the various ways within FFT to address the resistances that appear during the psychoeducation sessions. I have made a distinction between the overt behaviors that signify denial and resistance (e.g., medication nonadherence) and the underlying emotions and belief systems that motivate these behaviors (e.g., denial of the disorder, feelings of stigmatization, or grieving the lost healthy self). As you have undoubtedly noted, much of addressing these resistances involves normalizing and labeling them as healthy, understandable, and expectable reactions. However, the clinician continually points out the ways in which resistances interfere with the patient's ability to achieve his or her life goals, and the family's ability to cope with the consequences of the disorder.

The forthcoming chapters describe a different kind of psychoeducational intervention: the teaching of skills relevant to dealing with social stressors and improving family relationships (FFT Goals 5 and 6). I describe in the next two chapters the communication enhancement module, in which family members and patients are taught specific ways of listening, giving positive and negative feedback to each other, and negotiating change.

chapter 9

Communication Enhancement Training

Rationale and Mechanics

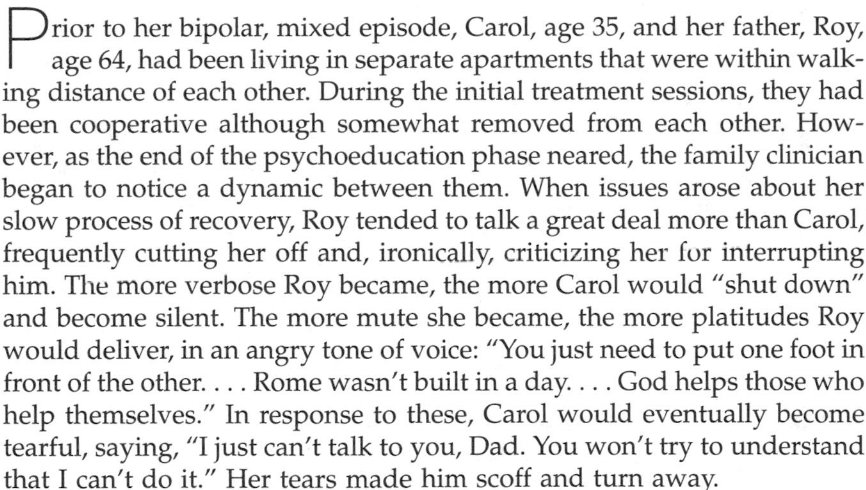

Prior to her bipolar, mixed episode, Carol, age 35, and her father, Roy, age 64, had been living in separate apartments that were within walking distance of each other. During the initial treatment sessions, they had been cooperative although somewhat removed from each other. However, as the end of the psychoeducation phase neared, the family clinician began to notice a dynamic between them. When issues arose about her slow process of recovery, Roy tended to talk a great deal more than Carol, frequently cutting her off and, ironically, criticizing her for interrupting him. The more verbose Roy became, the more Carol would "shut down" and become silent. The more mute she became, the more platitudes Roy would deliver, in an angry tone of voice: "You just need to put one foot in front of the other. . . . Rome wasn't built in a day. . . . God helps those who help themselves." In response to these, Carol would eventually become tearful, saying, "I just can't talk to you, Dad. You won't try to understand that I can't do it." Her tears made him scoff and turn away.

Chapter Overview

By the end of the psychoeducation phase, patients and family members have achieved a degree of understanding (if not acceptance) of bipolar disorder. It therefore becomes possible to address the sixth goal of FFT: reestablishing functional family relationships after the episode.

The next segment of FFT, usually begun by Session 8, is concerned with enhancing the quality and efficiency of the family's or couple's communication. This part of the program is assisted by structured exercises that in other literatures have been termed *communication skills training*. Jacobson and Margolin (1979) described these techniques in their manual on treating nonpsychiatric, distressed marital couples, as did Falloon et al. (1984) and Liberman (1988) in their manuals on psychiatric rehabilitation of the families of psychotic patients. We have adapted these techniques to the needs of the families of bipolar patients, which, as described in this and in previous chapters, are different from these other populations. The reason we use a somewhat different term—*communication enhancement training* (CET)—is that our focus is less on behavioral skill building and more on using these exercises to change the structure and function of family relationships. That is, we view CET as adding to the skill repertoire of various family members, but also as a way to regulate imbalances in the family system and strengthen alliance patterns.

This chapter addresses the rationale for CET and how to introduce it to the family or couple. It also discusses the mechanics of conducting structured role plays when teaching four basic communication skills: *expressing positive feelings, active listening, making positive requests for change,* and *expressing negative feelings about specific behaviors*. Chapter 10 addresses the handling of clinical issues stimulated by CET, including (1) treating the resistances that arise when conducting role-play exercises with the families of bipolar patients, (2) encouraging generalization of the new skills to outside settings, and (3) using CET directly or indirectly to alter disturbances in the functioning of the family system.

Objectives of CET

The family clinician introduced Roy and Carol to CET. She first presented two concrete communication skills: expressing positive feelings to another family member and active listening. She began by asking Roy to tell Carol something she had done recently that he had appreciated. Later in the same session, she asked Roy to listen actively (without interrupting or making suggestions) while Carol described her attempts to reconnect with several of her friends following her episode of depression. At the end of the session, Carol was upbeat, saying, "This is the first time we've ever *really* talked." For his part, Roy seemed surprised by what had transpired, although he stopped short of saying the session had been helpful. Nonetheless, he appeared for another session of CET the following week.

There are two primary goals of CET. The first and most obvious is to acquaint family members with new communication strategies they can bring to bear in the face of life stress. When a crisis occurs (e.g., the ill husband in a couple loses his job) or when severe family conflicts arise (e.g., the wife threatens to leave because the husband will not take his medication), the members of a couple or family often resort to past styles of communication (family homeostasis), which may be less than effective in resolving the crisis. Instead, they may be able to implement more constructive forms of communication, such as learning to listen to each other or to express what they wish for others in the family to do. In CET, participants learn new skills (or become reacquainted with skills they no longer practice) through modeling and rehearsal, and then practice these at home so that the skills generalize to other settings.

On the surface, the CET exercises seem rather simple, routine, and even mundane. However, as discussed in Chapter 10, their impact often goes beyond the application of narrow technical skills. Rather, the introduction of these skills often accomplishes a second goal: altering problematic relational patterns. Learning to communicate more clearly creates stronger alliances between members of a family; breaks taboos against talking about difficult, emotionally laden topics; brings out hidden agendas; and fosters a "collaborative set" and a sense of hope about the future. These improvements in the family's emotional climate can facilitate the patient's recovery process.

Families who are high-EE have a particularly hard time communicating effectively during the postepisode period (Simoneau et al., 1998). However, when patients and their family members adopt new communication strategies, patients are more likely to stabilize during the postepisode year (Simoneau et al., 1999).

Why Introduce Communication Exercises at This Point in Treatment?

CET is introduced, on average, at approximately 8 weeks into the FFT program. Why at this point in treatment? First, with the help of medication and the stabilizing effects of psychoeducation, the patient should be mostly remitted from his or her index episode. Thus, the patient and family members should be better able to handle tasks that are less didactic and more oriented toward changing preexisting patterns of behavior.

Second, the initial 8 weeks are dedicated to exploring the nature of bipolar disorder, which typically engenders at least some feelings of tension in the family. CET takes some of the pressure off the patient to admit that he or she is ill and replaces these discussions with tasks that are more mutual in nature (role-play exercises in which everybody must participate).

Third, although the patient is nearing a state of clinical remission, the family environment remains shaky. That is, conflicts may erupt at any time, preexisting marital conflicts may come to the fore, and earlier battles between parents and patients may recur. Family members are more forthcoming about the difficulties inherent in maintaining a low-conflict home environment. Specifically, they complain of difficulties in communicating with each other about illness- and nonillness-related matters, and in establishing balances in role relationships (i.e., who does what, who has power or the "final say," how to negotiate distance vs. intimacy). In some cases, these imbalances may be state-dependent and the direct result of the index episode, whereas in other cases, they are enduring features of the family that predated the onset of the disorder. Among recovering adolescents, issues regarding respect for authority or consideration for siblings often come up at this stage.

The directive, structured nature of CET is a useful antidote to these mounting levels of tension. It reduces the anxiety of the participants, provides a predictable organization for sessions, and offers participants a feeling of competence as they begin to master the CET skills. In contrast, simply asking the family "just to talk over" their problems while the clinician occasionally intervenes can lead to negatively escalating battles and the feeling in participants that theirs is a pathological, nonfunctioning family.

Fourth, whereas the goals of the psycheducation phase center on stabilizing the patient following his or her episode, the goals of CET center on the prevention of recurrences. That is, teaching new ways to communicate may help the family to cope better with future family conflicts and stressful life events. The family that adopts new communication styles may be able to create an environment that is protective against recurrences of the patient's disorder.

CET: Getting Started

Session Frequencies and Structure

CET generally requires about seven sessions. Thus, we recommend using Sessions 8–14 for CET. The first five of these are conducted weekly (Sessions 8–12) and the next two, biweekly. However, you may wish to modify this schedule depending on the existing skill level of the family, the length of the treatment contract, or the need for all versus only a subset of the communication skills. For example, some families benefit most from learning about active listening, in which case the entire module may be reduced to two or three sessions. However, in our experience this constitutes a minority of families. Even the best communicators have "communication setbacks" when coping with the stress associated with an illness episode.

Adolescents and younger kids rarely have the attention span to sit through seven sessions of communication training. For youth, consider having a few initial sessions of CET to familiarize families with role playing, and then move into the problem solving. You can then "sprinkle in" the communication exercises more informally as they fit the needs of a particular problem scenario. For example, Devon, age 15, complained that his parents were constantly asking him how his day went, which he experienced as intrusive and interpreted as their way of "checking his pulse." We used the exercises as an opportunity for the family to practice speaking and listening on topics unrelated to Devon's emotional problems: his father's recent disagreements with a colleague during a fishing trip, Devon's desire to assist in coaching his younger brother's soccer team, and how Devon could save money for a computer program he badly wanted. Each of these topics required that the family practice problem-solving skills (Chapter 11). As the family became more comfortable using communication skills for resolving relatively unemotional problems, they discussed ways that Devon's parents could stay informed of his mood state (for example, periodically examining his mood chart) without asking him directly.

Aiming CET at the Functional Level of the Family

You should attempt to mold the training to the needs of the particular couple or family. For example, some families are very accepting and have no trouble giving positive feedback, but have trouble dealing with negative emotions or requesting changes from each other. Other families deliver negative feedback frequently and even constructively, but family members have trouble saying anything positive. The stress of the post-episode recovery period tends to exaggerate these communication habits.

Before embarking on the CET exercises, review the family's skill assets and deficits, as revealed in the earlier functional assessment and psychoeducation sessions. In examining the communication behavior of family members, keep in mind the domains of functioning described in Chapter 5: What is the structure of the family's relational patterns? What is the affective tone of its interactions? How well does the family solve problems? What is the family's level of communication clarity?

Introducing CET to the Family

Some families will be suspicious of the introduction of CET. The psychoeducation module is more clearly congruent with the goals of the patient's drug treatment, with its emphasis on recovering from an illness episode and medical treatment adherence. Few could argue with the importance of learning the facts about a disorder with which one is faced. In contrast, CET is less focused on the syndrome of bipolar disorder and more on how family members get along on a day-to-day basis. As a result, some will see the introduction of CET as carrying the implication that the family is dysfunctional.

Their reactions are not unfounded. Early psychoanalytic views of schizophrenia placed substantial blame on mothers for "double-bind communication" and "schizophrenogenic mothering." None of these outdated notions are relevant to FFT. Although family members are unlikely to be aware of these theories, they may jump to the conclusion that you think they caused their son's or daughter's bipolar disorder through poor communication.

Offer the family a clear rationale for CET—even if it is a review—before proceeding with the exercises. Begin by distributing Handout 9, a flowchart explaining where CET fits into the relapse prevention process:

> "Remember a few sessions ago we talked about risk factors in bipolar disorder? Well, as you can see in this diagram, a person can be at risk for another relapse of bipolar disorder if the home environment is tense and there is much conflict. In contrast, good communication and problem solving within a family or couple can be among those 'protective factors' against stress that we talked about before. For a close relative, learning effective communication skills can be a way of decreasing one's level of tension and improving one's family relationships.
>
> "Now that you know some things about bipolar disorder, we think you'll appreciate the second major component of our treatment together, which is called communication enhancement training. We want to help you communicate in the clearest and least stressful way possible, so that everyone's voice is heard and problems get solved. We'll do a series of exercises called 'role playing.' This means we'll be asking you to turn your chairs to each other and practice new ways of talking among yourselves, such as praising each other, listening, or asking someone to change his or her behavior."

Note that, consistent with the vulnerability–stress model, you can frame the CET as a way of decreasing stress within the home, such that the patient is protected against recurrences. There is no implication that disordered family communication causes bipolar disorder in the first place. Finally, by alluding to the importance of effective problem solving, you plant the seed for the final module of FFT.

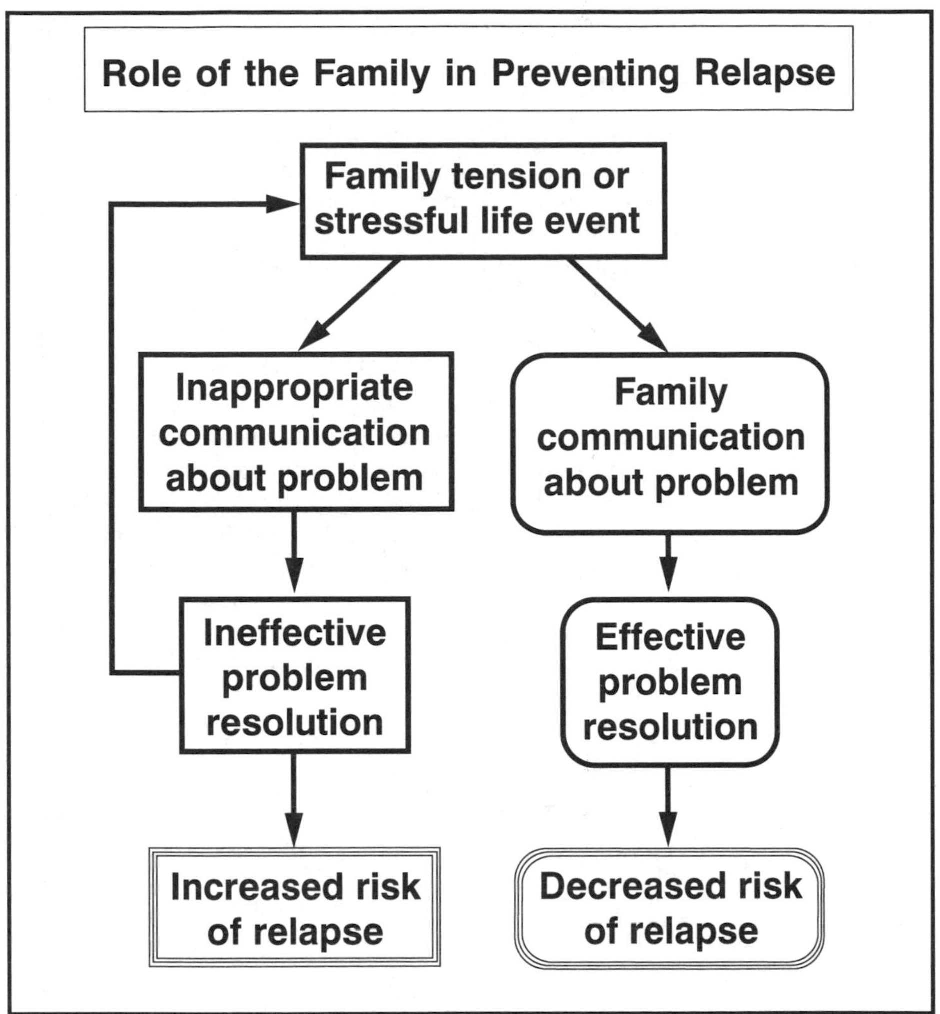

HANDOUT 9. *Source*: Adapted by permission from Falloon et al. (1984). Copyright 1984 by The Guilford Press. From *Bipolar Disorder: A Family-Focused Treatment Approach, Second Edition,* by David J. Miklowitz. Copyright 2008 by The Guilford Press. Permission to photocopy this handout is granted to purchasers of *Bipolar Disorder* for personal use only (see copyright page for details).

Addressing Initial Resistances

At this point, members of the family may raise questions about the relevance of CET to their family. They may argue that they really have no problems (see the discussion of these families in Chapter 7) and see no reason to role-play or to be trained in how to communicate. Examine the following interchange between the clinician, Roy (the father), and Carol (the patient):

ROY: What makes you think that we don't communicate well now? I don't think we have that many problems. We talk a lot, and we're pretty clear what we think about things.

CLINICIAN: I'm not implying that you're bad communicators, or that there's something wrong with your family. Instead, you're here because you've both dealt with Carol's illness, and the idea is to improve your relationship at home so that she can make the best recovery possible. After a bipolar episode, families often have to be able to access styles of communicating that they wouldn't otherwise have to use. [Frames the high-stress recovery period as an external factor that undercuts effective communication, and avoids labeling the family as dysfunctional.]

ROY: OK, that sounds like some of the things you've said before, and while I half agree, I still don't know how this will help her.

CLINICIAN: Well, to get personal for a second, it's easier for me when I'm anxious or upset to have a helpful conversation with someone I care about who listens, gives encouragement, and communicates that he or she is on my side. [Uses self-disclosure to normalize the value of good communication.]

ROY: Is that when you go to see *your* therapist?

CLINICIAN: (*Laughs.*) You got me! I suspect that's also true for the two of you. You've both been through this very stressful time, and although the worst is over you're both now trying to "regroup" and figure out how to get your family back to where it was before Carol got ill. Being able to communicate well leads to a calmer family environment, and gives you tools to use when things don't go so well in the future. (*to Roy*) It may also help you to feel less anxious about broaching important topics with Carol. [Again frames the goals of CET as relevant to ameliorating stress in the postillness recovery phase, and underscores the notion of longer-term prevention.]

You should expect that further resistances to CET will appear once participants begin role playing. However, at this point, forge ahead with the training and encourage the family to try these new communication styles before ruling out their usefulness.

Teaching the Four Basic Communications Skills

Previewing the Skills

As discussed above, we teach four basic communication skills to families, in the order listed in Handout 10. Falloon et al. (1984) have also described these skills in their manual on the behavioral family treatment of schizophrenia.

The rationale for this ordering is as follows. First, it is helpful to start the CET on an optimistic note, so begin with *expressing positive feelings*. Having family members turn to each other and offer praise or compliments defuses bad feelings, gives family members hope, and opens the door for more open communication about disturbing or conflictual matters. Next, introduce *active listening,* an essential building block for the other communication skills, and one that contributes to the feelings of validation participants experience when learning the first skill. Third, once you have promoted a cooperative atmosphere, participants feel more comfortable in negotiating conflicts, which requires two other skills: *making positive requests for change in the behavior of another member,* and, in the event that more diplomatic requests for change have not been effective, *expressing negative feelings about specific behaviors*. More is said about the specifics of each of these skills below.

First, offer the family Handout 10. In introducing the skills, proceed as follows:

> "We're going to acquaint you with four communication skills. They are expressing positive feelings, active listening, making positive requests for change, and expressing negative feelings about specific behaviors. When you try out these skills, they may feel a little artificial. This is entirely expectable, and most people we work with do feel a bit awkward at first. One way to think of these skills is like trying on new shoes. At first they may not fit and be uncomfortable, but they have the potential to work for you if you break them in. If after trying them for a while you still don't like them, you can always take them off. But sometimes you have to wear them for a while to see if they fit."

This message anticipates in family members a degree of discomfort and performance anxiety when first trying out new skills. It emphasizes how natural it is to feel this discomfort. The "new shoes" analogy tends to make family members feel more in charge of the CET process. They can select which styles fit, rather than having a clinician try to "make them over" to conform to his or her idealistic view of effective family communication.

The Four Basic Communication Skills

- Expressing positive feelings
- Active listening
- Making positive requests for change
- Expressing negative feelings about specific behaviors

HANDOUT 10. *Source*: Falloon et al. (1984). From *Bipolar Disorder: A Family-Focused Treatment Approach, Second Edition*, by David J. Miklowitz.

A Note on "Redirecting"

As I describe the role-playing and rehearsal strategies for teaching the four skills, you will notice that the clinician stays very close to the training agenda, even when participants raise problematic family issues. For example, during CET, spouses sometimes raise doubts about the quality of the marriage and question whether they should stay with the patient.

Although I strongly believe that you must address these more heated conflicts, the issue is one of pacing. These harder issues will be more easily tackled, through exploration and problem solving, once the tension level in the family has been reduced by positive experiences with face-to-face communication. Moreover, it may be dangerous to segue into major conflicts that generate a great deal of guilt or anger in a patient who is still symptomatic. Thus, it is often best to redirect discussions of potentially explosive family conflicts by encouraging the family to delay discussing them until they have mastered the basic communication skills. Later, you can address these issues in additional CET exercises or by breaking the issues down into smaller, more solvable conflicts within the structured format provided in the problem-solving module (see Chapter 11).

The Mechanics of Conducting Role Plays

The in-session role play is the core technique used to teach communication skills. Through this vehicle, family members practice new ways of communicating in a setting that is nonjudgmental and a reasonable approximation of real life. There are several steps to conducting role play exercises, as described in Table 9.1. In the sections that follow, you will see how each of these steps contributes to the learning process.

TABLE 9.1. Steps in Conducting Role-Play Exercises

- Model the skill for the participants.
- Set the scene.
- Ask the participants to role-play the interchange.
- Elicit feedback from all family members.
- Model alternative ways of delivering the message.
- Conduct new rehearsal with coaching.
- Offer praise for efforts.
- Give a homework assignment.

Note. Sources: Falloon et al. (1984); Liberman (1988).

Expressing Positive Feelings

Let's assume you begin with the first skill, expressing positive feelings. Begin by distributing copies of Handout 11, and briefly summarize the nature and purpose of the skill: It is a direct way to make other members of the family feel valued and appreciated, and to want to do something for you in return. Explain some of the components. For example, list the various ways to say "how it made you feel": Some family members have trouble distinguishing feeling "good" from feeling "valued," "relieved," "appreciated," or other emotions. Likewise, explain that this skill is used for the purpose of offering praise for relatively specific behaviors of other family members: "You're a wonderful person" may not be as meaningful to a parent or spouse as "I appreciate how you've been helping me with taking care of Jill (daughter)." Then, *model* the skill with your cotherapist (if one is available) or with one of the participating family members:

> "Let's imagine that I want to tell Wendy [cotherapist], that I appreciate the fact that she makes a long trip every week to help me conduct these sessions with the two of you. I might look at Wendy and simply say, 'Wendy, I appreciate how hard you've worked to arrange to come here at this time every week. I know it's a long way for you to drive. I find it very helpful to have you here.' Now that I've gone out on a limb here a bit, can you tell me, Roy, what you thought about how I just said that?"

It is entirely possible that the family member will say, "That was unnecessary" or "You laid it on too thick." Try not to be offended by this. Your willingness to be vulnerable and take constructive criticism makes family members feel less like they are on the hot seat and less defensive about their own communication styles.

Once you have modeled the skill, help the family members *set the scene* by turning their chairs toward one another and talking directly to each other. One member is appointed the speaker and the other the listener. Then, ask the dyad to *role-play the interchange*. Consider this example:

CLINICIAN: OK, let's have the two of you try it. What's an example? Have the two of you given each other a compliment in the past week?

ROY: Well, I gave you one, Carol. About the condition of your room.

CAROL: I don't remember.

CLINICIAN: Could you give her that compliment again now, only look at her and tell her specifically what she did that you liked, and how it made you feel?

Expressing Positive Feelings

- Look at the person.
- Say exactly what he or she did that pleased you.
- Tell him or her how it made you feel.

HANDOUT 11. *Source*: Adapted by permission from Falloon et al. (1984). Copyright 1984 by The Guilford Press. From *Bipolar Disorder: A Family-Focused Treatment Approach, Second Edition,* by David J. Miklowitz. Copyright 2008 by The Guilford Press. Permission to photocopy this handout is granted to purchasers of *Bipolar Disorder* for personal use only (see copyright page for details).

ROY: (*Looks at the clinician.*) Well, when I came over the other day, I said, "Carol, your room looks great. That was clever the way you got your roommate to do all your laundry. I wonder how you pulled that off?"

CAROL: (*sullen*) Whatever.

In the above vignette, the father is willing to role-play the skill with his daughter, for which the clinician (in the following exchange) is careful to praise him. However, as is immediately evident, this father has trouble expressing compliments without lacing them with implied criticisms. If this occurs, keep in mind that, given the family's recent history of severe conflict, it may be very difficult for family members to think about other members in positive terms.

With the aid of the daughter's feedback, the clinician normalizes the father's difficulties in expressing positive feelings, and then *models* the skill in a way that will be more pleasing to the daughter. With coaching, the clinician encourages the father to *rehearse the new skill*.

CLINICIAN: Roy, I appreciate the fact that you gave that role play a try. [Models expressing positive feelings.] Carol, how did you feel about what your dad said to you? [Elicits feedback from the target family member.]

CAROL: Not very good. He essentially insulted me by making me out to be manipulative or something.

CLINICIAN: Roy, I think it can be hard, in light of some of the problems the two of you have had lately, to think in these purely positive terms. And, Carol, I can understand why you heard it that way, especially because of some of your past discussions with your dad on issues like these. [Normalizes their reactions.]

ROY: She took it the wrong way.

CLINICIAN: Carol, was there anything you liked about what your dad said? Did he do any of the steps on this sheet? [Elicits positive as well as negative feedback.]

CAROL: (*reluctantly*) Well, he said he liked how I kept my room.

CLINICIAN: Yes, he did that. Now, Roy, let me take your part for a minute. What was it you really liked about how Carol keeps her room? [Coaches.]

ROY: Well, it looks tidy and nice.

CLINICIAN: And how do you feel when you see that?

ROY: I guess I'm glad she's able to maintain her apartment. It's a relief to me, one less thing to worry about.

CLINICIAN: Good. So, it sounds like what you really want to say is (*turns to Carol*), "It's pleasing to me that you are showing interest in your own place." [Models the skill.]

ROY: Yeah, something like that.

CLINICIAN: Could you turn your chair toward her and tell her again, in your own words? [Encourages new rehearsal of skill.]

ROY: (*Turns chair.*) Well, Carol, I'm glad you keep your apartment so clean, 'cause you're showing interest in your place, and 'cause it's one less thing for me to worry about, and you know I have a tough enough time keeping my own house clean (*laughs*)!

CLINICIAN: Nice job. Carol, how did you feel about it this time? [Praises efforts and elicits feedback.]

CAROL: Much better. Especially the last part.

The process of modeling, rehearsing, coaching, and feedback is an iterative process, which is repeated until you are reasonably sure the patient or family member has learned the skill, at least as applied to the specific example. Then, ask the other family member (or members) to be speakers in similar role plays so that they too can practice expressing positive feelings.

This process may take up to two sessions for each skill, depending on the preexisting abilities of the participants and the patient's clinical condition. However, remember that you're not shooting for perfection. If participants show rough approximations of the skill, praise them for their efforts and move on to the next skill. If you become too concerned that they perform exactly as indicated on the handouts, you can alienate them and weaken the impact of the CET.

It is best to finish by asking each family member to complete a *homework assignment* during the upcoming week, the Catch a Person Pleasing You task (Falloon et al., 1984; see Handout 12). In this task the participant is asked to record, for various days of the upcoming week, examples of positive, pleasing behaviors performed by a target member of the family (e.g., for a spouse: making dinner, bringing home flowers, offering a back rub, etc.), and exactly what the participant said to this family member to thank or praise him or her for these behaviors. This assignment requires the participant to practice the skill in the home setting. If family members complete the homework assignment, the examples they give become the basis for practicing the skills further in the next session.

Active Listening

An essential building block for good communication is the ability to listen. Family members coping with a recent episode of bipolar disorder or

Catch a Person Pleasing You

Day	Person who pleased you	Exactly what did he or she do that pleased you?	What did you say to him or her?
Monday			
Tuesday			
Wednesday			
Thursday			
Friday			
Saturday			
Sunday			

Examples

Looking good	Having a chat	Being considerate
Being on time	Making a suggestion	Going out
Helping at home	Going to work	Showing interest
Cooking meals	Offering to help	Taking medicines
Working in yard	Tidying up	Attending treatment
Being pleasant	Making bed	Making phone call

HANDOUT 12. *Source*: Adapted by permission from Falloon et al. (1984).

any other crisis have a great deal of trouble listening to the opinions, objections, feelings, or troubles of other members, especially if these family members have, in their opinion, been the source of the troubles. However, if members do not feel that others care enough to listen, they are unlikely to perform any of the other tasks essential to the postepisode recovery phase (e.g., keeping a low-stress, tolerant home).

Because it is in many ways the basis for other communication skills, active listening can be introduced before expressing positive feelings. However, we generally find that it is best to begin CET with a concrete skill that has a positive tone. Active listening is a more difficult skill to learn than positive feedback, especially if there has been recent, substantive conflict or if family members have trouble coming up with conversational content (see also "The Avoidant Family" in Chapter 10). Handout 13 lists the features of this skill.

Introduce active listening to the family as follows:

> "Now, this is a skill you're all probably familiar with, known as active listening. It's a skill that's useful anytime, but it comes in particularly handy in an argument—it's a way to defuse the argument, because whoever is talking to you feels heard and then is often willing to do the same for you.
>
> "There are a couple of components to it. If you want to indicate to someone that you're listening, usually you look at that person, nod your head, and ask some questions to clarify what you've heard, like 'When did that happen?' or 'How did that affect you?' It's also good to paraphrase what you've heard, or feed it back to the person who's been talking to you. Carol, when someone listens to you and asks you questions, how does it feel?"

When introducing the skill, briefly model its various components and solicit input from family members as to their understanding of and experiences with the skill. In the following vignette, the clinician illustrates the use of active listening with the patient.

CLINICIAN: Carol, can you give me an example of something that happened to you recently, something at work perhaps, and I'll show you what is meant by active listening?

CAROL: (*Pauses.*) OK. I'm at work, right? And my boss gives me this project to type that I'm supposed to share with these two other people. So for 2 days in a row they both call in sick. . . . And then when Wednesday came and it wasn't ready, my boss started yelling at me in front of the other people in the office.

CLINICIAN: Yeah. So he really took it out on you. [Paraphrases.]

Active Listening

- Look at the speaker.
- Attend to what is said.
- Nod head; say "Uh-huh."
- Ask clarifying questions.
- Check out what you heard.

HANDOUT 13. *Source*: Adapted by permission from Falloon et al. (1984).

CAROL: (*Tears up.*) Yeah. And called me names, and he just . . . I couldn't believe it because I felt like I was doing everything I could to get it done, and he was yelling at me when it's because these other people weren't there.

CLINICIAN: (*Nods.*) So he really blamed you for something that wasn't your fault. How did you react to him? [Asks a clarifying question.]

CAROL: I was really mad at him, and I really didn't know what to do because he did it in front of all those other people and it embarrassed me.

CLINICIAN: Yeah, I think that would make me mad, and embarrassed, too, if someone did that to me. [Paraphrases empathy.] OK, let's stop. Roy, right then I was doing some active listening. Can you tell me which of the components listed on the sheet you saw me doing? [Solicits feedback from the relative.]

In addition to modeling the skill, the clinician reviews the skill's components by asking the participants to attach labels (e.g., paraphrasing) to each of the clinician's listening behaviors. Next, she asks the family members to rehearse the new skill with each other, first regarding what appears (at least on the surface) to be a fairly neutral topic.

CLINICIAN: OK, Carol, why don't you be the speaker, and Roy, you be the listener. Again, turn your chairs toward each other (*sets the scene*) and let's pick something that doesn't have to do with the family to practice on. Carol, maybe something at work?

CAROL: (*Thinks.*) OK, it looks like I might be able to move to another job. A headhunter came by on Thursday and said he was looking for more programmers, and that I could switch to that one I told you about in Arapahoe County. (*Roy is silent.*) So that's about it.

ROY: Well, you know my feeling about this. Computer programming is not really for you. You can go get another job but it's still gonna be "been there, done that."

At this point, the clinician intervenes and coaches the father.

CLINICIAN: OK, Roy, a good start. Carol, what did you see your dad doing that time? Let's take a look at the handout.

CAROL: Well, he looked at me, and he nodded once. But that's about it. He got into his trip at the end.

CLINICIAN: Roy, I want to emphasize that you did certain things quite well there. You did keep good eye contact and you appeared to be attending. [Gives positive feedback.] But what else could you have done? Can you think of some questions you could ask?

ROY: Well, not much, she just needs to think of a different career.

As discussed above, it is not at all uncommon for structured role plays to degenerate into debates about certain emotionally loaded topics, such as the patient's career choices. Keep the role play task-focused, and remind the family that the purpose is to learn a communication skill, not to solve a problem. However, validate the feelings of the listener: He or she may have very legitimate emotional reactions to what is being said, even if you are asking him or her to temporarily inhibit the expression of those feelings.

CLINICIAN: OK, fine, but let's not get onto the topic of job choice—that's an important topic, but it's something we can deal with when we get to problem solving a few weeks from now. Let's focus on listening. Roy, I can think of a question you could ask, like "How would this new job be different from the one you have now?" [Coaches.]

ROY: Yeah, I could've asked that.

CLINICIAN: Let's try again. Carol, let's start from the top. [Encourages a new rehearsal of the skill.]

CAROL: Well, like I said, the headhunter told me I could get a job in the Arapahoe County office. I'm thinking about it.

ROY: How would that job be different from your job?

CAROL: Well, it would be basically the same thing, but there'd be more hours, some supervision of other employees, and stuff like that. But I'm a little nervous about taking on that much responsibility.

ROY: I don't think you're ready for that. Stick with what you know.

CLINICIAN: Roy, you have some very legitimate feelings about this issue. I think you're being very compassionate in wanting to help Carol keep her job stress down right now. But I'm asking you to hold on expressing your reactions for the moment and just try to understand what she's saying. [Validates father's feelings and frames his intentions as positive.] Can you think of a way to paraphrase what she just said?

ROY: What do you mean?

CLINICIAN: Well, paraphrasing is really just summarizing back to the person what you just heard. It helps make someone feel that he or she is being understood. For example, you might say, "So, you have another job opportunity, which is great, but it's more work and more responsibility, and that makes you a little uncomfortable." [Models.]

As in the case of practicing positive feedback, the clinician here continues the iterative process of modeling, rehearsal, feedback, coaching, and rehearsal until Roy demonstrates an approximation of the listening skill. Then, she switches roles and allows the father to speak while the daughter listens. Finally, she gives homework, the Communication Skills Assignment (Handout 14), to both of the participants. She instructs them to practice active listening with various persons in their daily lives, and to describe each instance on the homework sheet.

Active listening can be especially helpful in families including an adolescent. It is not unusual, however, for adolescents to say they find it annoying when their parents paraphrase them. It may remind them of the days when their parents took "Love and Logic" parenting classes. Worse yet, they may believe that their parents are trying to "one-up" them through using communication techniques that are more natural to parents than teens. Acknowledge to the adolescent that paraphrasing can indeed slow down communication and make ordinary conversations feel like therapy sessions. Nonetheless, remind them that this kind of collaboration, although perhaps forced and artificial at the beginning, will seem second nature as it becomes a part of the family's repertoire. I discuss resistance to CET in more detail in Chapter 10.

Making Positive Requests for Change in Another Family Member

The two remaining communication skills, making positive requests and expressing negative feelings about specific behaviors, address family conflicts related to the specific actions of one or more family members. Positive requests (e.g., "I would appreciate it if you would talk a little more softly") are considered the "first-line offense" in requesting behavior changes (Handout 15). Expressing negative feelings about specific behaviors (e.g., "It really makes me angry when you yell at me") is the last-line offense when positive requests have not achieved their desired effects.

It is easy to see how incorporating a skill like making positive requests might reduce the levels of tension and conflict in a family, particularly one dealing with an illness. Whereas criticisms (e.g., "I resent it that you stay out so late") are likely to generate defensiveness in other family members, stating requests in a more positive light (e.g., "It's very important to me that you come home at a reasonable time") tends to engender cooperativeness. Thus, positive requests offer family members a method for redirecting negatively escalating arguments, which tend to be common during the recovery period (see also Chapter 10).

There are two caveats to keep in mind when teaching positive requests. First, the request should be for another family member to *do*

Communication Skills Assignment

Day	Person you talked to	What you talked about	What positive feedback did you give?	What active listening skills did you use?	What positive requests for change did you make?
Mon					
Tue					
Wed					
Thu					
Fri					
Sat					
Sun					

Making a Positive Request

- Look at the person.
- Say exactly what you would like him or her to do.
- Tell him or her how it would make you feel.
- In making positive requests, use phrases like:
  - "I would like you to ___________."
  - "I would really appreciate it if you would do ___________."
  - "It's very important to me that you help me with the ___________."

HANDOUT 15. *Source*: Adapted by permission from Falloon et al. (1984).

something, rather than to stop doing something. That is, a positive request should not be a criticism in disguise. This distinction is not always easy to make, and you may be surprised at how defensive family members become when being asked to do something that sounds rather trivial. If this occurs, explore the emotional underpinnings of these reactions. Often, you will find that the positive request is tied in with a whole history of family conflicts. Nonetheless, you can help family members to make distinctions between these larger issues and the immediate, more specific requests that are being made of them.

Second, it is not essential that the target of the request agree to do what is being asked of him or her. This is particularly true when the target person is an adolescent, who may refuse simply because he or she is being asked! The request may be unrealistic or too difficult to perform during the postepisode period. So, once the family members have completed the positive request exercises, help them resolve any remaining disagreements using the problem-solving format (Chapter 11).

In the following vignette, the clinician has just passed out Handout 15 and introduces the skill:

> "Carol, what if Roy is doing something that you'd like to see him do differently, and you want to let him know without alienating him? Or, what if he can help you in some way—how can you ask him to do that? This next skill is called 'making a positive request.' As you can see in the handout, there are a couple of components to this skill—you look at a person, tell him or her what it is that you'd like him or her to do, and say how it would make you feel. Again, 'how it would make you feel' can vary anywhere from 'I would appreciate it if you would make dinner' to 'I would feel less anxious if you would call me when you've gotten home from work' or 'It would make things easier for me if you would clean up the living room.' Can you think of some times when you had to ask somebody to do something for you, and how you did it?"

The clinician has put the skill into the context of the patient's and family's day-to-day living. She reviews the skill components, and models different ways to use it. Then she elicits an example from the family that can be used to practice the skill.

CAROL: Well, the other day I asked Dad to stop coming over all the time. And he hasn't really honored that.

CLINICIAN: And how did you ask him?

ROY: It was something on the order of "Get out of here."

This topic is, of course, a high-risk one, because bipolar patients are particularly sensitive to issues of autonomy during the recovery phase, whereas family members become hypervigilant (Chapter 8). Nevertheless, the clinician views this example as a chance to support clearer interpersonal boundaries between these two family members, and uses it as the basis for a role-playing exercise. In this example, Carol becomes the speaker. The father is asked to use his active listening skills while she is speaking.

CLINICIAN: OK, let's work with that one. Carol, can you turn your chair toward your dad, and try to follow this sheet and say that same thing to him as a positive request? Roy, I want you just to follow the steps on your active listening sheet and listen—we'll get to the requests you want to make of Carol very soon.

CAROL: (*Pauses.*) OK, um, Dad, could you leave me alone more? That'd make my life much better.

ROY: (*defensively*) What do you mean, "Leave me alone"? I have no idea what you mean by that.

CLINICIAN: OK, Roy, what did you like or not like about what Carol said and how she said it? [Redirects, and elicits feedback.]

ROY: Well, it was better than what she actually said the other day, but I still found it insulting. The message that "my life would be better without you."

CLINICIAN: Well, Roy, I can understand that reaction on your part, although I suspect that's not how you meant it, Carol. [Validates father's perceptions but distinguishes them from the patient's intentions.]

CAROL: No, it's not at all! And this is one of the things we always fight about, he's so fatalistic about everything, and—

CLINICIAN: (*Interrupts.*) Let me stop you for a minute. I think it is sometimes hard to make the distinction between a positive request and a criticism. But I can think of another way to say the same thing that might be less offensive to your dad. For example, Carol, why is it that you want to be alone? [Coaches.]

CAROL: (*softly*) It's not that I don't enjoy his company . . . I do. But I'm a big girl, and I want to feel like my place is my own. If I knew when he was coming, that'd be much better, but as it is he just drops by and I'm in my bathrobe.

CLINICIAN: So, what you'd really like is for him to call and let you know he's coming over.

CAROL: Yeah! I actually like it when I know he's coming and I can clean the place up a bit.

At this point, the clinician has elicited the content of a positive request and the basis for the feeling statement. She then asks the dyad to role-play the interchange again.

CLINICIAN: OK, let's try it again. Carol, can you say to him what you just said to me?

CAROL: Dad, will you please call me before you're going to come over? That'd give me the chance to clean up first.

CLINICIAN: Good, Carol. And how would that make you feel? [Coaches.]

CAROL: I'd like it, and I'd probably feel grateful that you cared about me and what I need. It would also be nice to see you.

CLINICIAN: That was excellent. Roy, what did you think about what Carol just said?

ROY: Much better, easier to hear. And I might even do it (*laughs*)!

The clinician praises each of the participants for their efforts, and follows up this exercise with another in which the father practices the skill and the daughter listens. She then assigns homework: to practice this skill with persons inside and outside the family, and record one's efforts. The Communication Skills Assignment (Handout 14) can again be used for this purpose.

In the above vignettes, two goals have been accomplished. First, the participants have had the experience of practicing each skill from beginning to end. Second, they have had a taste of what it is like to have a higher-functioning relationship, which is its own reinforcer for the use of these skills.

Expressing Negative Feelings about Specific Behaviors

An exclusive focus on positive communication skills can leave family members with the impression that you do not recognize the realities they face on a day-to-day basis. They can begin to feel that life is being sugarcoated for them. It is one thing to try to maintain a low-EE, nonconfrontational atmosphere, but if another family member is consistently being unpleasant or annoying, how does one deal with this?

In many ways, expressing negative feelings is the most difficult skill to learn. Unlike the other skills, it involves delivering an unpleasant, negative message. Specifically, it is a way of telling another family member that he or she is acting in an unpleasant or distasteful manner. It offers family members a skill to use when making a positive request has been ineffective. Moreover, it is a useful segue into problem solving. Handout 16 lists the components of this skill.

Expressing Negative Feelings about Specific Behaviors

- Look at the person; speak firmly.
- Say exactly what he or she did that upset you.
- Tell him or her how it made you feel.
- Suggest how the person might prevent this from happening in the future.

HANDOUT 16. *Source*: Adapted by permission from Falloon et al. (1984).

In our experience, it is best to expose family members to this skill briefly (i.e., have them participate in one, or at most two, role plays each) and then move on. It is good to make family members aware of this communication strategy, even if they will rarely use it.

The clinician explains this skill to the family:

CLINICIAN: The final skill we want to expose you to is "expressing negative feelings about specific behaviors." It's not the same as telling someone off. It's a skill that's useful when someone is behaving in a way that bothers you, and you want him or her to stop and do things differently. How do you let someone know he or she is hurting your feelings?

As listed in the handout, the first thing you do is look directly at the person you're speaking to, say exactly what he or she did that upset you and how it made you feel, and suggest a way he or she could prevent it from happening in the future. For example, if a neighbor was playing his CD player too loudly, and you'd been unsuccessful in getting him to stop by using positive requests, what would you say?

ROY: (*Grins.*) Turn down the stereo or I'll come by with my shotgun.

CLINICIAN: Well, that might work. I had something a little less direct in mind, like "Your loud CD player is really starting to bother me, and I've asked you to turn it down before. I think you're not taking this very seriously. Let's talk about what we can do to keep us from having this discussion over and over again." Then, if he's cooperative, you might discuss with him what could be done—could he play it only when your car's not in the driveway? Could he play it lower after a certain hour?

The clinician models the skill. She makes it more palatable to family members by using an example involving a neighbor. This example helps alleviate a participant's concern that he or she will become the primary target of these negative messages.

In the following vignette, Gary, a married patient with bipolar disorder, had complained that his wife, Ellen, who had promised to meet him at the end of a bicycle race with food and water, had not shown up. The two began an argument that had spiraled into a rather unproductive debate about the expectations each held of the other. Rather than putting Ellen on the hot seat, one of the two clinicians treating this couple acted as the recipient of Gary's negative feedback, while the other clinician coached.

CLINICIAN 1: Gary, would you go over again what bothered you, only follow these steps on the handout involving expressing a negative feeling? Pretend Wendy [cotherapist] is your wife and look at her and say what it was that Ellen did that displeased you, how it made you feel, and what you would like her to do in the future. Try to be as specific as you can.

GARY: Well, Ellen, I was really hurting at the end of that race, I was waiting for water or something. I was mad because, just like last time, you weren't there at the end.

CLINICIAN 1: OK. Wendy, how did you feel being the receiver of that? [Solicits feedback.]

CLINICIAN 2: Well, you told me what I did wrong, and how you felt about it, but I wasn't sure what you wanted me to do in the future. [Coaches.]

CLINICIAN 1: Good suggestion. What could Ellen do in the future?

GARY: Well, any number of things, like come earlier, or get there at the same time as me.

CLINICIAN 1: OK, could you try it again, only this time say it directly to Ellen [involves spouse at this point], and try to get in all the components, including what she could do differently?

GARY: OK, Ellen, I was really hurting at the end of that race, I was waiting for water, and you never arrived. Do you think you could get there earlier next time and wait till I get to the finish line?

CLINICIAN 1: Good. Ellen, what was your reaction to hearing that? Was it useful feedback?

ELLEN: Yeah, that was better. To be honest, even though I got defensive before, I felt kinda bad about leaving him hanging like that.

The introduction of this skill helps you to transition to the final FFT module, problem-solving skills training. For example, this couple might have worked toward generating a quid pro quo agreement whereby, if the wife is considerate of her husband when he has a bicycle race, he agrees to do a special favor for her in return.

Handout 17, the Expressing Negative Feelings assignment, is given to family members once each member has had a chance to practice the skill. Again, ask family members to practice the skill in the upcoming week and record their efforts on the form. Family members should not look for or try to artificially generate examples of negative feelings to record on their sheets, but rather should rely on spontaneous instances during the week in which they were able to apply the skill with persons inside or outside the family.

Expressing Negative Feelings about Specific Behaviors Assignment

Day	Person who displeased you	What exactly did he or she do that displeased you?	How did you feel (angry, sad, etc.)?	What did you ask him or her to do in the future?
Mon				
Tue				
Wed				
Thu				
Fri				
Sat				
Sun				

HANDOUT 17. *Source*: Adapted by permission from Falloon et al. (1984).

Concluding Comments

The postepisode phases of bipolar disorder can have a strong impact on the functioning of the family unit, particularly its abilities to communicate productively and solve problems. Even families or couples that formerly communicated well have setbacks brought about by illness in one family member. However, if family members are able to employ communication skills in the face of life stress, they will create a milieu during the stabilization and maintenance periods that may speed up the patient's recovery and protect against recurrences of bipolar disorder.

The next chapter addresses how CET can be used to make changes in basic relational processes. As you will see, CET is most successful when it is applied with a "psychotherapeutic attitude," with an eye toward identifying and altering disordered patterns of interaction between family members.

chapter 10

Communication Enhancement Training

Clinical Issues

Mary Lou and Stephen had been married for 12 years, but Mary Lou had had her first manic episode only recently. The functional assessment and the psychoeducation module revealed a distressed marriage. In particular, Mary Lou admitted to having had a "one-night stand" during the height of her manic episode, when she impulsively drove to a city 200 miles away and seduced a man she met randomly in a bar. Stephen was understandably quite angry, resentful, and distrustful of her following this event.

The clinician noted that the partners rarely spoke directly to each other, preferring to address the clinician even on matters that clearly concerned the other partner. Moreover, when they did talk about emotionally laden matters, their discussions frequently escalated into "partner bashing" or explosive conflicts that did much damage. Mary Lou, guilt-ridden and angry, would complain that Stephen had become controlling and intrusive, and Stephen would counter that she was torturing him and eliciting this behavior from him. They were talking about separating.

CET introduced the couple to two skills: delivering positive feedback and active, reflective listening. At first, the couple was quite resistant, arguing that role playing was artificial and that they couldn't imagine talking this way in real life. But as they continued to participate in these exercises, each partner did admit to feeling more validated by the other. Occasional, spontaneous positive interchanges began to emerge. After the fifth session of CET, the couple noted that they were spending more time at home together and talking more. The avoidance of direct partner-to-partner communication observed in the early sessions had begun to wane.

Chapter Overview

CET is perhaps the most direct way to effect changes in the role relationships, dynamics, and transaction patterns of families including a bipolar person. When family members learn communication skills, their relationships change. However, in order to bring about maximal change in the family system, keep three therapeutic objectives in mind.

First, conduct role-play exercises in a careful and clinically intuitive manner. Like the resistances to psychoeducation, resistances to skill training are quite common. This chapter offers some suggestions for guiding the role-play exercises so that the therapeutic milieu is most conducive to learning.

Second, encourage the generalization of new skills beyond the treatment sessions. Many families of bipolar patients simply come to sessions and "perform" for you, and neglect to use the skills once they return home. Fortunately, there are a number of therapeutic maneuvers to encourage generalization, as described here.

Third, adjust the skill training to address each family's preexisting structure, hierarchy, and transaction patterns. An example was given in the previous chapter, where placing Carol (the patient) more frequently in the speaker role and Roy (her father) in the listener role created a more egalitarian power balance between the two.

I describe here some of the common transaction patterns we observe among families of bipolar patients during the recovery period, and how to individualize CET to address each pattern. Specifically, CET is implemented differently for families for whom conflict brews quickly and escalates ("short-fuse" families) than for those who avoid conflict altogether, or those who show the well-known "pursuer–distancing" pattern.

The Clinical Handling of Communication Enhancement Exercises

Keep in mind the ways in which bipolar patients and their families naturally communicate with each other, and how these styles may differ from those of other populations. Bipolar patients—particularly those who are always somewhat hypomanic, even between episodes—and their families often value spontaneity, humor, a degree of chaos, unbridled emotional expression, and fast-paced interactions. However, their interactions sometimes spiral into uncontrolled partner bashing or negatively escalating conflicts. Depressed patients, in contrast, often have difficulty in engaging with their family members, and frequently become the target of pursuer–distancing transactions. These transaction styles can become troublesome when you are teaching new communication skills: How can the family of a hypomanic patient maintain this sense of spontaneity but also learn to communicate in more productive ways? How can the family of a depressed patient achieve a proper balance between engagement and disengagement? Here, I describe the clinical principles for handling role-play exercises that can help address these resistances or styles of communication.

First, always keep in mind that family members should not be forced into doing anything they do not wish to do. Sometimes participants have had bad experiences with role playing (e.g., through high school acting classes or psychodrama) or simply feel uncomfortable with being put on the hot seat. Adolescents are particularly likely to refuse, and often don't give a reason. If a participant initially declines to role-play, encourage him or her once or twice ("Would you be willing to try it just one time?") or remind him or her that role playing, although awkward, is the best way to learn new communication skills. However, it is best not to push further. Try again during the next session after other members have tried it, at which point the participant may be more willing to comply.

Second, use your clinical skills to determine what level of stress each participant, and the family, can tolerate. Who should talk to whom? For example, if two parents and a patient are present, it may be safer to begin role playing with a dyad containing members who are already comfortably allied before moving to dyads in which there is much distancing and tension. What are appropriate topics to guide the role-play exercises? Early on, encourage the family to choose topics that are meaningful and not artificial (e.g., issues regarding care of the household, work, or time management), but that are not too emotionally laden.

Although conflictual, "hot" topics may appear most germane to the conduct of family sessions, they are not usually the best context for learning new communication skills. It is difficult to learn anything when one is defensive or upset. Thus, whether a couple should get a divorce and whether the patient's illness has ruined the family's financial stability are usually topics that are too emotionally charged for communication exercises. Wait until some degree of competence in a given skill has been attained, and then move on to more charged topics, either in further communication exercises or during the problem-solving module.

Third, learn to "head off at the pass" potentially destructive discussions that escalate. Occasionally, as was exemplified in Chapter 9, participants naturally segue from neutral topics to more conflictual ones. Participants may think that discussing these conflictual topics is what is expected of them, and that they are being better clients if they bring them up. Alternatively, they may be sidetracking themselves from the role-playing tasks in order to avoid the discomfort of communicating in a less familiar manner. You can redirect the communication exercises by interrupting emotionally charged discussions before they escalate. For example, you can say, "That is, of course, an important issue. We may want to get into this later, but how about something more immediate? We'll be better able to help you with that issue once you've learned some different ways to communicate."

A caveat, of course, is that sometimes one must depart from the skill training when participants react strongly to the issues raised during these exercises. Not all issues can be dealt with through role playing. For example, if a participant starts to cry or seems too angry to continue, it is best to stop the exercise and explore the nature of this participant's reactions. Once again, you can normalize the participant's reactions as reflecting a part of the recovery process (e.g., "I can understand why this is so upsetting to you. Given all that has happened, I imagine it is frightening to get back into these issues and talk with each other intimately again"). In families with adolescents or young children, it can be useful to take a 5-minute break when this happens.

Fourth, CET works best when you take an observing stance, with a focus on the "process" rather than the "content," or on the "hows" rather than the "whats" of communication. Keep the participants from being too content-focused. Sometimes, the content is so riveting or affectively charged that it takes over the attention of the participants and the clinician as well. In the role play between Roy and Carol (Chapter 9), it became difficult for Roy to depart from the content (his belief that she should switch jobs) long enough to examine his style of speaking and listening. When this happens, participants become confused about whether they are being asked to learn a communication skill or solve a specific problem. Refocus the discussion by saying, "I don't want to get us too far into trying to solve this problem—let's try to stick with learning this skill first, and then maybe later we can deal with the problem in more depth."

Fifth, when two family members are role playing, deal dyadically with the person learning the skill, rather than trying to structure the communication of two persons at once. For example, if you are training a speaker to use positive requests and the listener becomes defensive, refocus the exercise on the speaker. Say to the listener, "Your reactions to this are quite important. But first I want to help ____________ with how best to say this to you."

Sixth, when dealing directly with a speaker, it is best to keep him or her from going on too long or discussing several topics at once. The communication of the families of bipolar patients can become quite disorganized when structure is absent (Miklowitz et al., 1991). Thus, it is best to encourage in the speaker (whether a patient or a relative) a degree of succinctness, perhaps by asking him or her to break down statements into small chunks. For example, say to him or her, "I'm a little slow today. Could you say the first part of that again so I can follow along with the rest of you?" or "We're talking about several issues at once here. Let's hold on these others and stick with the first one."

Seventh, when dealing with families that seem to enjoy spontaneous, unbridled interchanges, dispense with the communication handout sheets. You can introduce such a family to the handouts when first describing the skill, and then take them away when the family begins to role-play. Prompting and coaching can still be offered verbally without any reference to the visual aids. Families with younger patients seem to do better without the handouts, preferring to adapt the skills to their spontaneous interchanges.

Finally, it is important to praise participants regularly. Emphasize even small steps toward the appropriate goal ("shaping"). Likewise, joke with family members when they are participating in these tasks, especially when things go awry (e.g., "I guess we're all talking about different things at the same time. Did I accidentally give you my shopping list instead of the handout?" or "My head is spinning and I'm having trouble following you. Maybe I need to work on my listening skills"). The skill training can be enjoyable for family members when it is conducted in a nonevaluative, friendly atmosphere.

Problems in the Generalization of Skills

It is one thing for families to agree to role plays and to show mastery of the skills in treatment sessions. However, it takes a great deal of motivation on their part, as well as careful planning and intervention on your part, to ensure that these skills go beyond the session room ("generalization"). Nongeneralization is usually reflected in incomplete homework assignments and/or statements in which participants admit they are not using the skills, even though they report instances during the week when to do so would have been to their benefit.

Your first task is to explore with the participants why the skills are not generalizing. Any number of issues may be in force: Is the patient too symptomatic to practice the skills? Did the participants misunderstand the rationale for the skill training? Do they not agree with this rationale? Could they not find a time to talk? Were the topics they chose to talk about too hot, and family members too angry, to make it safe to practice the skills? Do the participants not trust other family members to use the skills even if they (the participants) do?

The Performing Family

In our experience, a harbinger of nongeneralization is the family that appears to be "performing" during the communication exercises. Such families may be quite verbal and spontaneous in their ordinary interchanges, but once they begin role playing they show little emotion, stare at their handout sheets, say exactly what the sheets tell them to say, and then turn to the clinician as if to ask, "Did we do that right?" These families report, "We can do these things just fine here, but as soon as you're gone, things go back to the way they were." If you are treating such a family, you may feel that the role plays are phony or artificial, and do not fit in with the family's natural communication styles.

In part, the role-play exercises do require that people perform. The new skills are usually unnatural or uncomfortable for families or couples at first, and the participants appear to be going through the motions. In fact, we anticipate these reactions by using the new shoes analogy (see Chapter 9). However, most families become more comfortable with using the skills over time. If family members continue to approach the exercises in a superficial manner despite repeated practice sessions, then address the issues underlying their reactions.

In our experience, one of the following themes is usually operating: (1) The participants simply do not believe that employing the skills will in any way benefit them or their family; or (2) they are sitting on a great deal of conflict that could erupt at any moment, and their artificial communication during role plays protects them from confronting these issues (see "The Avoidant Family," below).

In the following vignette, Stephen and Mary Lou had just done an active listening exercise concerning the issue of how to keep the house clean. The clinician finds himself bored by the exercise, and Stephen and Mary Lou seem bored themselves. His first step in addressing this issue is simply to observe that the participants seem to be performing. Then, he explores the bases of this behavior before resuming the skill-training exercises.

CLINICIAN: OK, that was good, you were using the skills quite appropriately. But let me check something out with you. You both seemed as if you were just going through the motions, or just doing this for me. You seemed as if you were bored or thought this was silly. Am I right, or is this a misperception on my part?

STEPHEN: No, you're right. It does seem silly. We don't talk to each other this way. (*Laughs derisively.*) It sounds like the way therapists talk. But I can't imagine doing this at home.

CLINICIAN: What seems silly about it?

STEPHEN: It just seems artificial, like we're talking as if we're in a play or something.

CLINICIAN: Well, to some extent I am asking you to try some new things that are foreign to you. It may be a little like acting or performing, but it gives you some real life experience with these new ways of talking with each other. Eventually, of course, you'll want to adapt them to your own natural styles. But I can understand how they might seem forced.

STEPHEN: Yeah.

CLINICIAN: But let me check out something else with you. Are there any other issues or conflicts you're dealing with here that you're afraid will come out if we get into this training any further?

STEPHEN: Well, you know, we have our issues just like any other married couple. But I just can't see how this can help us if we feel awkward talking this way.

CLINICIAN: I'm sure it will feel awkward at first, but there is the possibility that the skills will become second nature if you keep trying them. Using them may lead to some real changes in your marriage. In fact, in some couples, people at first feel silly when they use these skills, and their spouses may even agree they sound silly. Yet a spouse may become more cooperative and more willing to do what he or she is being asked to do. Once this happens, then of course you can use more telegraphic ways of making your needs known.

The clinician empathizes with the participants' feelings about the discomfort of communicating differently, and revisits the purposes and goals of CET. Specifically, he makes clear that practicing the skills tends to bring about changes in the reactions of other family members, which in turn may allow the participants to talk more naturally and openly in the future. In fact, a goal of CET is to encourage family members to incorporate these rather foreign ways of communicating into their day-to-day, spontaneous dialogues.

The Family with Time-Budgeting Problems

Some families report being unable to find the time to practice the skills between sessions. Whereas in some cases this reflects a resistance to the communication tasks, in others it reflects a real problem in arranging schedules so that one member of the family can talk to another.

We have found that a three-pronged approach is useful in addressing this problem. First, validate the problem, empathizing with the difficulties one could have in finding time to complete assigned homework. Second, explore whether other issues interfere with finding time (e.g., is it because the communication tasks are difficult, unpleasant, or tension producing? Are there too many interruptions at home?). Third, encourage the family to schedule a *family* meeting: a half- to 1-hour time block during the week in which members practice the skills and complete the homework sheets. Help them to agree on the time of this meeting, and check with them in the next session to determine if it has occurred. Even this limited period of weekly practice will help the skills to generalize to the home setting.

The Family with Only One Cooperative Member

Among the families of bipolar patients, it is not unusual for one family member to complain that the skills simply "don't work." Upon exploration, you may find that this is because one member of the family is using the skills (and completing homework) and others are not. This one member may complain that he or she offers positive feedback to other members but these others do not do so in return, that he or she listens when others talk but no one returns the favor, or that the partner becomes angry and uncooperative when negative feedback is delivered in the suggested constructive manner.

One way to think of this problem is that it reflects processes within the family system as a whole. Does the one family member who cooperates represent the part of the family that wants to grow, whereas the others represent its desire to remain stable? If so, how is each member of the family contributing to this process? Are family members expressing hostility by not responding to each other's communication attempts? If so, are they seeking revenge for the times when they tried to make things different and other family members ignored *them?* You can explore and clarify these family dynamics by posing questions like "Why do you think your family is operating this way? Is this a common pattern, that Mom tries to do things differently and everybody else just stays the same?"

In some cases, the real issue may be the stability of the patient's disorder. Consider the following case of a family in which a parent used the skills but the patient, because of an unresolved clinical condition, did not.

The family consisted of a mother (Susan) and her son (Earl), who was recovering from a manic episode. During the CET module, Earl had been quite depressed and often unable to get out of bed. Susan began using the

Positive Request handout to get him up in the morning (i.e., "I'd appreciate it if you'd get up now and help me get breakfast ready"). However, she complained, rather bitterly, that he was not responding to her positive requests. Not only did he not get out of bed, but he consistently failed even to acknowledge that she was speaking to him. She therefore began to reject the communication enhancement approach.

The clinician began by praising Susan for her attempts to communicate differently with Earl. She also pointed to the various attempts made by Earl to improve his life condition: He had been looking at job listings, he had made an appointment to see a job counselor, he was taking his medications, and he had made some small attempts to talk with his mother in a more civil manner. However, the solution to this problem required a quid pro quo. First, Susan was to understand that Earl was still deeply depressed and was probably unable—at least for now—to communicate with her in the way she wanted. Second, Earl agreed to try to talk with his mother more frequently, and at least to acknowledge her attempts to use the skills, even if he could not use them himself. This agreement was aided by the scheduling of a half-hour weekly family meeting, in which they practiced the skills on fairly neutral, nonconflictual topics.

In this case, the clinician had to determine whether the son was being oppositional or was simply too ill to follow the skill-training procedures. She decided it best to let the patient off the hook until the symptoms had abated further and he was better able to engage with his mother verbally. Nevertheless, encouraging him to take small steps in her direction helped to unfreeze the situation and convince his mother to continue using the skills.

In other cases, the issue is that one family member is using the skills incorrectly, and other family members are becoming annoyed with or avoidant of him or her. In clarifying this possibility, it is best to have the participants replay a verbal interchange from the prior week, choosing an instance in which the cooperative participant complained of the lack of responsiveness of other family members.

CLINICIAN: So what kind of positive request did you make of Stephen? Can you replay it for us now?

MARY LOU: I said, "Look, if you're going to be sullen, could you do it in another room? I'd really appreciate you're not bringing me down any more than I am already."

Stephen's uncooperativeness becomes more understandable when one considers this kind of interchange. The clinician uses this example as an opportunity to coach them both on the delivery of positive requests, and encourages a weekly family meeting in which the partners practice this skill.

The Clinician's Countertransference

Sometimes the problem of nongeneralization can be traced to the clinician. If you feel uncomfortable teaching the skills, childish or awkward when conducting the role plays, or believe that the family's core issues are not being addressed, you may be implicitly communicating to the family members that they should give the homework tasks low priority.

We have experienced these reactions ourselves, and favor asking oneself the following questions. First, is this a general reaction I have to the treatment approach? Do I disagree with this way of working with families? If the answer is yes, you may wish to receive outside supervision or consultation, especially if your personal reactions begin to interfere with implementing CET. In addition, reacquaint yourself with the rationale for the skill-training module: to open up lines of communication, alter patterns of interaction, and create a lower-stress environment for the patient and other family members. Sometimes this is best done through a structured, didactic task format, which, although seemingly superficial, often accomplishes the same goals accomplished by other, more traditional family therapy techniques (e.g., encouraging two family members to sit closer together, reframing dysfunctional interaction patterns).

Alternatively, ask yourself, Are my reactions mirroring processes within the family? That is, am I bored because the family is strongly guarding against certain emotional conflicts, and as a result communicates in a rather stilted manner? Does it feel awkward to ask participants to compliment each other because these participants have trouble establishing intimacy? Do I feel removed because members of the family are removed from each other?

The answers to any of these questions, of course, are grist for the mill for your work with the family. These questions can be explored with the participants with the objective of identifying the unspoken issues (e.g., "You know, I'm feeling a bit awkward, as if we're sitting on something today. Maybe this is just my imagination. But is there anything going on today that makes you want to avoid talking with each other more directly?"). Sometimes self-disclosures of this kind lead to open family discussions of conflicts that otherwise would not have surfaced, but that may be essential to understanding the participants' difficulties in learning new communication skills.

Using CET to Modify Family Dynamics

How does simply asking two members of a family to turn their chairs toward each other and talk change the basic structure or functional dynamics of a family? In our view, these simple tasks have the effect of throwing a monkey wrench into the family's existing transaction patterns, leading to small changes that become bigger changes over time. These changes can occur even if only one member of the family alters the way he or she communicates.

In family systems language, CET introduces "first-order changes," those temporary alterations in family dynamics that are balanced out by the family's homeostatic (stability-maintaining) forces. However, repeated introduction of first-order changes can lead to second-order changes and growth, those more permanent alterations in the rules of the system or the interrelationships between different members.

In this section, I give examples of how CET can be employed to alter the family's preexisting dynamics. I describe three types of family systems problems we have encountered among the families of bipolar patients and discuss how CET can be used to modify these problems. These are exemplified by the *short-fuse family, the avoidant family,* and *the pursuer–distancing family.*

The Short-Fuse Family

Perhaps the most difficult family is one that has explosive patterns of interaction that interfere with meaningful communication. Such families have frequent negative escalation cycles, in which seemingly innocuous interchanges burgeon into angry back-and-forth debates that escalate in severity. These point–counterpoint volleys can be quite destructive to the family atmosphere and to individuals within the unit. In fact, negative escalation tends to destroy participants' motivations to learn new communication skills, because they think, "Why should I talk to him this way? He'll argue with me no matter what I do!"

Short fuses are quite common among families coping with bipolar disorder or schizophrenia (Hahlweg et al., 1989; Simoneau et al., 1998), notably in families of younger patients (Miklowitz et al., 2006). One way to understand this pattern is to think in terms of homeostatic mechanisms that are interrupted by the illness process. Every family has rules for how it operates, such as unspoken agreements as to who speaks to whom, how often and in what tone, or how close various members can get to each other. When one family member develops an illness, the family's rule structure becomes disorganized and unpredictable, and stress and conflict reach a maximum. Then, when the illness abates, family members try to restore their traditional styles of relating. But if the patient is still symptomatic during the postepisode period (e.g., highly irritable), he or she has different needs and correspondingly communicates quite differently. As a result, the old methods of relating do not work any more, and escalating conflicts result.

Family members' resistances to participating in CET exercises sometimes reflect their beliefs that the exercises will cause their communication to spiral negatively. Underneath these worries may be fears that they will be forced into sharing an intimacy that they find threatening. In fact, CET does encourage greater connectedness between family members, and one of its side effects is that it can ignite underlying conflicts. Certainly, you can make a significant impact on the short-fuse family through CET, but keep open to the possibility that close communication between members of a particular family dyad may be too difficult during the recovery phase.

Negative escalation can occur at any time. A basic tenet is to cut off the argument before it gets out of hand. In the words of the late Johnny Carson, "Never lose control of the show." There are several ways to retain control without alienating the family, as described in Table 10.1 and in the vignettes below.

The first step in changing this dynamic is to help the participants to be aware of when it is occurring. Consider the following vignette, again involving our couple, Mary Lou and Stephen. An issue that had surfaced earlier was Mary Lou's hypersexuality during her manic episode, which had included one tryst with an anonymous man. As she swung into a depressive episode, she became quite guilt-ridden about having done this, but also believed that Stephen was unrelentingly punishing her for it.

MARY LOU: And then as soon as I got home from work, he was on me. "Did you flirt with that guy at work? Did you talk to him?" And I don't even care about that guy.

STEPHEN: That's not true. And besides, why shouldn't I be able to raise that issue if it bothers me? It's not only your feelings that are important here.

MARY LOU: But it's always the same thing with you! You don't give people enough room!

TABLE 10.1. Interventions for Restructuring Negative Escalation Cycles in "Short-Fuse" Families

- Make a "process comment" to identify that a cycle has begun.
- Explore themes underlying the escalating argument.
- Reframe or comment on the reward value of the interchange.
- Use CET to restructure the interchange.
- Teach family members to ask for a "time-out."

STEPHEN: And you expect the world to revolve around you and your needs.

CLINICIAN: OK, let's call a halt to this. This is a pattern we've seen many times before, where one of you starts an argument, and the other continues it, and it just takes off and becomes explosive. Do you want to be doing this right now? Let's give each other permission to call it quits.

So far, the clinician has identified the pattern as it is occurring. He makes a *process comment,* a first step in redirecting the discussion toward the underlying emotions or beliefs that motivate this argument. Why do they react to each other so negatively? Are they expressing long-standing resentments in their relationship, or are their reactions unique to the recent period of illness and the raw emotions that have resulted from it?

CLINICIAN: Let's freeze this moment in time—what was happening just now and how did you get back into that old pattern?

MARY LOU: Same old stuff. No one respects my privacy. It's been that way all my life, starting with my parents. And now it's him who can't leave me alone.

CLINICIAN: Stephen, what was happening for you?

STEPHEN: Well, it's just that when I try to find out what's going on with her, she just bites my head off, even when I have good intentions. She seems to think that keeping everything to herself will make us get along better or something.

Here, the clinician begins to clarify the issues underlying the explosion: Mary Lou's need for boundaries, combined with her angry attempts to assert her independence; and Stephen's lack of trust and corresponding desire to cut through her secrecy. However, rather than getting into a historical examination of these relational processes, the clinician next *summarizes* this couple's communication patterns and *reframes* them.

CLINICIAN: You know, all families get into habitual patterns of communicating. So let me see if I can summarize the pattern you've shown here. The two of you start by discussing some fairly neutral topic, and then a button gets pushed, making you, Mary Lou, feel like your space is being invaded, and you, Stephen, feel like she's getting unnecessarily defensive and is trying to hurt you, even though you want to help. [Explores themes underlying the escalating argument.] (*Stephen nods.*) I know this has been going on for a long time. In some ways, it's probably very hard to impose a new way of communicating on this very old and familiar pattern.

MARY LOU: It's always been this way.

CLINICIAN: Tell me, is there anything good about communicating this way? Anything positive about it that would make it hard to give up? You've been doing it for a long time, so I imagine it must have some pluses. [Comments on the possible reward value of the interchange.]

MARY LOU: (*After long pause, chuckles.*) Well, neither one of us is exactly shy.

CLINICIAN: I think you're onto something there, Mary Lou. It's not *all* bad. At least the two of you get things out in the open, and neither of you is afraid to express your feelings. [Reframes.] But is it possible that in reacting to each other this way you're missing out on some other, more productive ways to talk that might make things less tense?

The effect of reframing is to relax the couple and encourage them to think of their interactional styles as having both positive and negative attributes. This opens the door for a discussion of how the couple can use communication skills to interrupt these cycles.

There are three communication skills that can be useful in helping family members to restructure negative escalation cycles. One is to encourage members to use active listening before responding to another member's statements (e.g., "Could you try to paraphrase what he just said, and then give your response?"). In addition to disarming the speaker, active listening allows family members to test for themselves their assumptions that the next statement from the speaker, no matter what has transpired, will be another criticism. It tends to build a sense of collaboration among members of a family or couple.

However, family members cannot always use active listening skills at these tense moments. To do so, they feel, means giving up ground to the other partner. In these cases, you may instead recommend a second option, using *time-out* (asking for space, escaping the unpleasant situation).

CLINICIAN: Let me ask you something. When you're in the midst of one of these arguments, can you imagine how you might use your listening skills to keep things from spiraling like they do?

MARY LOU: In theory, yes. I could've stopped and said back to him what he said, like you've been telling us. But it's very hard to do that when you're angry.

CLINICIAN: It certainly is. On the other hand, that very suggestion you just came up with would have helped a great deal. What about taking a time-out, would that have been easier?

STEPHEN: (*ruefully*) Well, we do that with Carrie [daughter] when *she* throws tantrums.

CLINICIAN: Well, I was actually thinking more about the kind of time-outs that football teams take. I mean, for example, saying to each other, "I'm getting really angry right now, and I want to be by myself until I cool down." [Models.]

The clinician then asks the participants to practice asking each other for a time-out. Often, this requires negotiation. For example, one member of the dyad may become anxious when the other partner asks to withdraw in this way, and may need an assurance that "we'll talk about this and resolve it later" or "this is important to me, but right now I can't deal with it."

Third, once family members have cooled down, encourage them to give each other positive feedback, however minimal. Later in this same session, this couple shows signs of relaxing. The clinician praises them for their efforts in the session and encourages them to end on a positive note by praising each other.

CLINICIAN: Well, you both worked very hard today. I'm impressed with your willingness to work through these things with each other. [Models giving positive feedback.] Is there anything positive you'd like to say to each other now to make peace?

STEPHEN: (*Laughs.*) Aw, no, not now!

CLINICIAN: Yup. We've got 5 minutes to go—it's not enough time for an argument, but it is enough time for another communication exercise.

MARY LOU: (*Thinks.*) OK, I've got one. Uh, Steve, I know I get on your case sometimes, but I never really told you that I appreciated the fact that you came to see me in the hospital every day when I was locked up in there. That made me feel a lot less lonely, and that you still cared about me despite all that's happened between us, and you know that it wasn't easy being in there with all those people.

STEPHEN: (*surprised*) Thanks. You never said that before.

The introduction of positive feedback at the end of a negative communication sequence significantly reduces tensions and tends to make family members feel that the discussions have been productive and even brought them closer together. However, the participants may be unable to do this after a heated argument, and it is usually best to observe the limits they set. Instead, suggest a family meeting later in the week, in which the participants practice expressing positive feelings in the home setting.

The Avoidant Family

In contrast to the short-fuse family, you may encounter the avoidant family, in which family members appear afraid to talk to each other. Their interchanges, those occurring during as well as outside the role-play exercises, are usually quite brief and seem "dead" and empty of content. Certain family members talk to each other and others do not. These families look different from "performing" families, who may communicate quite actively and spontaneously when no structure is imposed, but become self-conscious when asked to role-play.

The avoidant family is usually sitting on a mountain of conflict. It has adopted the defensive style of communicating in a stilted fashion, or avoiding communication altogether, as a way of preventing the introduction of painful, destructive, long-standing disagreements. Examples of these conflicts include marital infidelities, instances of abuse or violence, hidden alcohol or drug problems, histories of serious financial indiscretions, unacknowledged mental illness, and other problems.

Sometimes you will find that the core issue in avoidant families is a fear of precipitating a recurrence of the patient's disorder. In fact, the patient may be implicitly communicating that he or she will become depressed or manic if family members communicate openly and directly. If you sense this is an issue, and continue to feel that the patient is strong enough to handle open communication, then return to a psychoeducational stance and reassure the family members of the value of direct, honest family discussions. Help them make a distinction between being "open and direct" versus "conflictual and abusive," or between "keeping a low-stress family atmosphere" and "not talking." If you can carefully guide them through a single communication exercise in which a family problem is discussed productively, you will help assuage their fears about provoking symptoms of the disorder.

When treating an avoidant family, remember that the goal is not to resolve the underlying conflicts at the moment, but to give the family members the skills to address them when they feel ready. If you have only a limited time to work with the family, it is unlikely that opening up these deeper conflicts and examining them in an unstructured way will be productive. Nevertheless, you can give the family the hope that the issues can be resolved after the treatment has been completed, either with you or with another consultant.

The first step in treating the avoidant family is to obtain an assessment of why this avoidance occurs. In some cases, it may be wise to interview various family members alone. For example, why do the parents not talk to each other? Why does the patient focus everything on him- or herself? What is the function of the suppression of feelings, and why is it unsafe to reveal one's emotional world? Is covering up a good thing to do in this family climate?

Consider the case of a family in which neither parent talked to the other. The offspring was a 27-year-old woman, Laurie, who had had several manic and depressive episodes. This family was reluctant to participate in any of the CET exercises. The daughter appeared to be rescuing her parents by doing most of the talking and focusing the session content on herself. When the mother was asked to give positive feedback to the father, Dan, she gave a very terse, off-handed compliment ("I like your new briefcase"). The remaining attempts at role playing seemed flat, with "poverty of content."

CLINICIAN: I'm noticing that Laurie is doing most of the talking, and nobody else is saying anything. What's going on?

DAN: (*after long pause*) I don't really like to talk about my feelings. Laurie should quit trying to get me to talk.

CLINICIAN: Can you say more about what happens when the three of you try to talk?

LAURIE: Not much action here! Just a lot of looking and silence.

CLINICIAN: Any ideas about why that is?

LAURIE: No. Just always been that way.

CLINICIAN: Well, would you be willing to try something different now?

DAN: We can try, but I can't see that we're going to talk much more than we do now.

CLINICIAN: I don't necessarily think you should talk more. But I do think you might be able to increase how effective your communication is. Would this be good to try?

The clinician does not feel that the family is able to discuss the emotional conflicts that may be causing the avoidance behavior. Instead, she obtains an initial (albeit noncommittal) agreement from the family to work on its communication, and begins by working with the less conflictual dyads (mother–daughter and father–daughter). She reserves judgment about working directly with the mother–father dyad: The patient had not at this point indicated that her parents' relationship was a problem for her. So, the clinician first asks the mother to observe and offer feedback to the father–daughter pair as they practice the positive feedback and active listening skills.

CLINICIAN: Why don't we start with something positive? Last week we began talking about giving positive feedback to each other. Dan, was there a time in the last week when you appreciated something Laurie did?

DAN: (*after pause*) OK, she swept out the garage and fed the birds.

CLINICIAN: Good. Can you turn to her and tell her what she did and what you liked about it?

As this dyad becomes more comfortable with role playing, the clinician moves to the mother–daughter dyad. Each role play is balanced in such a way that both members of the dyad alternatingly serve as speaker and listener. This plan keeps the patient from constantly taking the hot seat.

In the continuing communication work with this family, it was necessary to move quite slowly. The clinician also decided it best to dispense with the handout sheets, which were adding a level of formality to this family's interchanges that was already present to excess. When the parents finally took turns talking with each other, the clinician chose very neutral topics (e.g., the father's business activity, the mother's horseback-riding lessons) and focused on active listening exercises. She avoided the "expressing negative" feelings skill altogether.

Avoidant families that have been approached in this careful manner often say that the communication training was the most helpful component of the FFT. Even though one's work with such families may not appear to be addressing the primary issues, there is often real change occurring owing to the strategy of opening up new lines of communication.

The "Pursuer–Distancing" Family

In Chapter 9, I described a "domineering parent" scenario in which a father (Roy) did most of the talking and advice giving, and Carol (the patient) would "shut down" whenever he spoke. This power imbalance commonly occurs in families, but if left unchecked, it can evolve into a "pursuer–distancing" relational process. This is especially likely if the weaker member of the dyad is depressed or otherwise low in functioning.

Consider the case of William, the 21-year-old man discussed throughout Chapter 6. His mother, Alyssia, was overprotective or at least prone to "overmonitoring." She dominated the sessions with her concerns about his well-being and a tendency to "psychoanalyze" him (his words). When she was asked to give William positive feedback, she went on at length about "how wonderful you are" and "you know I love you very much, but I know you're dealing with some issues that you should talk with me about." The more she spoke, the more difficulty William had in listening. When asked to paraphrase her, he gave quick sound bites (e.g., "You're worried about me again") but refused to look at her. His paraphrasing became even less frequent as she spoke more. This shutting down was punishing to her, and she reacted by anxiously and angrily increasing the frequency and intensity of her mind-reading statements. Thus, they exhibited many of the features of a pursuer–distancing relational process.

It is important when working with this family dynamic not to assume that one member of a dyad is more at fault than the other. In William's family, the fact that the mother pursued had to be balanced against the fact that he withdrew, possibly as a form of retribution. Furthermore, this dynamic was aggravated by William's episode, because his residual symptoms became a legitimate cause of worry for his mother. However, the pursuer–distancing pattern was an old theme in their relationship, one that both agreed predated the onset of his illness.

The clinician approached this case as follows: How could CET be used to (1) rearrange the power imbalance in this family, (2) get the patient to articulate his discomfort about his mother's boundary-crossing maneuvers, and (3) encourage the mother to verbalize the anxiety that generated her overmonitoring behavior? That is, how could CET become a forum for addressing some of the oldest conflicts in their relationship?

The first task was to give both members an opportunity to experience how their relationship could be different if they formulated their needs and desires more clearly and allowed each other equal air time. This was first done through an active listening exercise, with William's mother in the listener role. The father was to help coach the members of the dyad, without taking sides.

CLINICIAN: OK, William, let's go with you as the speaker. Can you say more about what makes you uncomfortable about talking with your mom? Try to be as gentle as you can. And, Alyssia, all I want you to do is listen, no matter how distressed you are by what William says. You'll get a chance to respond soon.

WILLIAM: (*not looking at Alyssia*) You have to stay off my case. You're always bugging me, always following me around the house and asking me stupid questions, and it doesn't help me. It makes me feel worse.

ALYSSIA: Will, I know you feel that way, and I suspect this reminds you of when—

CLINICIAN: Alyssia, I'm going to stop you for a moment. It's understandable to want to get to the root of what William's saying, and I imagine you're having some reactions to the way he said it, but can you just stay with the content? Paraphrase back to him what he just said. [Provides structure and remains present-oriented; encourages mother to try a different role than she is used to.]

ALYSSIA: (*bemused*) So, what do you want me to do? I thought I did what you asked.

CLINICIAN: What I'd like you to do is simply summarize back to him what he's said, for example, "So you feel I bother you too much, and that doesn't help you." [Models.]

ALYSSIA: Why should I just repeat what he said?

CLINICIAN: Well, when someone simply paraphrases what we say, or asks us questions to clarify our meaning, it makes us feel like that person is listening. [Reiterates the purposes and the components of the skill.] So would you be willing to try this again now?

The clinician in this case had to do several rounds of coaching the mother in her listening skills. However, as she began to listen more attentively, the patient became more verbal and assertive about his need for clearer interpersonal boundaries. The fact that his feelings were legitimized, as they were not on a day-to-day basis, temporarily changed his style of relating to his mother. Their relationship was undergoing first-order change.

Once the patient had been given an ample opportunity to express his desire for more room, the mother was asked to express her discomfort with his independence, in the form of a positive request. He, in turn, was simply to listen as she had done.

CLINICIAN: OK, your turn, Alyssia. Can you say a little about what makes you anxious about what William does? Why is it important for you to know about his internal state?

ALYSSIA: He's making me out to be a beast. I'm concerned about him! He's been sick, and I don't want him to get sick again. So, maybe I follow him around too much, but all he has to say is "I'm OK" or "Don't worry, I'm feeling fine," and I'll leave him alone.

WILLIAM: No, you won't.

CLINICIAN: Alyssia, I think what you just said was very helpful. I think your intentions are very positive—you're wanting him to get better, and when you monitor him, it's out of concern for his health. [Reframes.] But you've seen that it's possible to care too much.

ALYSSIA: (*sarcastically*) Yes, I'm certainly learning that.

CLINICIAN: Tell me something: Can you think of a way to phrase what you just said to me as a request for William? What would you like him to do differently and how would that make you feel? [Brings mother back to task.]

ALYSSIA: Well, William, you know I care about you very much, and I know you've been through a rough time, and I know you've been through some traumatic experiences—

WILLIAM: (*Cuts her off.*) There you go again.

CLINICIAN: Alyssia, let me give you some ideas. What, again, would you like him to do?

ALYSSIA: Just tell me, "I'm OK, I'm feeling fine," or better yet, "I'll let you know if I need your help."

CLINICIAN: And that would make you feel how?

ALYSSIA: Well, less tense, less worried.

CLINICIAN: Good. Now, can you turn to William and try it all out at once?

ALYSSIA: William, when I'm worried, all you have to say is, "I'm OK, I'll let you know if I need your help," and then I'll be less worried. That's all you have to do. And if you're feeling depressed yourself, you can—

CLINICIAN: (*interrupting*) OK, good! That's all you need to say. William, how did you feel about what your mom just said? [Solicits feedback from the recipient.]

WILLIAM: That was a lot better, but I just don't know if I can do it.

This family showed an ability within FFT sessions to experiment with different ways of communicating, but the clinicians consistently had to encourage each participant's use of the skills outside the sessions. The clinicians frequently asked them to replay in sessions the conversations they had during the week, and coached them on different ways to avoid the pursuer–distancing dynamic and maintain a better role balance when sending and receiving messages.

Concluding Comments

In introducing new communication skills to couples or families, one can alter the hierarchical structure, patterns of alliance, or habitual transactional styles of the unit. Families of recently ill bipolar patients are often motivated to work toward these changes, even if they are not always comfortable with putting new styles of communicating into practice. Thus, CET must be delivered with careful clinical handling and patience.

Once families have gained an understanding of the syndrome of bipolar disorder, and have been exposed to more effective ways of communicating, they are in a better position to solve day-to-day problems, particularly those associated with the illness. Problem solving is the topic of the next chapter.

chapter 11

Dealing with Family Problems

Walter, a 29-year-old European American man, appeared to be the model of a successful businessman. Prior to his hospitalization, he had successfully managed a sports car dealership, lived in a rented condominium in an elite part of town, wore expensive clothes, had an attractive girlfriend, and drove around town in a convertible. During his manic episode, however, he had "blown it all," as he put it—he had spent all of his money, lost his car to his creditors, lost his girlfriend following his numerous sexual indiscretions, and, of necessity, moved back into his parents' house.

When Walter was discharged from the hospital, he was full of grandiose plans for resuming his interests in the car dealership. He came to FFT sessions dressed in a three-piece suit and carrying a beeper, seemingly unaware of the damage his manic episode had done. During the psychoeducation sessions, his mother and father denied the realities of what had happened during the episode. For example, they cast the fact that he squandered much of his father's retirement money as a product of his "generous nature": "He's always done for others rather than himself, and that gets him into trouble." His father shrugged off any notion of illness, claiming that Walter was a highly successful businessman who had had a minor setback.

About 5 months after his hospital discharge, as the CET module was nearing completion, Walter claimed that he had obtained a job working for another car dealership. However, he was unwilling to give his parents his work phone number or tell them where the dealership was located. His charade lasted several months. When his stories about his new job were revealed to be untrue, his parents became quite enraged and threatened to kick him out of the house. He in turn threatened to discontinue all of his medications if he was forced to leave.

It was during this phase that problem solving was introduced to this family. The primary objective was to help Walter take small steps in resuming a productive work and social life and in repairing the damage he had caused when he was manic. This required that Walter, and his family, substantially revise their hopes and expectations for his recovery and eventual return to the preillness state.

Chapter Overview

The purpose of the problem-solving module is similar to that of CET: to reduce the family distress and tension that develops in response to life events, including an illness episode in one family member (Falloon et al., 1984). Its subsidiary objectives are to (1) open up a dialogue among members of the family about difficult problem topics and allow them a forum for expressing their emotional reactions to these problems and (2) offer patients and family members a framework for solving these problems.

Families of bipolar patients, like those of schizophrenic patients, vary in the degree to which they can effectively solve problems (Miklowitz et al., 1995; Chang, Blaser, Ketter, & Steiner, 2001). In this chapter, I discuss the specific problems faced by families during the aftermath of a depressive or a manic episode. I first discuss how to introduce the problem-solving module to families, and then how to encourage participants to define, generate solutions to, evaluate solutions to, solve, and implement solutions to problems (see Handout 18). As in prior chapters, I discuss how to deal with resistances to the approach. Finally, I offer several case vignettes illustrating how the specific problems of bipolar patients can be addressed using problem solving.

Problem Solving: Why at This Point in Treatment?

The problem-solving technique has been articulately described by behavioral and marital therapists (e.g., Jacobson & Margolin, 1979; Falloon et al., 1984). It is positioned as the final FFT module. Generally, this will begin at about the 15th session, or during the fourth or fifth month of FFT, at which point the treatment has been tapered to biweekly sessions. Based on our experience, we find that problem solving generally requires at least four or five sessions (i.e., Sessions 15 through 18 or 19). However, it can be compressed or otherwise adjusted to the needs of the family and the limits imposed by your clinical setting.

Solving Problems

- Agree on the problem.
- Suggest several possible solutions.
- Discuss pros and cons and agree on best solutions.
- Plan and carry out best solutions.
- Praise efforts; review effectiveness.

HANDOUT 18. *Source*: Falloon et al. (1984). From *Bipolar Disorder: A Family-Focused Treatment Approach, Second Edition*, by David J. Miklowitz.

Why do this module last? Falloon et al.'s (1984) argument was that families needed to have an understanding of the nature of psychiatric disorders, and to be able to communicate with each other on the most basic of levels, before problem solving could be successful. Certainly, we have found that the psychoeducation and CET modules engender among family members a more comfortable, collaborative emotional tone, which facilitates solving problems. Moreover, we often find that patients are too symptomatic in the first few months after an episode to act on proposed problem solutions, even when they have proposed these solutions themselves. For example, a depressed bipolar patient may be able to articulate verbally the steps involved in applying for a job, but cognitively and emotionally unable to carry out these steps. But once the patient is stable and has fewer residual symptoms, he or she may be ready to handle such challenges.

Nevertheless, there will be cases in which you see fit to conduct problem solving at the beginning of FFT, rather than at the end. For example, if your patient initially has no place to live and no idea of how to find one, it may be best to delay the psychoeducation module and begin with problem solving. If you are working with the family of a child who has been kicked out of school, you may want to begin by solving the problem of how the child can get back into this or a different school. If you are limited to only a few sessions with a family, you may feel that problem solving will be more beneficial to a particular family than CET or psychoeducation. In these cases, proceed with problem solving with an awareness of the limits imposed by the patient's clinical status.

What Kinds of Problems Do the Families of Bipolar Patients Have?

The case of Walter illustrates some of the dramatic ways that bipolar disorder creates life problems. Some of these were alluded to in prior chapters. In our experience, problems during the postepisode stabilization and maintenance phases typically fall into one of the thematic categories listed in Table 11.1. These problems can be summarized under the more general heading of adjusting to life in the aftermath of a bipolar episode. In addition to the difficulties inherent in coming to terms with the illness, the episode itself is a life event that often leaves much damage in its wake, in the form of great financial debt, ruined relationships, or losses of work (or, for children, school) opportunities.

Of course, a bipolar patient during the postepisode period may have any combination of these problems. For Walter, "life trashing" resulted in his premature attempt to resume his prior work and social roles, creating family relationship problems, which in turn fueled his desire to discon-

TABLE 11.1. Four Problems Areas Associated with the Postepisode Phases of Bipolar Disorder

1. Medication usage and adherence
2. Resumption of prior work, school, and social roles
3. "Life trashing"
4. Relationship/living situation conflicts

tinue his medications. In a later section of this chapter, I discuss each of these content areas individually, with illustrative case examples.

Conducting Problem Solving

Introducing the Problem-Solving Module

The first step is to offer the family a rationale for problem solving. We suggest the following:

> "Up until now we've been talking mainly about how you communicate with each other. Now we'd like to deal with some of the concrete problems of living you've all been alluding to. But rather than our just giving you suggestions about what to do about these—which probably wouldn't work that well anyway—we'd like to teach you a way of solving problems cooperatively, as a family."

At this point, pass around Handout 18, Solving Problems.

> "We think of solving problems as a series of stages. These stages are a little like what we all do naturally in our heads, but there are some tricks to doing it as a family that make things go better. First, there's a definition phase, in which you try to identify what the problem really is, and how it differs from other problems you may be experiencing. Usually, the more specific you can be about defining it, the better—breaking the problem down to very small chunks makes it easier to solve. Next, you try to come up with as many solutions as possible, without evaluating them yet—what we call 'brainstorming.' Then, together, you evaluate the pros and cons of each solution, and pick one solution, or maybe a couple of them, that you think will work. It's good to talk over the implementation of these solutions—how will you put them into practice? After trying the best solution, it's always a good idea to praise each other on a job well done, and determine whether you think the original problem was solved."

The procedure will seem rather abstract to family members at this point, and you should quickly help them identify a problem to practice on. Sometimes this is best done by reviewing with the family the problems members raised during the functional assessment period and determining whether these are still problems. Generating a list of problems—preferably by asking each family member to come up with at least one—gives you an idea of which of the four thematic problem areas the family is currently facing, if this is not already clear.

As is true in CET, problem solving works best when simple, rather nondistressing problems are chosen first and more difficult problems are introduced once the family appears to be grasping the method. The simpler and more concrete the problem, the more easily it can be solved. Thus, for example, one of our couples began by discussing where and when they would go on vacation; another began with use of the car for errands.

However, keep in mind a principal theme we have discussed throughout the book: Behind a seemingly simple problem are often more central, global conflicts, of which this problem is only one example. Thus, use your clinical skills in choosing problems to discuss: "Use of the home fax machine" (see the example of Neil and Julie below) may be a small problem in one family but a tremendous problem in another, especially if the family is struggling with issues about boundaries, personal consideration, or the importance of each other's careers. "Taking better care of the dog" sounded like a small problem when it was raised by one of our families that included an adolescent, until we learned that the teen was torturing the dog. Once participants have mastered the problem-solving method, you may be able to help them deal with these deeper, more distressing family problems using the same framework (see examples below).

The Mechanics of Conducting Problem Solving

As with the psychoeducation and CET modules, problem solving usually goes better if you adhere to a certain therapeutic stance. First, think of yourself as a coach or a referee. When problem solving is going well, the family should be doing most of the work. Once family members have learned the technique, it is not long before they can take themselves through an entire definition-to-solution sequence with no input whatsoever from you. In general, it is best not to offer the family your own definitions of a problem or your own proposed solutions, as these will often fail within a particular family system. If family members are struggling, you may have to do this kind of prompting at the beginning.

Second, help structure the problem-solving procedure. As we discussed in the chapters on CET, the love of chaos and spontaneity characteristic of bipolar families tends to interfere with discussions and resolutions of problems (Miklowitz et al., 1995). Thus, you should carefully guide family members through the problem-solving steps, keeping them on task and consistently praising them for their efforts, even if these efforts seem minimal. If the discussions get out of hand or irrelevant issues are introduced, encourage them to slow down and stick with the primary problem.

Third, encourage the participants to use their newly learned communication skills when discussing problems. Using these skills will help the problem-solving process go more smoothly, keep the family on task, and give family members feelings of validation. For example, the participants may be able to practice active listening while other family members share their definitions of a problem, or to practice making positive requests of other participants when generating solutions (see the example of Lew and Marianna below).

Fourth, keep in mind that the family may need to "ventilate" emotionally before going through the problem-solving steps. In the case of Lew and Marianna below, the clinician first encourages the couple to have an open discussion about the larger issues of trust and intimacy in their relationship, before addressing the more specific problem of the lack of physical affection between them. Often, such open discussions are an emotional release for participants and make them more ready to commit to solution-finding in regard to more specific problems.

An Example of Problem Solving

Lew, a 29-year-old Latino man, had been hospitalized for a manic episode and then cycled into a severe depression, for which he was treated with electroconvulsive therapy. About 4 months into the treatment, when he had begun to remit from his depression, a core relational problem emerged. His wife, Marianna, deplored the lack of intimacy in their relationship and, particularly, his lack of physical or sexual affection. Lew did not want to talk about this issue. His only comment was that he felt uncomfortable being close to her because of his depression and low self-esteem. After teaching this couple the basic steps of problem solving around a less emotionally charged topic (her work schedule), the clinician addresses this more difficult relationship issue:

CLINICIAN: I'd like to suggest you table the discussion of the trust issue for now—maybe we can't resolve it just yet. The thing I heard you talking about that is possibly solvable is the one about physical contact between you—let's deal with this issue first. Lew, how would you define this problem?

LEW: (*sullen*) I suppose I could break down and give a kiss now and then.

CLINICIAN: That may be a good solution, but maybe we could just stay for now with what the problem actually is. How would you describe it in your own words?

MARIANNA: I think it's really about trust.

CLINICIAN: I think you're right, Marianna, but I'm going to encourage you to be even more specific. How would you define the problem about physical affection? [Coaches couple to break the problem down into small chunks.]

LEW: She wants more touching and hugging, and I can't give it right now.

MARIANNA: It's not that I want to make him uncomfortable, but I just want to know that he wants me around.

Thus far, the clinician has obtained a partial *definition of the problem.* Then he encourages the couple to break down the problem even further. For example, when these conflicts arise, is it when they're alone versus in the company of their children? Is the issue about sex versus physical contact? Is the problem long-standing, or does it arise only during Lew's depression? The couple finally agrees on a definition, and the clinician summarizes and paraphrases it for them.

CLINICIAN: So the problem is that, Marianna, you want more physical contact during this period when Lew is recovering, particularly when the two of you are alone. You're not really concerned that much about sex, you're talking more about physical affection, like hugging. But it's difficult for you, Lew, to give it right now. You're just not feeling that good about yourself, and it's hard to feel good about someone else. So let's go the next step. Why don't you both throw out as many solutions as you can think of, and we'll hold off discussing them until they're all out on the table (brainstorming)?

LEW: (*long pause*) Well, like I said I could give a kiss, and with that usually comes a hug. But I'm not gonna make a schedule or anything, maybe just when she needs one real bad.

CLINICIAN: And how would you know if she wants one?

LEW: (*thoughtful*) She may be able to ask me. Other times I would just know.

CLINICIAN: So you've suggested two things so far, one is for you to just spontaneously give her a hug, and the other is for Marianna to ask you for one. Those are good suggestions. Marianna, can you think of any alternatives other than those?

MARIANNA: The biggest one is that if I feel the need for a kiss or a hug, to be able to ask for that and not feel like I'm imposing . . . (*to Lew*) it's not to grab onto you.

CLINICIAN: Good suggestion. Marianna, can you remember the positive request skill we taught you earlier? Can you think of how you might tell Lew that you'd like him to make it safe for you to ask? [Introduces communication skills into problem-solving exercise.]

MARIANNA: Well, Lew, I'd like you to, if you don't want to, just say, "I don't feel like hugging you right now, it has nothing to do with you, it's not that I don't love you."

LEW: (*Perks up.*) Kind of like a plan B hug. (*All chuckle*).

In this segment—the *solution-generation phase*—the clinician introduces structure into the discussions and keeps the couple on task. He encourages them to avoid the broader issue of trust in the relationship, a problem that would be difficult to solve in this manner. Note that the patient is becoming more activated as the exercise progresses.

Next, the clinician guides the couple toward generating more solutions. Once a number of solutions have been proposed, he encourages them to *evaluate the advantages and disadvantages of each.*

CLINICIAN: Let's start with the one you gave, Lew, that you'd just spontaneously give her a hug now and then. What's good about that and what could you see going wrong?

LEW: Well, it could make her feel better, and I want to do that. But it could make me feel worse. Sometimes I just don't feel like it. But I guess it could also make me feel better.

CLINICIAN: So we have two pros and a con.

LEW: (*Half smiles.*) Sounds like a winner. I'll take those odds anytime.

CLINICIAN: Marianna, any pros and cons you can think of?

MARIANNA: Well, it might make me feel better, but it'd feel pretty bad if he never did it.

At the end of this exercise, the couple chooses three solutions that they are both comfortable with. The clinician wraps up the problem-solving exercise by *summarizing the solutions and discussing their implementation.*

CLINICIAN: So you've come up with three solutions. One is for Lew to show you physical affection more spontaneously, at least when he feels comfortable with it. A second is for Marianna to ask you for a hug, and for you to either give her one or explain that it's uncomfortable for you to do it right now, but you'll do it if you're feeling better later in the day. And the third is for the two of you to have an evening out together once every 2 weeks, which might set things up so they'll occur more spontaneously.

LEW: There's the babysitter issue on the third one, but maybe we can work that out.

CLINICIAN: Good point, Lew. That's what I wanted to get to next. Do all these things seem doable? Can you actually carry them out? Or should we cross any off the list?

The following week, the clinician checked in with the couple about *the status of the original problem.* Aided by the gradual recovery from his depression, Lew had been more willing to express physical affection toward Marianna spontaneously, albeit in a limited fashion. He also noted being better able to express his affection for her verbally. Marianna, however, had been uncomfortable asking him for physical affection. Finally, the couple had scheduled one private event for the two of them. The original problem had not been solved, but important steps toward its resolution had been taken.

In addition to the actual implementation of the solutions, the problem-solving exercise achieved three goals with this couple. First, solutions to this relational problem were generated by the participants themselves, and what seemed at first like an insurmountable problem now appeared more workable. Second, the patient, who began in a depressed, rather withdrawn state, became more activated and verbal as he became more invested in the outcome of the problem-solving discussion. Third, both members of the couple expressed feelings of affection for one another during the exercise, an often positive by-product of such collaborative discussions.

The Problem-Solving Worksheet

Problem solving is aided by the introduction of a worksheet (Handout 19), where problem definitions, proposed solutions, pros and cons, and implementation strategies are each recorded. You can give this sheet to the participants before beginning an exercise and appoint one member of the family as secretary. It's best to assign this task to (1) a member who seems uninvolved in the discussions of the problem or (2) a verbose family member who frequently takes discussions off-task (including a symptomatic patient), as this puts more responsibility on him or her to ensure that the task is completed.

Introducing the worksheet is most helpful for families that have a great deal of trouble staying on task, because it offers an external structure. However, there are other times when you are better off dispensing with the worksheet and allowing a more free-form discussion. When discussion topics are heavily laden with affect, or deal with very personal issues, the worksheet adds an unnecessary element of formality. In the

Problem-Solving Worksheet

Step 1: Define: "What is the problem?" Talk. Listen. Ask questions. Get everybody's opinion.

Step 2: List all possible solutions: "Brainstorm." List all ideas, even unrealistic ones. Get everybody to come up with at least one possible solution. Do not evaluate any solution at this point.

(1) ________________________________

(2) ________________________________

(3) ________________________________

(4) ________________________________

(5) ________________________________

(6) ________________________________

Step 3: Discuss and list the advantages and disadvantages of each possible solution.

Advantages	Disadvantages
____________	____________
____________	____________
____________	____________
____________	____________
____________	____________
____________	____________
____________	____________
____________	____________
____________	____________

(continued)

HANDOUT 19. *Source*: Adapted by permission from Falloon et al. (1984).

Step 4: Choose the best possible solution or solutions, and list. (May be a combination of possible solutions.)

____

____

____

____

____

____

____

Step 5: Plan how to carry out the chosen solutions, and set a date to implement them. Date: ______________

A. Specifically decide who will do what. List.

____

____

____

B. Decide what resources will be needed, list, and obtain them.

____

____

____

C. Anticipate what can go wrong during implementation and decide how to overcome the problems.

____

____

____

D. Rehearse the implementation of the solution.

E. DO IT! (Implement the chosen solution on schedule.)

Step 6: Review the implemented solution and give positive feedback to all participants.

Step 7: If the implemented solution was unsuccessful, go back to Step 1 and try again. Do not become discouraged.

HANDOUT 19. *(page 2 of 2)*

example of Lew and Marianna above, the clinician avoided using the worksheet.

Homework and Generalization

As members of the family or the couple become increasingly familiar with the problem-solving format, encourage them to generalize this new skill to their home setting. For example, once they have identified and defined a problem in a session, ask them to use their weekly family meeting to generate solutions to and attempt to solve the problem. Alternatively, ask them to meet once during the week and arrive at an agreed-upon definition of a problem, and then use the next FFT session for the solution-generation phase. Encourage them to bring to the next session completed problem-solving worksheets detailing their between-session efforts.

It is especially important to encourage this week-to-week practice among families of adolescent or younger patients. We have observed that many families of teens come to FFT sessions with a "conflict of the week." For example, one week the issue will be the teen's lack of homework completion, the next, her late night hours, the next, her disrespectful tone, and the next, her eating habits. You may have the impression that you are just putting out fires rather than making any real changes in the family. Getting the parents and teen to choose a time each week to practice the problem-solving method beginning to end, without the influence of a therapist, may go a long way toward instilling these skills in the family's repertoire. As in the proverbial story of teaching a man to fish rather than catching a fish for him, knowledge of the problem-solving method can give the parents a sense of control over the chaos and repeated family conflicts generated by their child's disorder.

Dealing with Resistance

Therapeutic Approaches to Resistance

As with the other FFT modules, the families of bipolar patients often meet problem solving with a degree of resistance. Here, I define resistance rather broadly, as an unwillingness to define or solve a problem despite the apparent presence of skills to do so, or as difficulty in following through during the solution-implementation phase. Table 11.2 lists common expressions of resistance to problem solving.

Problem-solving discussions, like trains, can get stuck on the tracks, become derailed, collide with other trains, or fail to reach their intended

TABLE 11.2. Family Members' Expressions of Resistance to Problem Solving

- Complain that the problem-solving process doesn't work for them or that it is silly.
- Sidetrack the discussions and bring up irrelevant issues.
- Remain stuck at the problem-definition phase and cannot transition to discussing solutions.
- Cross-complain or bring up separate problems to counter those raised by other family members.
- Fail to complete homework or follow through on solutions they have selected.

destinations. Here, I describe some of the approaches you can take to get families back on track (see also Falloon et al., 1984).

First, participants may not believe that problem solving is a useful procedure, or that the myriad of problems they face can be addressed using such a structured format. In such cases, you may need to reiterate for them the purposes of problem solving. However, you may also have to assess the origins of their resistances: Why are family members having trouble solving this particular problem? Are they clear about what the problem is? Do the suggested solutions seem contrived, or externally imposed on them? Is there an underlying, larger problem that is not being addressed? Is this larger problem brought about by the unusual demands of the postmanic or postdepressive period, or is it a long-standing issue?

If you encounter resistance, first "take the blame" for the family's inability to solve the smaller problem they began with (see example below). If it seems appropriate, admit that you have encouraged them to solve a problem that is not really central to their concerns. For example, if a couple is really struggling with whether they should continue living together, problem solving about who washes the dishes will seem mundane and unimportant. Taking the blame yourself takes the pressure off the participants and makes them less likely to feel they have failed.

Next, try to clarify with them the larger, underlying conflicts or disagreements fueling their resistances (e.g., trust, personal consideration, boundaries between family members). Allow them time to ventilate about these larger problems in as constructive a manner as possible. Determine with them whether the larger problems can be broken down into more manageable units. Then, the participants may be better able to return to the problem-solving framework to address the specific manifestations of these problems.

Turning Resistance into Productive Problem Solving: A Case Example

Neil, a 32-year-old electrician, had always been a "caretaker." He felt natural in the role of helping someone who was ill, something he drew from a childhood of dealing with a very ill mother. So when his wife, Julie, 30, was discharged from the hospital and returned to their house severely depressed, he quickly grasped onto the role of "doctor" in their relationship. He became hypervigilant about her symptoms, took over most of the household tasks, and began dispensing her medications to Julie. For the time being, this role for him seemed comfortable for both of them.

About 5 months into FFT, Julie began to stabilize on a combination of Divalproex, Quetiapine, and Ritalin. She returned to her secretarial job. But it was not until the family clinician initiated the problem-solving module that this couple began to raise problems relevant to their relationship. Interestingly, it was Julie who brought up the majority of these problems. She said that several issues had been "baking" all along, but that she didn't feel she had the strength to address them when she was symptomatic. It became clear that they had significant problems with relational boundaries: Julie needed more space, and Neil did not know when to back off and let her do things independently.

In the second problem-solving session, Julie said that she and Neil could not agree on the use of the home fax machine. This struck the family clinician as a good example for a problem-solving exercise. However, as soon as the couple began to define it, the problem grew bigger and bigger, encompassing other issues such as borrowing each other's belongings and the use of their two cars. The clinician encouraged them to stay on the task of solving the fax machine problem. However, neither could do so, and each of the solutions generated by one member of the couple was unacceptable to the other.

How do you address this logjam in the problem-solving process? The clinician begins by questioning whether the couple is reacting to the problem-solving procedure itself, and then explores the underlying issues.

CLINICIAN: When we were talking about dealing with your in-laws last week, you both took to this problem-solving procedure quite well. This week you're having some trouble. Is it the procedure itself, or is it the problem we're discussing?

NEIL: I think it's this particular problem. I think it's kind of superficial.

CLINICIAN: Well, it may seem that way, and my thinking in encouraging you is that sometimes you have to gain some confidence from solving small problems before moving on to bigger ones. [Reiterates the rationale for problem solving.] Julie, why do you think you're having so much trouble with this problem?

JULIE: Well, sharing clothes and food are the issues with him, space is the issue with me—I need to be alone more, and this applies to my fax machine and my car. I feel like I'm being told what to do. *(Voice rises)* I feel like I'm being totally invaded. Like my job interview, you told me how to act, not to get my hopes up, you acted like I didn't know what I was doing. [Cross-complaint.]

NEIL: Sorry. Didn't mean to do that.

CLINICIAN: I think maybe I'm the one who should apologize—I've guided us in the wrong direction here. Maybe this problem is really a part of a larger problem that we first need to clarify. [Takes responsibility for the logjam in the problem-solving exercise.]

The clinician believes he has tapped into an underlying relational process. But of what nature? Why is Julie feeling so intensely that she is being invaded and controlled, a feeling she had not raised in the first 5 months of treatment?

CLINICIAN: It sounds like this is a larger issue about sharing space—sharing a household—it's about boundaries, how much is yours, how much is mine. When we get married, do I have to give up my individuality? Does everything become yours—where do I stop and you begin? [Begins to clarify the nature of the larger problem.]

JULIE: Yeah! It's especially bad with Neil because we're so close to each other, and it's something I feel real offended by. . . . Where does he get off telling me what to do?

CLINICIAN: How do you see this issue, Neil?

NEIL: Well, I'm not trying to boss her around, and this is the first time she's brought this up.

CLINICIAN: You know what I think is happening? Neil, you've been in the position of taking care of Julie for the last 5 months, and Julie is feeling better now and not needing as much help, and is starting to resent you staying in the role of caretaker when she feels confident. [Begins to clarify underlying issues.] On the other hand, for you, Neil, I think starting to act differently toward Julie must be hard to do, particularly when you've felt that taking care of her has been expected of you all along. [Normalizes the role confusion Neil is feeling.]

NEIL: (*to Julie*) I just feel like you're mad at me now, I don't know what to do. You always ask me what to do; like on your interview, you asked me for my advice.

JULIE: But I just wanted to ventilate how nervous I was about the interview. I didn't want advice. (*to clinician*) I think Neil does want to take care of me, but I think he also resents the fact that he is taking care of me, I think he hates me for it.

NEIL: I think we're still in a mixed place. She's still overtly asking me to take care of her, and in some ways I think she hates me for it. I still get her medicine. In a lot of ways our whole relationship is based on this illness.

The clinician now has a hypothesis: that Neil, who has been taking care of Julie since she became ill, has not fully recognized her clinical improvement and corresponding need for independence and feelings of self-efficacy. He may fear that he won't have a role in the relationship once she is well. Julie, in turn, has not expressed her needs directly, or perhaps has given him mixed messages about his role as caretaker. Their relationship has not grown with Julie's improved condition, and there is much resentment over the confusion of roles and expectations. The clinician further clarifies this dynamic for the couple.

CLINICIAN: So I guess the resentment goes both ways. Neil, you may resent having had to take care of Julie in these very difficult situations where you wanted to be helpful but didn't know what to do. But maybe you, Julie, feel resentful that you had to ask Neil for help, when you really wanted to take care of things yourself. But I agree with you, I think he does care about you a great deal. (*to Neil*) Julie's been in a lot of trouble before. It's hard to know when to back off. [Clarifies further the underlying relational dynamic, and attends to underlying affect.]

JULIE: (*to Neil*) If you don't like that role, why don't you just get out of it? (*Neil is silent*.)

CLINICIAN: Perhaps what you both really want is for your relationship to grow in a different direction. You can't use the old methods you used to use when you were sick and you were the caretaker. That isn't going to work anymore because you're not sick anymore, and in fact, you're really getting your life back together. This requires a dialogue and some collaborative work between the two of you. [Redirects couple back to problem solving.]

The clinician next encourages the couple to generate solutions to the larger problem of how their relationship can adapt to Julie's improved condition and greater need for independence, and how they can be clear with each other about their individual expectations. He encourages them to use their communication skills to enhance this process. For example, Neil practices asking Julie whether she wants him simply to listen to her versus give her advice when she raises personal problems, and Julie practices being more direct with Neil about her increasing need for independence. Later, the clinician guides the couple back to the original problem of the home fax machine, which is now easier for them to solve, given their recognition of the underlying relationship conflict.

This case example shows how the problem-solving procedure can be adapted to large as well as small problems, as long as you and the family can be flexible about its application. However, larger problems are usually not solvable in a single session. Rather, exploring and clarifying the underlying issues for each participant makes it easier, in subsequent sessions, to break large problems down into smaller ones.

Resistance to Problem Solving as a Cost–Benefit Decision

Some families of bipolar patients, in nearing a solution to a specific problem, suddenly express the sentiment that the problem itself is of minimal importance and/or that other problems are of more immediate concern. Alternatively, family members may agree to deploy certain solutions and then return for the following session explaining that the solutions did not work, or that the original problem solved itself, without anyone's effort.

One way to think of these dynamics is that the solutions to the problem are more costly than the problem itself. Certainly, solving a problem can carry certain costs, such as having to plan one's day differently, capitulating to another person's needs, or having to do things that are foreign or unnatural. Compared with these costs, the initial problem may seem rather minimal.

In one family, a parent raised the problem that her two teenage sons, both of whom had bipolar illness, did not clean up around the house. The sons complained that they did not know what was expected of them and when. The family agreed, with some coaching from the clinician, to develop a weekly schedule that listed each person's daily housecleaning tasks. The next week, the family had scrapped the schedule and the problem remained. They laughed about how messy the house had become and how chaotic the week had been, and admitted that the schedule felt like a "straitjacket." The clinician joined in their humor, and then reframed solving the problem as a cost–benefit decision:

"Your family prides itself on spontaneity. This is a good thing about your family—people are spontaneous and impulsive at times. Maybe this makes for an exciting atmosphere at home, and I may have been reining you in too much with this schedule idea. [Takes responsibility for the failure of the solution.] I guess a schedule is a high price to pay because it would interfere with your family's natural habits."

The clinician here points to a positive aspect of the family's dynamics. This family enjoys not knowing everyone's comings and goings and rebels against any externally imposed structure. The clinician gives the family "permission" to ignore the original problem by saying, "This problem is not necessarily something you have to solve, unless we can think of some ways to solve it without interfering with your spontaneity." This is an important message to give: Family members may need to know that they are not dysfunctional just because they choose to solve certain problems and not others.

The Problems of the Families of Bipolar Patients: Are There Good Solutions?

At the chapter's beginning, I outlined four key problems affecting the families of bipolar patients. Now that you are familiar with the problem-solving process, I offer clinical examples of how problem solving can be used to address these difficulties.

Medication Usage and Compliance

You will recall that in psychoeducation the core issues about medication concerned the patient's or family's over- or underidentification with the disorder, problems regarding independence and autonomy, and the stigma of taking medications. In problem solving, you can address these issues on a more concrete, behavioral level. Specifically, nested within the compliance issue is often the problem of overmonitoring by family members. The patient may believe that he or she should take medications, but is put off by his or her parents' or spouse's repetitive questions about whether he or she is complying or has gone to have blood drawn. In some cases, the patient will continue to take the medications but torture the family by being evasive about whether or not he or she is really doing so. Thus, the dilemma in problem solving becomes, how can the family be assured of the patient's compliance without the patient feeling that his or her independence is being sacrificed?

In our work, we have found that good solutions to medication nonadherence problems can be identified if you keep in mind two principles. First, the family should be encouraged to define the problem as "How can we all agree on or be comfortable with ___________'s medication habits?", rather than "___________ won't take his or her medication." The former definition reduces tension by underlining that this is a family rather than an individual problem. Second, you can set up quid pro quo contracts between patients and their relatives that strike compromises between the relatives' need for reassurance and the patient's need for autonomy.

One of our patients, Alicia, a 25-year-old African American woman who lived with her father, argued persuasively that she was taking her medications and that her father was needlessly annoying her about them. Her father argued that she had no right to oppose him on this issue, because he had "been through hell" in dealing with her hospitalization and now needed assurance that she was going to take care of herself. This family, after generating various viable and nonviable solutions (e.g., that she would move out, that a member of the extended family would be in charge of dispensing her medications, that her father would be allowed to discuss medications with her only by telephone), agreed to the following contingency contract: Her father would be allowed to ask Alicia whatever questions he had—whether these were about her compliance, side effects, or blood monitoring—but only on a once-per-week basis, over Friday night dinner. She, in turn, was to remain compliant with her regimen and answer his weekly inquiries as best she could.

Bart, an 18-year-old European American male, constantly needled his mother by leaving lithium tablets around the house, including on the kitchen floor and behind the toilet. His behavior, while immature, masked an emotional issue similar to that of Alicia: He was willing to take medication only if he could be assured that it was his decision to do so. This family finally agreed that Bart's mother would put a plate containing his four tablets by the kitchen sink every day. He was to agree to take them each day, and she was to inquire about his medication only if she found any pills around the house or on the plate when she went to bed at night.

Both of these examples concern patients for whom the core issue was the family's overmonitoring behavior. However, many other issues motivate noncompliance, and some of these can also be addressed using problem solving. For example, if the issue relates to the patient's shame over the social stigma of mental illness, you can use problem solving with the family to determine which members may talk about the patient's illness or medications outside the family, to whom they may talk, and how much information they should convey.

Resumption of Prior Work and Social Roles

The financial realities for patients who have had an episode of bipolar disorder—the medical bills, the costs of new living arrangements, and the money spent irrationally during the episode—usually require that the patient return to work or school as soon as possible (see the example of Walter, in the chapter's opening case). Spouses and parents quickly grow tired of footing the bill for everything and become resentful of the patient's inability to produce anything for the family. In other cases, family members may underestimate what the patient can actually do during the postepisode phase, and "float" the patient for a time by paying all of his or her bills. This arrangement takes the immediate pressure off the patient but can lead to complacency over the long term.

Your task in problem solving is often one of helping the patient to rein him- or herself in and set realistic goals for functioning during the stabilization and maintenance periods, goals that reflect a compromise between goals of the patient and those of the family members. In other cases, you can use problem solving to help motivate the patient to take the first steps toward a functional recovery.

Consider the example of a 22-year-old Asian American patient, Tina. Once her manic episode had largely resolved, she insisted on going back to work full-time. In part, this was because she owed considerable money and had had to move back to her parents' house. She also wanted to take several evening courses to complete her bachelor's degree. Her parents doubted that she could do each of these things, especially because she was still symptomatic. Rather, they wanted her to apply for disability payments, an option that was anathema to her.

The clinicians encouraged this family to generate solutions to the problem of how professionally active Tina should be during this post-episode phase. The solutions they produced included going back to work full-time, going half-time, not working at all, or only going to school. A compromise was struck in which Tina did go back to work full-time, an arrangement facilitated by her employer, who was aware of her condition. However, in return, she agreed not to go back to school for 3 months, at which point, if she were clinically stable, she could take one evening class.

In the case of Alicia above, the problem was the reverse. She appeared to have recovered from her episode, but was immobilized when it came to getting back in the job market. Her father had been initially supportive but became increasingly frustrated with her. He owned a business and felt the best solution was for her to come work with him, an option she was unwilling to consider.

Problem solving centered on her taking small steps toward entering the workforce, including developing a resume and calling the college she had attended to see if she could complete her teaching certificate. However, she arrived at the sessions not having completed these assignments. When the clinicians explored this issue with her, it became clear that she was unable to do more than one of the assigned tasks per week. Therefore, in subsequent sessions more limited goals were set. When FFT sessions were finally tapered off to monthly, the clinicians buttressed the problem-solving exercises with weekly phone calls to Alicia to determine whether she had implemented any of her (or her father's) proposed solutions. This additional structuring was quite helpful to her.

Often, your challenge is to help the patient and family realize that, indeed, the patient has been ill, and may now need to pursue goals that on the surface seem mundane and low level. Remind the family that people with bipolar disorder take longer to recover their prior level of functioning after an episode than to recover from their symptoms (Keck et al., 1998). Keep in mind that if problem-solving exercises produce expectations of the patient that are too high, you can inadvertently set up a failure experience for him or her. If this occurs, take responsibility for the negative outcome and encourage the participants to try again, this time with more limited goals.

Life Trashing

Walter "trashed" much of his life and accomplishments during his manic episode. He had alienated most of the people he knew: His girlfriend no longer wanted to see him, nor his business partners to work with him. In fact, the illness brought him back, rather awkwardly, to his childhood home, and under the care of his parents. His primary question, and that of his family, was "How do I get my life back?"

Many patients damage their lives during manic or depressive episodes and must regroup and make amends during the postepisode phases. Sometimes the destruction has been financial (e.g., running up enormous credit card or medical bills, failing to pay rent and losing one's apartment), legal (e.g., destroying property, wrecking a car), or social–emotional (e.g., ruining a romantic relationship). For relatives, the key reaction is usually one of intense anger, because often their lives have been damaged as well.

Although one cannot undo these events, problem solving helps patients and families to address some of the problems these events have created. In some cases, it can be used to develop preventative plans so that the next episode is not accompanied by the same level of destructiveness (see discussions of the relapse drill in the next chapter).

In Walter's case, we encouraged his parents to discontinue bailing him out financially. Instead, we encouraged the family to problem solve about how he could make arrangements with his credit card company to steadily pay off his bills; how he could find a used car; how he could stick to a financial budget that, although limited, would be within his control; and how he could develop plans for paying his father back for the losses to his retirement income.

Walter was at first defensive when these issues were discussed. He felt these discussions represented an attack on his self-concept, given that his own goals centered on regaining his business and former level of income. However, as he remitted from his manic episode, he became more realistic and began to appreciate the structure of the problem-solving interventions. In fact, he began summarizing the recommended solutions at the end of each session (e.g., "So I should call this number about the car, and call this guy about the credit cards"). The problem-solving exercises tended to "stick" better as he became more fully remitted.

Another form of life trashing is exemplified by the patient who has alienated many people—including friends, family members, lovers, or coworkers— during a manic or depressive episode. Children with the disorder are particularly prone to this situation: Their behavior during a symptomatic period ruins peer relationships or gets them thrown out of school. For instance, a 14-year-old boy cursed out his favorite teacher on a particularly bad day, and then went back to apologize the next day. However, she no longer wanted him in her class.

One patient, Amanda, 27, had embezzled money from her employer during her episode. In addition to the legal issues she faced, she wanted to address whether she could mend fences with her employer. With issues such as these, we have found it useful to combine certain aspects of problem solving with CET. Specifically, you can use problem-solving exercises to help patients evaluate the pros and cons of discussing the episode with alienated friends or family members, and CET exercises to rehearse within sessions appropriate ways to do this. For example, Amanda agreed to talk with her former employer and explain her manic episode and its meaning, as well as apologize for her behavior. We used in-session role-play exercises—with her husband pretending to be her employer—to help her practice ways to do this. Although she did not ultimately get her job back, she did feel that she achieved some understanding and closure regarding her role in causing an unfortunate situation.

Relationship and Living Situation Problems

Resuming a relationship with a spouse, sibling, or parent is quite difficult for a bipolar patient during the postepisode period, and equally difficult for his or her family members. As I have discussed previously, relationships go awry during the postepisode period: Family members become too enmeshed or too distant; the recovering patient is viewed by others as overintrusive or, in contrast, too avoidant; imbalances emerge in the degree of control some members hold over others (e.g., Neil and Julie); trust is disrupted (e.g., Walter and his parents); or physical and sexual relationships deteriorate (e.g., Lew and Marianna). In addition, problems emerge as to how members will live together: Families or couples may disagree on basic rules such as how the house will get clean, who will cook dinner, or even who will live in the household.

Anita, a 35-year-old European American woman, lived with her father. After her bipolar, depressed episode, she became extremely dependent on her father, wanting him to spend all of his time with her. He became increasingly irritated with her and finally insisted that she move to a board-and-care home. However, she was desperately unhappy in this new setting and began calling him at work several times a day, until he refused even to come to visit her.

Problem solving identified two separate issues: the participants' disagreements over where she should live, and over how much contact they should have. The clinicians encouraged more mutual definitions of the problems, rather than the participants' original complaints of "He wants to get rid of me" and "She's too needy." The living situation problem was addressed first. The dyad generated the following possible solutions: Anita should move back in with her father, stay in her board-and-care home, move to a different home, or try to live in her own place. Her father agreed that he could save enough money—between his job and her disability payments—for her to have her own place, but he required that she stay in the board-and-care home for the next 2 months. In a quid pro quo contract, Anita agreed to limit her face-to-face contacts with him to once per week, and her telephone calls to once per day, none of which were to be to his workplace.

In the case of a couple, we addressed a living situation problem: the issue of when and how to feed the dogs. The problem as it was first introduced to us seemed superficial. However, as the couple explained it further, we became concerned that this was potentially a more serious problem than it had first appeared. Carrie explained that she and her husband, Alan, could not agree on when and how much the dogs should be fed. The result had been that one of the dogs had been coming into their room and waking her up in the middle of each night. As a result, her sleep–wake cycle had been disrupted, and she was becoming increasingly irritable.

The couple generated, within an atmosphere of levity, a number of solutions (e.g., they would feed one of the dogs more than the other, one member of the couple would feed one dog and the other would feed the other dog, or they would teach the dogs to open the refrigerator themselves). With the clinician's encouragement, they were able to listen to each other actively and ask clarifying questions during the solution-generation phase. They finally agreed on what constituted full meals versus snacks for the dogs, when they would be fed, and who would do the feeding. If the dogs awoke them at night, Alan was to get up and feed them.

Of course, not all relationship and living situation problems can be dealt with so easily. However, the problem-solving procedure—particularly if you can combine it with certain aspects of CET—gives you an avenue by which relational problems can be concretized, troubleshot, and resolved.

Concluding Comments

Problem solving, the final module of FFT, is introduced when patients are largely remitted from the mood disorder episode that brought them into treatment. It provides the patient and relatives with a template for defining, generating solutions to, and implementing solutions to problems faced during the postepisode period. When resistances to solving problems arise, there are steps you can take to work this resistance to your advantage. Often, discussing resistances leads to exploring larger relationship problems that may not otherwise have emerged and that interfere with day-to-day functioning.

The next chapter addresses the emergencies and crises that arise during the course of FFT. You will notice that we frequently introduce problem solving when addressing these emergencies, providing a structure the participants usually need.

chapter 12

Managing Crises in Family-Focused Treatment

Kathleen, a 24-year-old European American woman, lived with her husband, Jerry, in a trailer park. She had a long history of bipolar disorder, marked by several severe manic and depressive episodes and psychiatric hospitalizations. During her depressive episodes, her conflicts with her husband, Jerry, almost invariably escalated. She had begun to threaten suicide after these arguments. Jerry soon tired of these threats, began to ignore them, and withdrew from her. When he had avoided her long enough, she would make a parasuicidal gesture (e.g., a superficial slashing of her wrists), and he would, rather resentfully, take her to the hospital. This pattern had led her psychiatrist to diagnose her as "borderline" as well as bipolar.

Kathleen and Jerry were reasonably cooperative with FFT. However, shortly after the introduction of CET, Kathleen slipped into a depression. After one particular quarrel during this period, they considered separating. This led to another of Kathleen's suicidal episodes, which was psychiatrically managed on an outpatient basis.

During their next FFT session, Jerry reported feeling "thrown for a loop" and was quite withdrawn. He expressed a great deal of anger about what he termed her "punishments" and "manipulations" of him and her "unwillingness to take care of her own problems." She, in turn, complained that he didn't care about her and was inattentive during her depressive periods, when he could have been of most help.

Bipolar disorder is an illness associated with frequent psychiatric crises. Some of these crises are the direct result of the disorder (relapses of mania or depression), some are more clearly the result of comorbid personality or other psychiatric disorders, and some are associated with substance or alcohol abuse. As the case of Kathleen and Jerry illustrates, you will often have to depart from the FFT agenda to keep these crises from spiraling out of control, or to deal with their aftermath. However, within FFT you have leverage that other clinicians working with bipolar patients do not have: You can conceptualize the crisis in terms of co-occurring processes within the family and use family members as allies in treating and resolving it.

Chapter Overview

In this chapter, I explore the use of FFT to address specific psychiatric crises. How do you treat psychiatric emergencies among bipolar patients within the framework of providing psychoeducation, CET, and training in problem-solving skills? How do you use the core FFT techniques, after a crisis has resolved, to help prevent similar events from occurring in the future? The chapter deals with four types of emergencies that often arise in this population: manic relapses, depressive relapses, suicidal episodes, and substance/alcohol abuse. It also discusses briefly other types of crises: impending divorces or separations, and child abuse or partner violence. Throughout, it gives examples of how to deal with crises among child and adolescent patients.

Within the section on manic relapses we discuss the rather difficult problem of hospitalization: how to use the family sessions to help the patient and family accept the necessity of short-term hospital care and to arrange for it. Although depressive episodes may also require hospitalization, we have found that arranging hospitalizations for manic episodes is far more difficult.

Suicidal episodes are sometimes associated with the onset of major depressive episodes, but not invariably. Moreover, depressive episodes are not always associated with suicidality. Therefore, I discuss suicidal thoughts and actions in a separate section. I discuss ways for the family to communicate about the patient's suicidal feelings, understand where these come from, and put into practice steps for intervening during and following the suicidal crisis. As you will see, suicidality is understood as a symptom of the disorder that, like other bipolar symptoms, is strongly affected by both biological predispositions and life circumstances.

In the section on substance and alcohol abuse, I describe intervening with the family to clarify the underpinnings of abuse, and engaging family members as allies in arranging for ancillary substance abuse care. Remember that FFT is viewed as only one component of a comprehensive treatment program, which, in addition to pharmacotherapy, may include self-help groups (e.g., AA), motivational enhancement therapy, drug rehabilitation programs, or even detoxification.

General Principles for Managing Crises within FFT

The first basic principle of crisis management with bipolar patients is that you have the most leverage during the period before the crisis spirals out of control. When a patient is fully manic or acutely suicidal, there is not much you can do beyond getting him or her into the hospital. It is when the patient is beginning to cycle (or becomes suicidal or starts to abuse drugs or alcohol) that your interventions will have their maximal impact. In parallel, you have the most leverage in preventing future crises if you intervene after the most recent crisis has resolved. After a hospitalization, the family and patient are highly motivated to prevent another one from occurring, and they are more likely to see the value in developing relapse prevention procedures.

In younger patients, the prodromal period prior to the acute crisis may be very short—even just a few hours. Likewise, there may be a very short postepisode remission before the child cycles into another episode. It can be quite challenging to distinguish symptom exacerbation from the continuation of an existing episode or even from the youth's temperament or personality. Yet you can still encourage family members to develop a relapse and/or suicide prevention plan when the child is well, so that they can immediately put it into action when the child begins to cycle. For a thorough discussion of relapse prevention plans for teens, see Miklowitz and George (2008).

A Four-Pronged Approach to Emergencies

It will not surprise you that I favor an approach to addressing crises that contains the following four elements: assessment, psychoeducation, communication enhancement, and problem solving. Table 12.1 summarizes the steps of dealing with the onset or aftermath of crises. You can think of these steps in the following terms: What is happening to the patient and family members? How do they understand it? How will they talk to each other about it? What will they do to fix it?

Keep in mind that you may wish to implement these core interventions in a different order, depending on the demands of the crisis situation. For example, you may think it best to begin with problem

TABLE 12.1. A Four-Pronged Approach to Crisis Management

1. *Assess* the nature of the crisis: What is going on?
2. *Educate* the family about what the crisis means within the vulnerability–stress model.
3. Encourage family members to *communicate* to each other their feelings, worries, or thoughts about the meaning of the crisis.
4. Encourage the family to *develop and implement solutions to the problems* the crisis has generated.

solving, before conducting any psychoeducation or communication exercises. Alternatively, you may determine that much can be accomplished through direct communication between family members, before educating them about the broader illness context surrounding the crisis.

Assessment

Your first task is to find out what is going on, and what needs to be done immediately. Is the patient developing a new episode? If the problem is escalating mania, is this escalation the direct result of medication discontinuation, and/or did family tensions or life events contribute? If the patient has become suicidal, what were the precipitants, and what are the immediate consequences? Did the crisis come out of the blue, was it associated with a major depression, and/or was it in response to a relationship event (see the case of Kathleen and Jerry earlier in this chapter)? Does the patient need to be hospitalized, and if so, how can the family be engaged in this process? If the patient is abusing drugs or alcohol, does this abuse reflect acting out against the family? Does he or she need to be hospitalized for detoxification or because of danger to him- or herself or others?

Psychoeducation

It is often at times of emergencies that family members come to understand the nature of bipolar disorder more fully. Crisis management often requires restating for the family members the material presented during the psychoeducation module, but making this material relevant to the specific crisis they face. Can they view a manic or depressive relapse as an expected event in the course of this recurrent disorder, and hospitalization as an important part of treatment? Can they think of the patient as having a biological predisposition to react with suicidal thoughts or actions, and identify the psychosocial precipitants that evoked these vulnerabilities? Can the patient understand that his or her cocaine abuse triggers a neurophysiological predisposition to bipolar episodes?

Communication Enhancement

Encourage the family to use its new communication skills in resolving the crisis. Can the relatives express to the patient why they think he or she should be in the hospital? Can the suicidal patient communicate his or her despair to a spouse? Can the spouse communicate compassion for the patient and concern for their lives together? Can an increasingly depressed patient explain to his mother why he can't get out of bed in the morning?

Problem Solving

What can the family members and patient do to solve the problems relevant to the crisis? Through using the problem-solving steps, you can help them generate a list of "who will do what." How will they undertake the steps that a hospital admission requires? Who is going to call the patient's physician? Who will drive the patient to the hospital? Does the school need to be contacted? Who will find out when the next AA meeting is? During what time frame will these tasks be undertaken? Who will make sure they happen? Remember that most persons—psychiatrically ill or not—are relieved by the introduction of an external structure when handling a crisis.

The Clinical Handling of Crisis Management Sessions

FFT sessions may turn into crisis sessions with little warning. For example, you may begin with an agenda of conducting a CET session, but if a patient arrives having gone off his or her medication and obviously alcohol intoxicated, a different agenda must ensue.

The first rule in conducting FFT crisis sessions is to *keep calm yourself*. A relaxed presence communicates to the family members that you have seen problems of this kind before, that their family is not unusual in having them, and that you know how to handle such emergencies. Take heed of Samuel Shem's (1978) advice to new doctors treating patients with cardiac arrests: "The first procedure is to check your own pulse" (p. 50).

Second, *be flexible* in structuring and determining the appropriate content of the session. You may wish to see the whole family together, the relatives without the patient, or the patient by him- or herself. Depending on the needs of the family and what your setting will allow, you may decide to have a short or a long session. You may wish to explore issues that at first glance do not seem relevant to the stated crisis. Having a cotherapist is particularly helpful at these times.

Third, when appropriate, *normalize the crisis* by indicating that it is expectable, given what is known about the nature of bipolar disorder. Explain that manic, depressive, and/or suicidal episodes, although painful for the patient and everyone in the family, should be expected to occur at some point during the life course of the disorder. Likewise, hospitalizations can be framed as an essential and, often, predictable component of the treatment process, not a shameful admission of one's (or one's family's) inability to cope. You can say, for example, "I can understand why this hospitalization is so upsetting, but let's remember that recovering from an episode usually goes along with some setbacks."

Fourth, if this is true within your setting, *make it clear to the patient and family members that they can continue to see you after the crisis is resolved*. Some family members will believe that they cannot come back after the patient has been in the hospital, or that the patient's suicidal crisis signals the failure of the family treatment. Be clear that you will support them after the hospitalization (or other crisis event) and help them pick up the pieces.

Finally, *communicate regularly with the patient's physician*. He or she may not know that the patient has discontinued medication and is relapsing, requires hospitalization, or is suicidal. The physician also may not know that the patient is using drugs or alcohol. Changes in medication regimens are often a key component of resolving crises, and the physician is often centrally involved in the process of hospitalization.

Manic Relapses and Hospitalization

Juan, a 21-year-old bipolar Latino man, had missed several FFT sessions. He arrived late for the next scheduled session, accompanied by his mother and his older brother Albert. He had clearly cycled into a full-blown mania. He had brought with him an electric keyboard and frequently interrupted the session by playing loud, eerily synthesized music. He spoke forcefully and quickly, laughed inappropriately, talked about his childhood when questions were addressed about the present, and behaved in an overtly hostile manner toward his brother. His mother and brother were ready to hospitalize him, but were unclear how to proceed. Juan did not feel there was anything wrong with him and refused to contact his psychiatrist.

You may encounter manic relapses at any stage of escalation. If the patient is acutely manic, the primary goal of an FFT emergency session is to help the patient and family to arrange a hospitalization or, at minimum, an emergency outpatient evaluation. In other cases, the patient may be hypomanic, and careful planning during family sessions may help prevent further escalation and hospitalization. After the acute manic episode has passed, you can help the family make sense of what happened and review the procedures for preventing future episodes. I deal with each of these issues in this section.

Keep in mind that manic patients—particularly if, like Juan, they are elated and grandiose—rarely see themselves as ill. In contrast, those in the family or social network are usually painfully aware of the patient's escalation. Thus, the manic relapse reignites the "patient rejects/family accepts the illness" conflicts outlined in Chapter 8.

Mania Requiring Hospitalization

Juan had cycled into mania, but it was unclear whether he needed to be hospitalized, or whether his episode could be handled on an outpatient basis. This, of course, required an assessment.

The family clinicians first saw Juan and his relatives in separate rooms. The clinicians asked each of them to express what they understood to be happening to Juan, and assessed the degree to which he was showing the core symptoms of mania. The assessment revealed that Juan was manic to the point that he should at least be evaluated for a hospitalization. For example, he had taken the family car and run over a neighbor's free-standing mailbox, which he had thought was quite funny.

After bringing the family back together, the clinicians asked each of the participants to express to each other what they thought was happening to Juan, and encouraged them each to speak in turn and not interrupt each other. The focus was simultaneously on two issues: (1) Did Juan need to be hospitalized? (2) Could each member of the family clarify what issues were at stake for him or her?

CLINICIAN: I think all of you have your own ideas about what's happening here. Why don't you say what they are? Let's start with you, Juan.

JUAN: (*speaking rapidly*) I just think they want to control me. There's nothing different about me—they just want me to take more medication. They know what's best for me, as a child! But I'm no longer a child.

ALBERT: (*angry*) What you mean there's nothing wrong with you! You took the car and ran over Russ and Marlene's mailbox!

JUAN: Albert's all pissed off because of the car, because it was his car, and that's what he really cares about.

ALBERT: I'm not pissed off about the car! I'm pissed that you could've killed yourself or somebody else!

The family was revealing a dynamic that was a recurrent theme in their treatment: the tendency to voice concern in a hostile way, such that it lost its intended meaning. But how could the brother communicate his concern without sounding hostile?

CLINICIAN: Juan, I wonder if you're missing something here. Albert has expressed feeling very concerned about your welfare. Did you hear him say that?

JUAN: Not really.

CLINICIAN: Albert, I think you're really worried about Juan, and we certainly hear that, but Juan thinks you're just pissed off. Could you express the same sentiment in a way that might make Juan feel less defensive? About why you're concerned about him?

ALBERT: (*Pauses; looks at Juan, still angry.*) Well, yeah. I'm worried about you! I don't want to get a call from the police and find out you've been killed.

This use of direct communication is often an important prerequisite to the crisis resolution. Members of the family need to feel that their positions have at least been given credence. At this point, however, the clinicians are becoming more convinced that Juan needs to be hospitalized, and target the session at that objective. They are not optimistic that Juan will agree to a voluntary hospitalization. They begin by educating him, and the rest of the family, about what they believe is happening.

CLINICIAN: Juan, we think you're probably having a manic episode. Think back on what we taught you about manic episodes. Right now, it looks like you're experiencing some of the signs: You're having racing thoughts, you're not sleeping, and you're doing some dangerous things [psychoeducation]. It may be that you'll need to go into a more controlled environment for a week or two, in order to be safe and protect yourself as well as other people.

JUAN: No way.

CLINICIAN: Well, let me share my view of a hospitalization before you throw out the idea all together. First, I don't think it's the most horrible thing that can happen to a person. In fact, sometimes it's the best thing. If nothing else, it gives you a chance to catch up on your sleep and have your medications reevaluated. It's a safe place where you can protect yourself, be taken care of, and give your family a break as well. And, of course, we'll continue to see you when you get out, and then maybe we'll be able to figure out what we can learn from all of this. [Reframes hospitalization as a normal part of the treatment process, and emphasizes continuity of the therapeutic relationship.]

Although this way of characterizing the hospitalization is welcome to his relatives, Juan continues to resist the idea. Therefore, the clinicians depart from discussions with Juan about whether or not he is really ill, and discuss the practicalities of arranging an involuntary hospitalization. They emphasize the realities of what will happen if Juan does not seek voluntary treatment.

CLINICIAN: I think it's pretty clear that Juan won't go to the hospital on his own, and won't call his doctor either. So, let's talk about what the two of you [brother and mother] will do if he has to go to the hospital against his will. What will you do to get him onto the inpatient unit?

MOTHER: I don't know. That's one of the reasons we came in.

CLINICIAN: Do you remember the relapse drill we did a few weeks ago? About the steps of dealing with a hospitalization?

ALBERT: Yeah, we could call the police. Or one of us could drive him to the emergency room. But he's not gonna go voluntarily.

JUAN: Wait just a minute.

Sometimes the loss of control implied by a forced hospitalization has a way of cutting through the patient's denial. The healthy parts of the patient are afraid of being dragged into a hospital, and at this point a degree of cooperation—at least with the crisis evaluation process—may emerge.

Supporting the Relatives

If the acutely ill patient is refusing to acknowledge his or her illness, the real target of your interventions becomes the relatives, and educating them about how to deal with the emergency. Encourage them to problem solve about how to take the patient to the hospital; how to contact the doctor; what role you, as the family clinician, can play; and so forth. For example, Juan finally agreed to be walked to the emergency room by the family clinician, and his mother agreed to call his psychiatrist. In a separate session with Juan's brother and mother, they agreed that after Juan was discharged, his brother would give him access to the car keys only if he had seen his doctor that same week.

An important message to give relatives is that there are certain things they can and cannot control. That is, they can learn as much as possible about the illness, they can keep their own reactions from getting out of control, and they can communicate to the patient their desire to help and/or their frustration over his or her lack of acknowledgment of the disorder (see Handout 8, How Can the Family Help?, in Chapter 7). However, relatives cannot single-handedly force the patient into the hospital, control his or her mood swings, or make him or her take medications. They have more control if the patient is a juvenile, but even then their options are limited. Understandably, these limitations are not always clear to relatives.

You can help relatives determine which actions on their part will help during a manic relapse and which will not, as well as what they can delegate to you, the physician, or the other treatment personnel. Moreover, encourage them to take care of themselves during crises—to come in for FFT sessions without the patient, talk to friends or their own therapists, or make use of reading materials that will help put their reactions into perspective (e.g., *Contagious Emotions*; Podell, 1993).

Hypomania Not Yet Requiring Hospitalization

You may be able to help the family avert a hospitalization when the patient is just beginning to escalate. If Juan had been hypomanic rather than manic, the clinicians would have been in a stronger position to handle the crisis on an outpatient basis. A good message to convey to the patient and family during such times is "You have a certain amount of control now over what happens. But that control can disappear quickly if your [his or her] symptoms escalate."

Although the psychoeducational and communication interventions discussed above can also be introduced in cases of upward-cycling hypomania, we generally find that problem solving is the most powerful intervention at this stage. Specifically, you can help the patient and family members to make a list of what each person will do in the forthcoming days to prevent a full-blown episode from occurring.

The emergency maneuvers listed in Table 12.2 can be quite useful. For example, the patient can try to keep to a regular sleep–wake cycle and

TABLE 12.2. Emergency Maneuvers for Patients with Escalating Mania or Hypomania

- Call the physician for an emergency visit to evaluate medications.
- Take medications previously recommended for escalating symptoms.
- Stay home from work/school and catch up on sleep.
- Regularize daily schedules and sleep–wake habits.
- Avoid caffeine, street drugs, alcohol, large amounts of sugar, or other mood- or sleep-altering substances.
- Arrange for a family member to monitor the patient.
- Encourage the patient to take a trusted companion along when going out at night.

daily routine. A relative may have a flexible enough work schedule that he or she can stay home with the patient for part or all of the next few days. Another member of the family may be able to help the patient to keep track of his or her medication usage. If the patient is prone to hypersexual behavior or other forms of impulsiveness, encourage him or her to take a trusted companion along when going out at night.

It is important that an action list be developed by the family as a whole. Preferably, each family member—and certainly, the patient—plays a part in the solution.

Prevention Efforts Following the Manic Relapse

Once the manic or hypomanic episode begins to resolve, which may follow a course of inpatient treatment, reinstitute some of the exercises recommended in the psychoeducation chapters. Try to do a "postmortem" on the episode, with special reference to the relapse drill (Chapter 7). What were the first signs and symptoms of mania this time? What were the precipitating events? Were there observable changes in the patient's sleep—wake patterns, levels of activity, or mood? Then, review the family members' implementation of the relapse drill, with attention paid to *what went wrong:* Did they remember the drill at all? If so, did the patient or relative not notice the prodromal signs, or not think to call the physician? Was the patient too belligerent to cooperate with the steps outlined in the procedure? Then, reintroduce the drill as a new problem-solving exercise, with the objective of developing and rehearsing new and, it is hoped, more effective strategies.

For example, perhaps a relative had trouble telling the patient that he or she was getting manic. You can ask this relative to practice making this observation to the patient (e.g., "I'm noticing you're sleeping less and you're getting irritable with me a lot. Maybe you're starting to cycle again. Would you mind if I called your doctor?"). In return, encourage the patient to express what would and would not be helpful when in these states. One teenage girl told her mother, "It's important to remind me to take my medications, because it's really difficult for me to tell (when I'm getting manic). I won't like it, but you should do it anyway."

During the postmanic phase, there is a high probability of a recurrence or a swing into a depressive episode. During this phase, check in with the patient more frequently about his or her mood and associated symptoms, and, if necessary, encourage him or her to reinstitute the self-management strategies outlined in Table 12.2. Try to get the patient to track his or her day-to-day fluctuations with a mood chart (Chapter 7).

Depressive Relapses

Depressive relapses are typically more gradual than manic relapses, although they can also necessitate emergency interventions. If a patient comes to FFT with worsening symptoms of a major depression, your task is twofold: (1) to help the patient identify those things he or she can do to alleviate this condition and (2) to give the relatives the tools for helping to activate the patient behaviorally. Once again, the task involves assessment, psychoeducation, communication enhancement, and problem solving. First, just how depressed is the patient? Is he or she worse than last week? Were there any losses, events, or conflicts within the family that precipitated this change in mood? How have relatives reacted to the patient's mood and/or tried to make him or her feel better?

Second, remind the patient and family of the symptoms of major depression, and of the biological bases of this condition. Make it clear that the patient has not willfully produced his or her symptoms: The patient may be unable rather than unwilling to get out of bed each morning.

With adolescents, depression often hides behind hostility and angry outbursts. Some adolescents acknowledge depressed feelings to their parents directly; others require considerable prompting. Although it is not critical that the adolescent acknowledge depression, it is important that parents do so. Encouraging the parents to recognize that an increase in irritability—along with other symptoms of a downward-spiraling mood—may signal depression, as opposed to mania. This is an important component of psychoeducation during a crisis.

Third, encourage the patient to communicate to the family how he or she is feeling, and why. This is especially critical in cases in which the family thinks the patient is faking it, or is being lazy. In other cases, family members may wish to verbalize their concern about the patient's emotional state, especially if he or she is actively rejecting their attempts to be supportive. Coach them to say to the patient, for example, "I know you think that when you're depressed it's just a personal issue and no one else's business. But I think it's really a family problem, and I'm concerned and want to help."

Most important, problem solve with the family about what to do next. If hospitalization appears to be necessary, follow some of the steps recommended for manic relapses. If it appears that the depression can be handled on an outpatient basis, encourage the family to help the patient become more engaged with his or her world. For example, one member of the family may be able to encourage him or her to get out of bed, take walks, or eat properly. Similarly, the patient may agree to undertake one or more behavioral assignments each day that will be pleasurable or at least motorically activating (see Beck, Rush, Shaw, & Emery's, 1987, "pleasant events scheduling"). As always, you can negotiate a contract between the patient and family members about who will call the patient's physician.

The Suicidal Crisis

Shortly after her suicidal episode resolved, the family clinician explored with Kathleen and Jerry its meaning. The notion that Kathleen had a biochemical imbalance was familiar to Jerry, but he had not seriously considered the possibility that her suicidal behavior was not done with the explicit intention of exacting revenge on him. The family clinician instructed him to listen to Kathleen articulate her feelings of despair about her life, while he paraphrased and asked her clarifying questions. The clinician also encouraged Kathleen to make specific, positive requests of Jerry: "When I'm feeling this way, will you stay home with me? Would you take the pills away so I don't overdose on them? Would you drive me to the hospital if need be?" In turn, Jerry voiced his frustration about not being able to help her, and made clear his desire for her to stay alive and remain married to him.

With the help of problem solving, Kathleen and Jerry developed a contingency contract for managing future suicidal episodes. Specifically, Jerry agreed to check in with her more frequently about her emotional state. She, in turn, agreed to take more responsibility for getting herself psychiatric help when her suicidal feelings recurred. They agreed to schedule emergency family sessions if they had the types of arguments that in the past precipitated her self-destructive behavior.

Clare, age 17, had bipolar I disorder and thought about suicide almost daily. She had made two prior suicide attempts, both by Tylenol overdose, and both following loss experiences (for example, a breakup with a boyfriend). She had managed to hide both attempts from her parents. The clinicians encouraged Clare to talk about her impulses with her parents, who were not nearly as surprised nor as punitive as she had feared they would be. The knowledge that her self-destructive impulses had a biological origin made her parents less likely to accuse Clare of being manipulative.

FFT sessions focused on problem solving to develop a safety plan: Was Clare willing to tell her parents when she became suicidal? Could Clare call her own doctor and therapist, or was it better to tell her mother and ask her to make the call? Was it safe for her to be alone when she was thinking this way, and if not, what kinds of responses from her parents would she experience as supportive? Could her parents keep their pain relievers in a place where she could not find them?

Clare's safety plan involved a detailed list of early warning signs, an action plan for Clare (e.g., paging her father, reviewing a list she constructed of reasons she wanted to live) and a separate action plan for her parents (contacting her doctor, checking with her by phone every hour when she was home alone). Subsequent sessions of communication and problem-solving training did not eliminate Clare's suicidal thinking, but she and her parents felt better about having a list of alternative courses of action to follow when she felt most desperate.

Suicidality raises a unique set of issues in the FFT of bipolar patients. It is quite a common occurrence in this population. In fact, the risk for suicide among bipolar adults is about 30 times that of the nonpsychiatric population (Harris & Barraclough, 1997). Adolescents with bipolar disorder are at higher risk for attempts or completions than adolescents with any other psychiatric condition (Brent et al., 1988). Risk factors for suicide include substance and alcohol abuse, anxiety symptoms, a family history of suicide, illness of recent onset, a depressed or mixed affective illness phase, being single, and a prior history of attempts (Jamison, 2000). Keep these risk factors in mind when evaluating the level of suicide risk posed by your patient.

We have found that keeping patients in an intensive family program like FFT, with carefully administered pharmacotherapy, keeps them from feeling socially isolated and creates a "holding environment" that may help prevent them from acting on self-destructive impulses. However, this environment is not always adequately protective, and despite your best efforts, you can expect suicidal episodes to arise in some of your patients.

In most cases, suicidality is best explored as openly as possible within the family. Communicate to the patient and family that you are not afraid of his or her self-destructive impulses, that you have seen them before in other patients, and that you want the family and patient to solve this problem mutually. Use words or phrases like "suicide" and "wanting to kill (or hurt) yourself" rather than "those bad feelings" or "when you get that way."

Although FFT employs standard suicide prevention procedures, you are in a more powerful position if you can engage each family member as an ally in the prevention process. Both Kathleen's and Clare's suicidal impulses would have been much tougher to address if their relatives were not engaged in treatment. Open up a dialogue with each family member about the meaning of the current suicidal behavior within the family context, and help elicit that person's ideas about how to prevent it from recurring.

Assessing Suicidality

Some of your patients may be so acutely suicidal that hospitalization is your only option. Little productive work can be done with the family at this stage. However, most bipolar patients do not arrive at your sessions in this state, but, rather, present as depressed and with suicidal thoughts. As in any psychosocial treatment, assess the lethality of the suicidal impulses: the presence of a plan, a means, and a stated intent. Being bipolar increases lethality risk, especially if the mood is unstable, the patient has a history of suicide attempts, and there is current substance or alcohol abuse.

It is important to clarify for yourself, and for the family, the degree to which suicidal feelings reflect a worsening state of depression versus a temporary reaction to recent life events. Table 12.3 lists some of the many reasons why bipolar patients—and other psychiatric patients—become suicidal. None of these motivating factors are mutually exclusive of the others.

In assessing your patient's suicidality, ask yourself difficult questions such as the following: Does the patient truly wish to die? Is there evidence of this wish from past attempts? Do his or her attempts occur frequently, and are they apparently dissociated from depressive periods, life events, or family conflicts? Alternatively, does his or her suicidality reflect a worsening state of depression? Are other symptoms of a major depression present, and if so, might the patient require changes in his or her medication regimen? A structured interview, like the Hamilton Rating Scale for Depression (Hamilton, 1960), can help you make this judgment.

In addition to the patient's associated symptoms, does suicidality reflect a family dynamic issue? Kathleen, for example, was more likely to become suicidal when having a depressive episode, but her suicidal feelings were never fully separable from her reactions to relationship events. What is the nature of these precipitating events? Does the patient believe that others will be better off if he or she dies ("altruistic suicide")? Do the suicidal feelings reflect despair stemming from fears of abandonment by members of the family (as in Kathleen's case)? Has the patient's family or

TABLE 12.3. Factors Motivating Suicidal Behavior among Bipolar Patients

- A true wish to die
- A worsening state of depression
- A desire to be altruistic to others
- A desire to punish or manipulate others
- A desire to escape intolerable feelings or situations
- A desire to communicate a message that is difficult to communicate verbally

life situation become so intolerable that he or she wishes to escape, and dying seems to be the only way to do so? Is he or she primarily angry at family members over repeated conflicts, criticisms, or hostility, and thus wants revenge? Alternatively, are suicidal impulses more related to issues outside the family, such as romantic losses (as in Clare's case)?

We find it useful to conduct a "chain analysis" (Linehan, 1993), in which we determine the sequence of events that preceded the onset of the suicide attempt (if there has been one) or the most recent thoughts or impulses, as perceived by the patient and each family member. For the patient, what events, followed by what thoughts and feelings, produced the suicidal behavior? For the relatives, how did they intervene (or fail to intervene) at each step of this process? What did each member think and feel at various times? Did relatives perceive the episode as coming out of the blue, or did they see it building? After the episode, what did each family member do? Was the patient in any way rewarded for his or her behavior (e.g., with more attention or displays of concern)?

The identification of "antecedent–behavior–consequence" patterns will help you design family interventions to interrupt these sequences. For example, you can encourage relatives to use active listening skills with the patient during the early phases of the suicide sequence, so that the patient at least feels understood and validated. You can help them determine when a call to the patient's psychiatrist will have the most impact on the outcome.

Based on your assessments, you may decide to structure the FFT session in any number of ways, including seeing the patient alone, the relatives alone, or all of the participants together. If the patient is severely depressed and resistant to coming to your office, consider making a visit to the patient's home. You may decide to accompany the family and patient to the hospital emergency room if the threat of completed suicide seems imminent.

Psychoeducation

Family members and patients need a context for understanding where suicidal behavior comes from. The family may already have such a context from your previous psychoeducation sessions and are sometimes on the lookout for suicidality in their ill relative. In fact, some will have already called the physician and arranged for an emergency medical visit even before they speak with you.

Other relatives are less clear on how to understand suicidal thoughts or actions. They can readily identify the stress precipitants of the episode, or the contributions of the patient's personality attributes (see the case of Kathleen and Jerry), but have a harder time understanding that biological processes play a role in stimulating self-destructive impulses in a vulnerable patient. As a result, some relatives blame the patient for his or her suicidal behavior, which they view as manipulative, willfully produced, and due to a character weakness or moral failing.

We recommend treating suicidality like any other bipolar symptom. That is, (1) provide psychoeducation about the underlying biological changes that precipitate these crises, (2) address the meaning of the eliciting life or familial events, and (3) explore and help clarify the patient's resulting feelings of despair and hopelessness.

As a beginning, normalize the patient's suicidal behavior and put it in the context of the patient's diagnosis:

> "Quite a lot of people have suicidal thoughts and impulses, feeling that their lives are not worth living. These impulses are in themselves symptoms of bipolar disorder. And although I know you're dealing with some difficult life circumstances and events within your family, let's remember that you're probably also dealing with biochemical imbalances that get automatically set off by those life circumstances. You're certainly not alone in reacting this way."

This intervention has two purposes. First, it recognizes that the suicidal individual feels quite isolated. He or she may derive comfort from understanding that these feelings are not necessarily crazy, and that there are other people who feel this way. Second, it brings the family back to the vulnerability–stress model. For most bipolar patients, suicidal despair is at least in part a product of the uncontrollable, significant biological changes associated with the cycling of the mood disorder.

Exploring the psychological factors associated with the episode is perhaps the strongest hand you can play. The participants need to clarify the meaning of the events that have occurred, and why the patient feels that ending his or her life is the only solution. We often find it helpful to interpret the suicidal behavior as an escape response to unpleasant emotions or life circumstances; for example, "I don't think you really want to die. I think you want to escape from some pretty awful feelings. Let's talk about some of those feelings first, and why dying seems to you like the only way to get rid of them."

You should also tell the patient and family that suicidal episodes tend to be temporary rather than permanent. When a person feels suicidal, he or she is unlikely to be able to see the way out of the fog. Although he or she may not believe you, the family will be relieved to hear that the patient is reacting to negative life circumstances and/or is in the throes of a depressive episode that will eventually remit. However, avoid being cornered into making promises about how long the suicidal feelings are likely to last.

Communication Enhancement

When managing a suicidal crisis, ask yourself the following questions: Does the suicide threat reflect a message that cannot be verbally conveyed? If so, can the patient put this message into words? In our experience, the "caption" underlying the suicidal threat is often one or more of the following: "I no longer feel a part of this family," "I feel terribly guilty about the damage I've caused to my own and everyone else's life," or "I feel others would be better off if I weren't around." However, your task is not necessarily to restructure these negative self-statements, the way you might in cognitive therapy. Rather, use the CET strategies to help the suicidal patient clarify for the relatives his or her fears, wishes, and needs. In turn, try to use these same strategies to encourage the relatives' expressions of reassurance and concern for the patient.

Consider the case of Cliff, a 25-year-old male bipolar patient with a severe depression. His mother, with whom he lived, could not tolerate his lack of motivation or action and had become quite hostile toward him. He was beginning to have suicidal thoughts. We asked him to try to communicate his internal despair to her, while she listened actively without interjecting suggestions, criticisms, or advice. He was able to say, "It's not that I'm lazy. I'm lying in bed all day because I feel like I can't do anything . . . that I've let you down . . . that life isn't worth living." Although hearing this did not keep his mother from feeling angry, it did diminish her hostile tone in her subsequent interactions with him.

For Kathleen and Jerry, the challenge was to get her to explain the role that marital events played in her suicidality. With coaching, she was able to communicate her underlying abandonment fears: "I'm afraid when you get angry you're going to leave me, and that's when I want to kill myself."

It is equally helpful is to teach family members to inquire directly about the patient's suicidal feelings. However, teaching family members to make such inquiries raises for them the question of whether doing so will precipitate such a crisis. Direct this question to the patient: "If your mother [father, spouse, sibling] asks you if you're feeling suicidal, will that make things worse?" More often than not, you will find that patients appreciate it when their relatives check in with them and voice concern. Then, you can coach relatives on appropriate and inappropriate ways to address these questions, such that the patient will not perceive them as intrusive or threatening.

Even more powerful are communication exercises in which the relative voices his or her desire for the patient not to commit suicide, or his or her despair about not being able to help more.

CLINICIAN: Can you turn your chair toward Kathleen and tell her how you feel when she threatens to kill herself?

JERRY: It's like, I don't know, how come you wanna do that?

KATHLEEN: It's 'cause it seems like nothing's working, between us or anything else.

JERRY: So you think killing yourself's a good solution?

CLINICIAN: Let's stop for a minute. Jerry, how would you feel if she actually did kill herself?

JERRY: Terrible! Awful, of course. I want to, I don't know, I don't know what to do.

CLINICIAN: Can you tell her that directly? How you'd feel?

JERRY: Well, I don't know. Hon, I'd miss you if you died. I don't want to see you hurting yourself.

Interchanges like the above tend to help families or couples get beyond the anger and guilt produced by suicidal episodes and focus instead on their underlying worries, fears, and concerns. When they do so, the emotional attachment between the members emerges, and patients are less likely to feel unwanted by or burdensome to others.

Problem Solving

Next, help the family members or couple construct a plan for how they will deal with the immediate suicidal behavior and its likely future recurrence. Start with questions of the form "If you're concerned that Kathleen is getting suicidal, what are you going to do, Jerry?" "Kathleen, what are you going to do if you feel suicidal again?" Then, break these questions down into a series of component questions, all of which can be addressed (individually or simultaneously) in problem-solving exercises. Examples of these questions are listed in Table 12.4. If you use these questions as starting points, families can develop individualized plans for coping with suicidal episodes.

For example, after her suicidal episode had resolved, Kathleen and Jerry agreed that she would initiate telling him about her self-destructive thoughts only if she felt she was in real danger. Otherwise, during these high-risk periods, he was to inquire about her suicidal thoughts at least once each week. More important, he was to inquire about how she felt her life was going, even when she was not suicidal. They also agreed that if she became acutely suicidal, Kathleen would call the physician and the family clinician. Finally, they agreed that Jerry would stay home from work with Kathleen at times when she felt the worst and drive her to the emergency room if necessary.

TABLE 12.4. Questions to Stimulate Problem Solving about Suicidal Episodes

- Is the patient willing to tell relatives if he or she becomes suicidal, and if so, in what way?
- When feeling suicidal, what kinds of encounters with relatives will the patient experience as supportive?
- Is it safe for the patient to be at home alone? If not, who can stay with him or her?
- Who will call the physician and arrange a medication reevaluation?
- How else can the patient or family get help?

It is particularly important to rehearse the implementation of these strategies. Take the family or couple through role-play exercises in which, for example, the patient makes specific requests for help from a relative (e.g., for Kathleen, "Will you sit up with me tomorrow night if I can't sleep?"; for Clare, "Dad, is it OK if I page you at work?"). If the relative or patient is uncomfortable with calling and telling you or the physician about a suicidal crisis, ask him or her to role-play with you such telephone calls, and respond the way you or the physician might respond.

Alcohol and Substance Abuse

Mark, 29, worked at night as a keyboard player in a barroom jazz band. He had smoked marijuana since he was a child and currently traveled in social circles where it was widely available. Because his use had been so constant, it was not always clear whether it directly contributed to his mood swings. He "took a few tokes" immediately before he performed with his band and before he went to bed at night, but did not feel compelled to smoke during the day. He was compliant with his Depakote and Wellbutrin regimen, and for several years his illness had been well controlled.

After his wife, Wendy, had their first baby, Mark's marijuana smoking increased dramatically. Because she had a rather demanding day job and they had little money for child care, they agreed that he would stay at home most of the day. He began to smoke marijuana from the moment he got up in the morning until dinnertime. One day, he left a lit marijuana cigarette near the baby's bassinet, and on another day fell asleep while he was supposed to be watching her. In response to these events, Wendy became enraged and accused him of being an incompetent and irresponsible father. As they began to argue more, he began to smoke more. In part because of his excessive marijuana use, he became amotivational, irritable, and agitated, and experienced sleep disturbances.

Substance and Alcohol Abuse: How Much of a Problem Is It?

Lifetime substance and alcohol abuse or dependence characterizes about 61% of all bipolar patients (Regier et al., 1990). Adolescent patients have rates of substance abuse that are about five times higher than rates among nonbipolar controls (Wilens et al., 2004). A patient who begins to drink heavily or use drugs is in a psychiatric crisis, because the use of substances greatly worsens the course of bipolar disorder, interferes with the effects of prescribed medications, decreases treatment compliance and consistency, and increases the chances of his or her suicide or early mortality. Prolonged abuse of alcohol and sedatives causes severe depressive symptoms. Likewise, central nervous system-activating drugs like cocaine can precipitate mania.

Dependency and abuse problems are harder to treat than depression or suicidality, particularly if these problems are long-standing. Much as in mania, the substance-abusing bipolar patient sees little wrong with his or her behavior and is usually not motivated to change it.

Although FFT is not designed to serve as a primary treatment for substance or alcohol abuse, it can be quite useful in addressing the family issues that interact with these problems. In the following sections, we consider patients who show gradual or sudden increases in their drug or alcohol use. You will observe that our four-pronged approach is more difficult to implement with these patients, but not impossible.

The Interface between FFT and Self-Help Groups

In our experience, FFT is most helpful in treating substance or alcohol abuse or dependence when there are proximal causes (i.e., the abuse reflects a direct reaction to family conflict or a recent life event) and less effective when there are distal causes (i.e., a long-standing pattern of drug abuse dating back to childhood or adolescence, severe personality problems, a heavy genetic loading for substance or alcohol abuse). Particularly in these latter cases, we refer patients to AA, Narcotics Anonymous (NA), or other substance abuse programs during their participation in FFT.

Despite their utility, many patients refuse to attend self-help groups. In fact, in our experience, only a minority of the bipolar patients we refer actually attend one or more group sessions. When we feel strongly about the necessity of support groups or other substance abuse treatments (e.g., for patients with long-standing alcohol dependence), we explain that we will not work with the family unless the patient enrolls in one of these adjunctive treatments. We offer the rationale that the coping strategies for dealing with bipolar disorder will be largely irrelevant until the substance problem is controlled.

We also believe, however, that you can be too trigger-happy in referring patients to AA or NA. Not every patient will be comfortable in subscribing to the set of beliefs associated with these programs, or with discussing his or her problems in front of a group of people. Thus, if the patient's substance or alcohol abuse is not life-threatening and is clearly related to proximal causes (e.g., family conflicts), you may wish to begin with FFT and introduce the referral to support groups later on. Also consider other chemical dependency programs, such as motivational enhancement therapy (Miller & Rollnick, 1992), cognitive-behavioral therapy (CBT), or individual 12-step programs.

If the patient does agree to attend a self-help group, be sure that FFT and the group do not have conflicting goals. For example, if the patient gleans from a self-help group that "all drugs are bad" (whether or not this was actually stated), he or she may use this argument to rationalize discontinuing psychiatric medications. In such cases, educate the patient about the differences between drugs of abuse and psychiatric medications, and the risks to him or her of medication nonadherence (see Chapter 8).

Ideally, refer the patient to a treatment group with a "dual-diagnosis" emphasis, in which the parallels between recovery from substance or alcohol abuse and recovery from bipolar episodes are drawn, and skills for coping with both diseases are emphasized. A recent randomized trial found superior effects of an "integrated group therapy" over standard drug counseling groups in controlling alcohol abuse among bipolar patients (Weiss et al., 2007).

Assessment

If your patient begins to abuse drugs or alcohol, try to address a core question: What is the underlying function of the abuse? Is it primarily to "self-medicate" his or her affective symptoms? Bipolar patients frequently use substances to relieve depression, mixed affective states, or rapid cycling (Weiss et al., 2007). Thus, substance or alcohol abuse may be a prodromal sign suggesting the onset of a new affective episode. When this is occurring, help the patient arrange to get his or her medications reevaluated.

The self-medication of symptoms is only one function of drug or alcohol abuse. Like suicidality, substance abuse can be a form of acting out against or withdrawing from uncomfortable family dynamics (as in Mark's case, above). For example, one of our patients, an 18-year-old who lived with his parents, smoked marijuana to excess whenever his father—a former police officer—became more strict in his discipline. Likewise, some patients use alcohol or drugs to cope with recent, severe life events or to withdraw from uncomfortable life circumstances (e.g., a job in which they feel overstimulated, persecuted, or incompetent).

Another possibility is that the patient has always abused drugs or alcohol, even before the onset of the bipolar disorder. For some patients, you may even suspect that substance abuse triggered the first manic or depressive episode. Of course, patients with long-standing habits can also be using substances to self-medicate their current mood problems or deal with ongoing stressors, much as they did in childhood or adolescence.

When assessing the factors motivating substance or alcohol abuse, keep in mind the family and social context, from the viewpoint of the patient and all key relatives. When and why does the patient drink or use drugs? Who is there at the time? Do family members know when the patient is drunk/stoned? Does the patient use substances openly and in ways that mock family members, or is his or her use reclusive and secretive? Does a teen get stoned only when peers are over, or does he do it when alone as well? Can the patient discuss his or her usage openly with family members, without fearing their punishment?

Once again, conduct a chain analysis: When the patient does abuse alcohol or drugs, what are the immediate precipitants? Arguments with a spouse? A rejection experience? A stressful interaction with a child? In parallel, what happens after the patient indulges him- or herself: Do one or more family members confront him or her? Does anyone pretend that nothing happened? Is the patient rewarded in any way, even if negatively? Does getting drunk or stoned end for him or her an aversive family interaction?

Psychoeducation

Mark was not surprised to hear the family clinician say that drugs were bad for his bipolar disorder—this was no different from the many "Just Say No" messages he had received from mental health professionals over the years. He was clear that he used pot to self-medicate a depressive state. He had not considered, however, the possibility that marijuana might interfere with his sleep–wake cycle and how smoking therefore put him at risk for a manic episode. Although he did see his marijuana use as a reaction to family tensions, he did not believe it impaired his performance as a father. In fact, he claimed it improved his parenting because "I get mellower, less likely to get upset when things don't go well."

Start your intervention by offering the patient and family information about the biological interactions between drugs, alcohol, and mood disorder. For example, say, "I'm concerned about the effects of this drug (or alcohol) on your nervous system. We know you're biologically predisposed to episodes of bipolar disorder, and you're putting yourself at greater risk if you continue to take them." Tell the patient and family that substance or alcohol abuse may aggravate illness-based neurophysiological dysregulations and interfere with the efficacy of the patient's medications. Give them examples, as we did in Mark's case, of the ways in which drugs can affect social and circadian rhythms, increase the patient's exposure to stressors (e.g., through family conflicts), and diminish his or her most effective coping mechanisms. However, *avoid making moral judgments about whether people should or should not use substances*. You will maintain a better rapport with the substance-abusing patient if you empathize with his or her need for pleasure, escape, or stimulation, and simultaneously communicate concern about his or her health.

In our experience, patients usually reject at first the notion that substances put them at greater risk for a mood disorder episode, arguing, "I can handle it." However, many come around to accepting this notion as time progresses. Sadly, patients often have one or more recurrences associated with substance or alcohol abuse before this association seems real.

Communication Enhancement

Drug and alcohol abuse is often an expression of the underlying pathophysiology of bipolar disorder, but it can simultaneously reflect an implicit communication to the therapist and the family. Encourage the patient to express, while members of his or her family listen actively, the unmet needs, insecurities, or anxieties that alcohol or drugs temporarily relieve. Begin with a statement such as "Can you tell your mom and dad what's going on in your life that makes [name of drug] [alcohol] so important to you?"

Patients vary tremendously in their ability to answer this question. Some appear unable to address the issue at all: They may simply say, "I like to get high" or "It makes me feel better," but they cannot identify the underlying states they are trying to alleviate. Help them along with probing questions: In what ways do they feel better? Can they explain to their relatives how drugs provide an escape, and if so, from what? What activities are easier to perform if the patient is stoned or drunk? Do any of these involve the family? What would happen if he or she tried to perform these activities without drugs or alcohol? In other words, cast the substance abuse problem as a symptom covering up less obvious, more deeply rooted family or interpersonal problems.

In parallel, encourage family members to express their own discomforts with the patient's drug or alcohol abuse. To what extent do they feel angry at the patient (e.g., "You're never there for me when I need you") versus worried about something (e.g., "I'm afraid you'll accidentally hurt the baby")? Help them make the distinction between these two affective states. If necessary, encourage them to use the expressing negative feelings CET exercise from Chapter 9 (e.g., "I got really angry that you kept smoking weed on our vacation. What should we do next time? Should I go away and do something else while you get high?"). Once you feel that the family has had a reasonably open discussion about these issues, steer the discussion toward problem solving.

Problem Solving

After exploring his marijuana use further, Mark concluded that he needed to escape from the stresses associated with being a new parent. In parallel, smoking marijuana had provided an escape from a miserable family situation when he was a teenager. He was not confident about his ability to get through a day with the baby without smoking, but also refused to enroll in any drug rehabilitation program or self-help group. In response, the clinician voiced his fear that the child would be in danger if Mark's marijuana abuse continued. Problem solving with this couple focused less on his marijuana abuse and more on how he could be relieved of his nearly full-time parenting role. How could he break up the day? Was part-time day care affordable? Was it realistic for him to be a full-time parent and also work nights? Could he get together with other people who were at home during the day with young children? Could Wendy's work schedule be altered so that she could relieve him more frequently?

Treating substance or alcohol abuse problems within a family context involves addressing two subsidiary problems, the solutions to both of which require the family's cooperation. First, by what other means can the patient obtain the pleasures, or the escapes, currently provided by drugs or alcohol? Second, under what conditions will the patient agree to enroll in ancillary substance abuse programs, and how can the family facilitate this process?

Problem Solving about Escapism

In introducing the first of the problems, you can say to the patient, "You get pleasure from drugs, and of course you deserve to have pleasures in your life, especially given what you've been through with your illness. But can you think of any other ways in which you could get pleasure?" In most cases, patients will agree with this basic sentiment, although the notion that they could get pleasure from sources other than drugs or alcohol will probably seem an abstraction.

Encourage the participants to define the substance abuse as a family problem rather than only the patient's. In the case above, the two participants settled on the following definition: "Mark is unable to stay away from weed (their words), and Wendy is confused as to how to help him do so." Next, coach them on developing solutions that address the underlying functions of the substance abuse: How could the patient get more tangible rewards out of his life? If the purpose is to escape, are there other ways to escape? Are there other ways to get the stimulation currently provided by drugs? If a contributing factor is the patient's social milieu (e.g., Mark's employment facilitated marijuana use), how could he find different social outlets? How could he modulate exposure to the social cues (in Mark's case, child care) that lead to abuse?

A good preliminary solution is to encourage self-monitoring. For example, the patient can keep a schedule of his or her daily drug or alcohol abuse and its association with his or her sleep–wake cycles and mood states. If an association is revealed, the patient may agree to a time-limited experiment in which he or she abstains for a few days (during which time the spouse or parent removes all drugs or alcohol from the house) to determine the resulting effects on his or her sleep and mood.

Problem Solving about Adjunctive Treatments

In cases in which self-help groups or drug rehabilitation programs are strongly indicated, help the patient and family identify the steps involved in obtaining these kinds of treatments. However, do not overwhelm them with a long list of behaviors they must perform in a single week, as this will set them up for a failure experience. In our experience, you are doing well if you can convince patients and family members to make even one move toward exploring these treatments in a given week. For example, a patient may agree to attend one AA or NA meeting in a period between FFT sessions. Alternatively, he or she may agree only to have the spouse find out when and where the meetings are held.

In the next session, check in with the family or couple about whether the task was completed. If it was, encourage a second step, such as attending an AA meeting together. If they do not follow through, explore their resistances: Were they simply going along with your recommendation so as not to seem oppositional? Did they forget? Is there no motivation to solve the substance problem, and if so, how will they cope with it in the future? You can then introduce a second problem-solving exercise with more limited goals.

Of course, the patient's need for adjunctive treatment may be more dramatic than illustrated by the case. Some bipolar teens and adults need detoxification, live-away drug rehabilitation programs, antabuse protocols, methadone, or other treatments. You can sometimes help the family most by having connections with programs offering these treatments and arranging evaluations for emergency care when the patient needs it most.

Other Psychiatric Crises

There are many other types of crises associated with bipolar disorder, and space limits an extensive discussion of these. I discuss here two other emergency situations we sometimes encounter with bipolar patients. First, separation or divorce can be a precipitant *or* a sequel of manic episodes (Coryell et al., 1993; Kessing, Agerbo, & Mortensen, 2004). Second, as in any psychiatric disorder, severe episodes of bipolar disorder can be associated with child abuse or partner violence (Post & Leverich, 2006).

Divorce or Separation

Clearly, the CET and problem-solving modules of FFT are intended to help prevent marital failures. Nevertheless, there will be cases in which, despite your best efforts, couples decide to separate. In these cases, I recommend conducting conjoint or, less preferably, individual sessions that focus on problem solving. Within the structured format that problem solving provides, you can encourage the members of a couple to make temporary decisions about where each of them will live; if there are children, what kinds of short-term custody and visitation arrangements will be made; what kind and amount of contact they will have with each other; how they will manage finances; and whether additional marital counseling or divorce mediation is desired from you or another provider.

For the patient, be especially vigilant for signs of medication discontinuation, drug or alcohol abuse, high-risk behaviors, or mood disorder exacerbations during the period after the separation. Usually, these reflect direct reactions to the stress of the loss experience (along with the likely changes in sleep patterns and daily routines), but can also reflect covert attempts to bring the spouse back into the picture. If possible, ask the couple to contract for a limited number of FFT sessions after the separation, to discuss new problems that develop and clarify what each wishes to do next.

Adolescent patients are prone to mood recurrences and suicidal episodes following the marital failure of their parents. Of course, a recurrence can serve the temporary function of bringing the parents back together to coparent, but we have found little value in exploring such systemic realignments. Instead, focus your efforts on how the parents can put their marital battles aside long enough to obtain help for the child. They will need to do this kind of cooperative coparenting after the divorce, and the sooner they learn to master the difficulties inherent in postdivorce arrangements, the better recovery the child will make. In the short run, the adolescent usually needs assurance that both parents are still emotionally available to him or her.

Child Abuse and Partner Violence

State laws mandate that cases of suspected child abuse be reported to Child Protective Services. Some local jurisdictions also have procedures for reporting partner violence. In developing intervention plans for the family, try to determine the degree to which the disorder itself contributed to the abuse: Was the patient manic when hitting his or her child (or spouse)? Did a severe depression make it impossible for a bipolar patient to take care of his or her children properly?

In some cases, we have successfully implemented problem-solving strategies with child/partner abuse or child neglect problems. This usually requires allying with the healthier members of the family in developing temporary intervention plans. Help the well spouse of a child-abusive patient to identify the determinants of the abuse and take immediate steps toward implementing a "safety plan" for the child. Often, the healthy spouse of a relapsing patient, or perhaps a friend or neighbor, must take care of the children while the patient is in the hospital or otherwise incapacitated by symptoms (recalling that Child Protective Services will need to be notified if no adequate arrangements can be made).

Explore the options available to a spouse who believes she is at risk for physical violence from the spouse with bipolar disorder. Can she arrange to go to a shelter or the house of a friend or other family member? If the abusive behavior reflects a patient's incipient relapse, encourage the healthy family members to undertake the aforementioned relapse drill procedures, with treatment for the abuse to commence once the patient has recovered.

When addressing these complex problems, be especially attuned to the various ways to structure FFT sessions. For example, in cases of partner violence, it is usually best—at least at first—to see the endangered spouse and the patient separately. Likewise, in cases in which the patient has committed an act of child abuse or neglect, interview the healthy spouse separately. If possible, involve the patient's psychiatrist in these sessions.

Finally, independent of whom you actually see, be aware that abusive persons often have violent outbursts immediately after psychotherapy sessions. Check in with family members after sessions that have been emotionally heated, and set up mechanisms by which they can contact you and the police if they feel at risk.

Concluding Comments

The course of treating bipolar disorder is like the course of the illness itself: There are peaks and valleys, during which much work is accomplished and much is undone. You can expect that certain crises will surface among many of your patients during FFT. However, well-planned assessments followed by psychoeducation, CET, and problem solving provide a framework for addressing clinical emergencies. Furthermore, encouraging the patient and family members to avail themselves of other clinical services—including hospitalization, emergency sessions with the psychiatrist, or adjunctive self-help groups—promotes better resolutions to these crises.

chapter 13

Termination

Chapter Overview

This chapter addresses the issues involved in terminating FFT for bipolar disorder. As in other psychosocial treatments, the final sessions of FFT provide an opportunity to review the course of treatment, identify areas in need of future work, and help the patient and family to plan for future treatment needs. However, there are special issues that arise in terminating family treatment with bipolar patients.

Termination of FFT does not have a specific length, although in the modal case we recommend using the final two or three sessions (Sessions 19–21) for this purpose. Consider the family's status in terms of the six FFT goals (see Chapter 1). Table 13.1 presents a series of questions to ask yourself in evaluating which of the FFT objectives have been realized and which may require further work. The answers to these questions provide important guidelines as to how to focus the termination sessions.

Terminating FFT: Two Examples

Let us consider two families that participated in our 9-month program of FFT, which are at different places according to these outcome criteria. For one family (in the case of Phil, below), the therapist answered all but one of these items affirmatively, namely Item 3, a and b. Thus, much of the termination work focused on family issues related to the patient's desire to discontinue his medications. In the second case (Maria, below), issues related to Items 5 and 6 (handling stress and restoring functional family

TABLE 13.1. Evaluating the Impact of FFT

Have the patient and relatives come to understand the following:

1. The nature of bipolar disorder and the precipitants of the most recent episode?
2. That, despite the patient's recovery, he or she is at risk for fully syndromal recurrences and subsyndromal mood fluctuations?
3. a. The role of medication in the treatment of acute episodes of bipolar disorder?
   b. The need for continuing medication to prevent recurrences?
4. The distinction between enduring aspects of the patient's personality (or, for a teenager, "being a normal teen"), as contrasted with signs of his or her disorder?
5. More effective ways of identifying and managing external stressors?
6. How to maintain a positive, cooperative emotional tone in their family relationships, by employing effective strategies for direct communication and conflict management?

relationships) were more salient and guided the focus of those termination sessions.

The Case of Phil

Phil, a 23-year-old European American man, had his first manic episode during the middle of his senior year in college. He was extremely aggressive during the manic state, destroying property in his parents' home (where he resided) and threatening his parents with violence. Finally, after much ambivalence, his parents called the police and asked them to take Phil to a psychiatric unit. Although Phil resisted, they did transport him, in handcuffs, to a local hospital where he was admitted.

Phil, his parents, and his teenage sister Kim entered the FFT program shortly after Phil's hospital discharge. The early sessions were very tense, because Phil was still irritable, resistant to the idea that he had bipolar disorder, and particularly resentful that his parents had involved the police in forcing him to go to the hospital. However, the North family rarely missed a session. The psychoeducational sessions were moderately useful in reducing family tension, but it was the CET sessions that stimulated major changes in family relationships. In particular, they benefited from sessions in which Phil and his family members shared their thoughts and feelings about that traumatic evening when they called the police. By the end of treatment, the family had changed markedly in the openness of the members' communication and in their sense of connection with one another. As they subsequently put it, "We are closer as a family than we've ever been."

During the 9-month treatment, Phil remained compliant with his lithium and had no return of his manic symptoms. Toward the end of the recommended 21 sessions, the clinicians suggested termination. Phil thought it was a good time to terminate, but also expressed his desire simultaneously to stop his medications. His parents expressed a certain reluctance to terminate, as they enjoyed the family sessions and feared that without the support of the clinician, the improvement in their family relationships might disappear. They were also rightly concerned that Phil would be at a greater risk for a recurrence if he was not protected by his medications.

The family clinicians focused the termination sessions on medication issues. In a conjoint session involving Phil, his parents, and his psychiatrist, the family clinician explored in some depth Phil's wish to discontinue his lithium. However, Phil's mind was made up, and scheduling additional sessions to convince him otherwise seemed counterproductive. At this point, the participants all agreed that it was appropriate to terminate FFT. However, as with all families, the door was left open for future contacts in the event that problems arose—including the development in Phil of the prodromal symptoms of a new episode. Follow-up sessions were scheduled for 1 month, 3 months, and 6 months.

Let us contrast the course and termination of treatment with Phil's family with that of Maria and her family. The contrast highlights some very significant issues in ending the FFT of bipolar disorder.

The Case of Maria

In her early 20s, Maria had immigrated to the United States from a Latin American country with her father and three siblings. Her parents were divorced, and her father came to the United States to find a business to invest in. Maria had had an episode of bipolar, manic disorder in her native country, was hospitalized there, and was treated only with medication and released to her mother's care. Her mother was unable to deal with Maria's difficult behavior, which included numerous suicidal threats and at least one serious attempt, and insisted that the father take her with him to the United States. Reluctantly, her father moved with her, her older sister, and the two younger children, one of whom was severely physically disabled.

Maria had been studying at a Latin American university at the time of her first manic episode and was unable to return there afterward. As a result, her father withdrew financial support for her further education in the United States and assigned Maria the role of housekeeper and caretaker for her younger sister and brother. Maria intensely resented this role and her father's denial of support. Her father, on the other hand, believed that Maria was destined to be a "chronic mental patient" and not capable of much, educationally or occupationally.

Within 2 months of arriving in the United States, Maria relapsed and was hospitalized with manic and psychotic symptoms. Shortly after her discharge, Maria, her father, and her older sister were informed of the availability of a program of FFT coordinated with her medication management, and they agreed to participate.

When Maria started attending sessions, it was clear that she was still symptomatic. She was mainly depressed, very irritable and testy, and somewhat impaired cognitively. Her hostility toward her father was almost palpable, as was his disdain for her. Her older sister attended one session but refused further participation.

The psychoeducational sessions involving Maria and her father seemed effective in reducing the general level of family tension, although her father had difficulty accepting the idea that Maria could potentially function at a higher level. Maria, in contrast, accepted her diagnosis but struggled to find some signs of acceptance and encouragement from her father. She got very little of this initially.

During the CET sessions, the tension rose again as Maria sought positive feedback from her father, which he found difficult to give. When the skill of making positive requests was the focus, Maria used it to express her desires to return to college and resume her education. This required considerable financial support from the father. He was very reluctant to spend the money on her, given her past history of breaking down during her university studies. Finally, he agreed and she entered a community college, signing up for a full load of difficult academic subjects.

Although Maria appeared to be doing quite well in her first semester of junior college, her ability to function was seriously challenged when she showed the prodromal signs of another manic episode. Close consultation with Maria's psychiatrist resulted in an increase in her medication, and the family clinicians worked out a plan with Maria and her family to focus her efforts on the courses she could pass, while asking for "incompletes" in the others. She handled this effectively, and over a 3-week period her symptoms receded and hospitalization was averted.

In the last 3 months of treatment, Maria was mostly asymptomatic, although there were occasional flare-ups of symptoms, mainly of impulsiveness and irritability. Her father seemed to soften his view of her possibilities and agreed to support her return to college for the spring term. Although Maria was no longer heading toward another major episode, she was still not quite stable. Therefore, when the 21st session was reached, it was suggested that the family treatment continue for a while longer. In fact, sessions continued for another 3 months on a biweekly basis, during which time she continued her schoolwork without incident.

In the final weeks of treatment, Maria came to grips with the realization that she would never get the full acceptance from her father that she desired, and that she would have to seek this acceptance from people outside her family. Although never able to praise Maria directly, her father was extremely complimentary about the clinicians' efforts and claimed that Maria was in the best shape psychologically that she had been in recent years. The clinicians' view was that Maria had improved markedly, but was still in need of future treatment. They felt her current problems were best addressed in an individual therapy relationship, a point with which Maria agreed. In the last FFT session, a relapse drill was repeated, a follow-up session was arranged, and Maria was strongly encouraged to remain on her mood-regulating medications.

FFT is a time-limited treatment with a modal number of 21 sessions. But, as the above cases illustrate, sometimes families can terminate treatment readily at this point (or even earlier), and sometimes treatment has to be extended until either a reasonable degree of clinical stability is achieved in the patient or until certain critical family issues are resolved. Alternatively, you can schedule "booster sessions" every few months to maintain treatment gains and help ensure ongoing use of the skills.

The Structure of Termination Sessions

The termination sessions are often accelerated problem-solving sessions in which problems likely to arise in the near future are identified and feasible solutions explored. We have found it useful to structure these sessions around the following themes: reviewing the course of the treatment, anticipating future problems, evaluating future treatment needs, and arranging for follow-up visits.

Reviewing the Course of Treatment

As in the termination of any psychological treatment, you should review with the family members what they have and have not accomplished. Start this process, as the clinicians do with Maria and her father, by asking each of the family members to look back on how things were when they entered treatment and to indicate what they gained over the course of the sessions:

CLINICIAN: We've been meeting for 9 months on and off, and I was wondering what you found useful from this experience.

FATHER: I really appreciated those information sessions. I was never aware that Maria had bipolar disorder and that she couldn't control some of the things she said and did when she was in the middle of one of her episodes. I was very doubtful that she could ever recover, and now I feel more hopeful. I also found it very helpful that when it looked like Maria was getting sick again, you scheduled those special sessions and worked out a plan to lower the pressure on her.

MARIA: I didn't particularly enjoy those same sessions that Dad liked 'cause I felt on the spot, as if you were talking about me as an object or something, but I do have to admit they did clear some things up for me—especially that model about biology and stress and stuff. I found the role-playing sessions hard, but it was good that you made my father sit still and listen to what I had to say—that's a first in my life!

CLINICIAN: What about the relapse drill?

MARIA: I found it hard. It's very difficult to think that this thing could happen again, and I didn't want to think about it. But when I started getting manic a few months back, it was good that I knew how to recognize my symptoms and called you and my doctor right away. I think that when I showed that I could see what was happening to me and did the right thing to keep from getting sicker, my dad had more confidence in me.

CLINICIAN: How about things between the two of you?

FATHER: Well, Maria is easier to get along with, but I'm still not sure she can handle the stress of college. I'm willing to pay for one more semester, but only that. I wish she'd help more around the house.

MARIA: Well, you can see that he still doesn't value me the way he values my older sister. But at least now he understands about my problems and doesn't blame me when I get down—you know, depressed or agitated or whatever. But I've tried to make more friends at school. So things are better, but I still have this illness and nobody but me can solve that problem.

As revealed in this interaction, things are better in the father–daughter relationship but far from ideal, and Maria has come to recognize that dependence on her father, emotionally and financially, cannot be the answer for her. In contrast to Phil's family, in which much progress was made toward more functional family relationships (FFT Goal 6), Maria and her father have achieved a truce but not much more. The recognition of Maria's bipolar disorder softened her father's criticism of her, and the gradual improvement in her clinical status increased his willingness to support her reentry into college. Interestingly, Maria and her father fully accepted her vulnerability to future episodes and need for mood-stabilizing medications (FFT Goals 2 and 3), whereas Phil never fully accepted his need for treatment.

A critical point in the treatment was when Maria started relapsing during her first semester and her father saw a validation of his pessimism. It was only strong support by the family clinicians and by Maria's psychiatrist during this crisis period that headed off a major failure experience, which could have led to a significant deterioration in their relationship. The family clinician's use of many of the crisis intervention principles, outlined in the previous chapter, played a major role in helping Maria and her family to weather this difficult episode. When reviewing the course of treatment, both Maria and her father mentioned this phase of the treatment as a turning point in the course of her illness and in their relationship.

Anticipating Future Problems

One way to solidify the gains of treatment is to ask the family members to consider how they will deal with future problems. How will they cope with new stressors when they no longer have FFT sessions to focus their efforts?

In the termination sessions, a general principle operates: *Whenever possible, use the elements of FFT to resolve the feelings of the family members about ending family treatment*. The elements of psychoeducation, communication enhancement, and problem solving can all serve as instruments for facilitating the termination of FFT. This not only is helpful to the family in resolving concrete issues surrounding termination but reinforces individual family members for the use of these elements in their everyday lives. In one of the final sessions with Phil's family, the clinician inquires about the participants' concerns, which leads to this interchange:

CLINICIAN: You have really worked very hard during this treatment program, and now that we're ending, I was wondering if you had some concerns about how things would go for you as a family without these sessions.

MRS. NORTH: Well, I must admit I'll miss the sessions. We've grown so much closer as a family that I am afraid we'll go back to the way we were before.

PHIL: (*facetiously*) I'll be able to stay home and watch the big screen instead of coming here! (*all laugh*) No, honestly, I don't think we'll slip back. Things are much better.

CLINICIAN: Well, in what ways do you think you could make it more likely that the good things you've learned could continue—how could you use the skills on your own? Let me ask you to use your problem solving one more time and work out how you could continue to use some of the things you found valuable in this program.

The family then problem solves as a group as to how they will keep the regular family meetings going, who might take the leadership role in making them happen, how they can remind each other to use communication skills in providing open and honest feedback to each other, and how to continue working together in an organized way to solve family problems. At the end of this part of the session, the participants feel more optimistic that they can continue their positive interactions independently of the family clinicians.

Evaluating Future Treatment Needs

The third major goal of the termination sessions is to assist the patient and the family to evaluate future treatment needs. Because FFT is time limited, it will not address all of the needs of a patient with bipolar disorder. Certain issues likely to arise at this point are (1) the need for continued maintenance medication, (2) the need for more and possibly a different type of family therapy, (3) the desire for individual therapy, and (4) the desire of patients and relatives to participate in some form of support group with others who struggle with bipolar disorder.

The Need for Continued Maintenance Medication

As the family treatment draws to a close, there is a strong tendency for persons with bipolar disorder to conclude that this is also the time to discontinue their medications. There are many good reasons for these feelings: The patient is usually doing much better at this point and cannot see the need for continued maintenance medication, or may simply want to see what life is like without it. Younger patients having experienced their first or second episode are particularly likely to feel this way. Nevertheless, you should take a strong stand on the need for continued medication adherence in the final family sessions.

If compliance is an issue for the patient (as in Phil's case), address this material in a conjoint session involving the patient's psychiatrist, so as to present a solid front on the issue. Then you have an excellent opportunity to take a psychoeducational stance and remind the patient of the facts regarding the risk for relapse if medication is stopped. However, approaching the issue from a purely cognitive or informational point of view is usually insufficient. Once again, explore the underlying emotional issues for both patients and relatives. These may involve the themes addressed early on in the treatment program, such as feelings of stigmatization because of using a psychiatric medication, a desire for autonomy, a distaste for the sensations produced by the medications, and other issues.

Very often, these discussions stimulate more dormant family conflicts. Family members who have been through FFT are frightened of a subsequent relapse, whereas the patient may still deny or minimize the risk. This was a very important issue for Phil and his family in their last sessions.

PHIL: I realize that what you're saying about relapse may be true for some people, but I don't think it applies to me. I think I deserve to know what I'm like without my medication.

MRS. NORTH: For God's sake, Phil, how can you do that? You're doing so well, how can you take that chance? Don't you remember how awful it was when you were hospitalized?

MR. NORTH: Well, son, I just want to say one thing—you don't even have any health insurance and, if you do relapse again, I'll be damned if I'll pay for you to go to some pricey hospital. It's the county hospital for you! Think about it.

CLINICIAN: Well, it's pretty clear that this is a very hot issue for all of you. Mr. and Mrs. North, you don't want to see Phil get ill again, particularly because he's doing so well and you are all much closer as a family. Phil, you can't quite believe that the risk is as great as science tells us, and evidently you're willing to take a pretty significant chance on your belief. Maybe you can tell your mom and dad why you are willing to take this risk—what's so good about your alternative.

Sometimes the patient can be influenced to stay on his or her medication. Often this is best achieved when a specific time period is suggested, such as for one more year. Young people in particular may not be able to accept the notion of long-term reliance on prophylactic mood medications, and it is best to focus on small time periods and renegotiate the issue at the end of each period. But Phil, despite hearing all the facts and figures, had made a very firm decision. He reiterated his desire to be normal like other young people and how taking medication is inconsistent with this image.

What can you do when such a decision appears immutable? You will see how the family clinician deals with this issue in Phil's case, reinvoking the principles of the relapse drill described in Chapter 7.

CLINICIAN: Well, Phil, it sounds as if the decision to stop your medication is pretty firm. As I've told you a number of times, the risk for relapse is quite high if you stop your medications, and particularly so if you do it abruptly. So, I hope you will work with your psychiatrist on a schedule to reduce your dose gradually over time to limit the risk to some degree. Mr. and Mrs. North, your concerns about Phil's doing this are very understandable—you don't want Phil or the two of you to go through all this again. You want to protect yourselves emotionally and financially, which is a real issue, given Phil's lack of health insurance. But, ultimately, whether or not to continue on a medication is a personal decision, and if you, Phil, have made it, we now have to devise a strategy to minimize the damage should another episode happen.

MRS. NORTH: Like what?

CLINICIAN: First, we think it's very important, Phil, that you maintain regular contact with your psychiatrist so that she can monitor your clinical status. If the early signs of your disorder appear, she can encourage you to restart your medication. But beyond this, you need to use your relapse prevention principles to work out a plan as a family to minimize the likelihood of this happening.

The clinician then encourages Phil and his family to go through the relapse drill again, reviewing early warning signs of a manic recurrence and settling on some agreements as to who will be contacted if the early signs appear. Although there are still many uneasy feelings at the end of this discussion on the part of the family as well as the clinician, there is a sense of reduced tension and a plan of action is in place.

In general, we have found that, despite many mishaps, if clinicians do take an accepting stance toward medication discontinuation and set up a relapse prevention plan for the patient and his or her relatives, the patient will be more likely to reach out early in the prodromal phases of a relapse. In fact, about 6 months after leaving family treatment, Phil called his family clinician and said that he felt he was getting manic again—he had racing thoughts and was not sleeping much, symptoms that had preceded his last episode. The clinician asked Phil to come in immediately and, upon meeting with Phil, recognized that he was probably correct about his clinical state. The clinician used the principles of crisis intervention to explore what stresses, if any, were important in Phil's life at this point and explored with him ways to minimize their impact. The clinician also strongly encouraged Phil to see his psychiatrist immediately to resume a course of medication. He did so and was prescribed lithium and an atypical antipsychotic, which reduced his symptoms substantially over a 2-week period.

At the end of this period, Phil decided to stay on the lithium "for a while longer," as he put it. The near-miss experience of a relapse played a big role in his decision. The fact that Phil was able to reach out on his own was very encouraging to his mother and father and led to more improvement in their relationship.

Phil had carried out an experiment on himself to become more convinced of the reality of his illness. He needed to do this to accept the reality of his illness and its long-term prophylaxis with medications.

The Need for More or a Different Type of Family Treatment

In one of the original models developed for schizophrenia patients, Anderson et al. (1986) suggested that, after a course of psychoeducational family therapy, certain families come to recognize that there are significant long-standing issues in their relationships that would be profitable to explore. These issues, the writers suggested, were better approached using more conventional family therapy techniques such as structural or strategic approaches. This point is also applicable to families coping with bipolar disorder.

Many families showed marked improvement in family communication after FFT (Simoneau et al., 1999). In our experience, it is rather uncommon that families request or respond to therapists' suggestions for additional family treatment after completing the 9-month protocol. But when pursued, additional treatment can be extremely beneficial. As we have illustrated in several of our case studies, FFT sometimes only serves as a holding function to permit the patient to recover in the most favorable family environment, while masking long-standing, deep-seated family problems. Sometimes the positive changes experienced during FFT raise all family members' consciousness of unresolved family conflicts, which they now feel more ready to address.

Among spousal families in which one member is the patient, there is often a recognition of the need for continuing work on the marriage. Among patients living in parental families, issues relating to childhood abuse sometimes arise during FFT, and the patient or his or her family members may wish to pursue the significance of these experiences for their future relationships. If this need arises, you can work out a new treatment contract with the family to focus on these topics, or a referral can be made to other family therapists. If a referral is made, it is extremely important that the new family therapists be well educated about bipolar disorder and feel comfortable operating within a vulnerability–stress model, including the importance of medication management.

The Desire for Individual Therapy

After completing FFT, neither Maria nor her father wanted any further family treatment, but Maria did want to continue on her medication and have individual psychotherapy. As she put it, rather bluntly, "I need somebody to talk to who can help me straighten out my feelings about my G-d-damned father and my bitchy sister. I need some help to find a reasonable goal in life for me and to figure out how to get closer to people." She was referred to an individual therapist following the termination of FFT and has profited from the relationship.

In contrast to the relatively low numbers of families who request additional family therapy, many bipolar patients express a desire for individual therapy near the time of the termination of FFT. This is particularly true of young adult patients who face many of the normal developmental tasks of the postadolescent period, including separation and individuation from their primary family group. Older adolescent patients may express this desire as well.

The orientation of FFT is first to assist a person to come to terms with his or her bipolar disorder, but then, by concentrating on communication and problem solving, the focus changes to more general issues in coping with interpersonal relationships. Because of this, many patients come to recognize the need for individual therapy to deal with a multiplicity of conflicts, only some of which are related to bipolar disorder. How to resume one's education or career, how to develop greater independence from one's parents, how to develop successful intimate relationships or whether or not to continue in a particular one, how to improve relationships with one's children, and how to handle the hassles of daily life more effectively—these are all relevant issues for persons who have achieved remission from a bipolar episode. In those cases in which marriages or other intimate relationships have ended prior to or during the course of FFT, there is a strong desire among patients or key relatives to explore relationship concerns in individual psychotherapy. Finally, some patients—those in spousal as well as parental families—still want to explore the significance of their bipolar disorder with a psychotherapist, particularly those patients who still suffer from a kind of posttraumatic stress disorder regarding prior manic or depressive episodes (i.e., flashbacks, recurrent nightmares, or persistent, intrusive worries about the return of their symptoms).

If patients or their relatives—who also sometimes become aware of psychological issues they wish to pursue—do request individual therapy, it is again important to make referrals to therapists who are knowledgeable about bipolar disorder and who appreciate the importance of combining medication with psychological treatment. We have seen a lot of good work undone when patients found psychotherapists who did not want to recognize the patients' bipolar disorder, were hostile to the use of maintenance medication, and sought to "cure" the patients on their own.

The Desire for Participation in Support Groups

We strongly encourage the participation of relatives and patients in mutual support groups, such as those offered by the National Alliance on

Mental Illness (NAMI; *www.nami.org*) or the Depressive and Bipolar Support Alliance (*www.dbsalliance.org*). Chapter 4 includes the phone numbers for these national support groups for bipolar patients and their families. Many relatives in our program have expressed a desire to participate in such support groups after they finish FFT, and some have requested referral even during the program. We have not experienced any difficulties in achieving the goals of FFT if the relatives are concurrently attending support groups. Moreover, family members may solidify some of the educational gains they have made if they continue to interact with other families coping with bipolar disorder. NAMI's "Family to Family" classes seem particularly useful for parents and spouses.

Many patients also express a desire for some type of support group. A group therapy program for persons with bipolar disorder could serve a very important function for a patient, particularly if the group addresses a broad spectrum of issues ranging from medication concerns to relationship problems. A recent study found that group psychoeducation in combination with medication led to better outcomes of bipolar disorder than participation in standard support groups (Colom et al., 2003). Some communities have support groups that involve a trained clinician leader and focus on positive and negative interpersonal behavior styles, as these are expressed within the group. Other groups consist solely of patients with the disorder and do not include trained clinicians, as a means of providing mutual support and education.

In order to be maximally beneficial, these psychoeducation groups should be age graded as much as possible. Relatives of young, recent-onset patients do not respond well to groups composed largely of relatives of older, more chronic or severely ill psychiatric patients. Similarly, older patients do not feel that young persons with relatively short histories of bipolar disorder are their reference group. Unfortunately, support groups based on age are difficult to find, but they do exist. If your setting permits, perhaps you can initiate such groups.

Arranging for Follow-Up Visits

Although termination usually implies that the FFT program is not to continue on a formal basis, some kind of follow-up agreement is frequently very useful in easing the transition for the patient and relatives. We recommend that a specific follow-up session be set up with the patient and family, usually about 3–6 months after termination. This session is often oriented toward evaluating the patient's clinical status since ending FFT, the ease or difficulty of obtaining desired follow-up care, the patient's attempts to reenter the school or working world, and the need for any new referrals.

We also schedule a second follow-up roughly 1 year after termination to examine the same issues. After this, no further appointments are scheduled, although we indicate that we can be contacted in the event of a crisis. Naturally, if the patient or family members are in treatment with other professionals, these follow-up sessions must be handled in a fashion that does not undermine their current therapeutic relationships.

Concluding Comments

The termination sessions of FFT offer a valuable opportunity to review the course of treatment and establish future treatment needs. Continued use of mood-regulating medications is emphasized as a means of maintaining stability after FFT has ended. Once the major goals of FFT are realized—a stable clinical state for the patient and more effective interaction between the patient and his or her relatives—the time may be right to pursue other forms of psychological treatment that address a broader set of goals.

Keep in mind that treating bipolar disorder is often an indefinite process. Once you have successfully treated a patient and his or her family, you can expect to hear from them again, whether this is because of an incipient crisis, the desire for a referral, or just the wish to reestablish contact. The parents of a bipolar teen may call you to say that the young adult has now started college or is living independently. In having these contacts, you will often be impressed by the trust you have built among these patients or family members, even among those who were the most resistant and difficult during FFT. But this can be one of the joys of working with persons with chronic mental illness and their family members—the feeling that you have made an impact on and a difference in their lives.

References

Aagaard, J., & Vestergaard, P. (1990). Predictors of outcome in prophylactic lithium treatment: A 2-year prospective study. *Journal of Affective Disorders, 18,* 259–266.

Akiskal, H. S., Bourgeois, M. L., Angst, J., Post, R., Moller, H., & Hirschfeld, R. (2000). Re-evaluating the prevalence of and diagnostic composition within the broad clinical spectrum of bipolar disorders. *Journal of Affective Disorders, 59*(Suppl. 1), S5–S30.

Altman, E., Rea, M., Mintz, J., Miklowitz, D. J., Goldstein, M. J., & Hwang, S. (1992). Prodromal symptoms and signs of bipolar relapse: A report based on prospectively collected data. *Psychiatry Research, 41,* 1–8.

American Psychiatric Association. (2000). *Diagnostic and statistical manual of mental disorders* (4th ed., text rev.). Washington, DC: Author.

Anderson, C. M., Reiss, D. J., & Hogarty, G. E. (1986). *Schizophrenia and the family.* New York: Guilford Press.

Anderson, C. M., & Stewart, S. S. (1983). *Mastering resistance: A practical guide to family therapy.* New York: Guilford Press.

Angst, J. (1978). The course of affective disorders: II. Typology of bipolar manic–depressive illness. *Archiv für Psychiatrie und Nervenkrankheiten, 226,* 65–73.

Anthony, W. A., & Liberman, R. P. (1986). The practice of psychiatric rehabilitation: Historical, conceptual, and research base. *Schizophrenia Bulletin, 12,* 542–559.

Beck, A. T., Rush, A. J., Shaw, B. F., & Emery, G. (1987). *Cognitive therapy of depression.* New York: Guilford Press.

Birmaher, B., Axelson, D., Strober, M., Gill, M. K., Valeri, S., Chiappetta, L., et al. (2006). Clinical course of children and adolescents with bipolar spectrum disorders. *Archives of General Psychiatry, 63*(2), 175–183.

Brent, D. A., Perper, J. A., Goldstein, C. E., Kolko, D. J., Allan, M. J., Allman, C. J., et al. (1988). Risk factors for adolescent suicide: A comparison of adolescent suicide victims with suicidal inpatients. *Archives of General Psychiatry, 45,* 581–588.

Brodie, H. K. H., & Leff, M. J. (1971). Bipolar depression: A comparative study of patient characteristics. *American Journal of Psychiatry, 127,* 1086–1090.

Brown, G., & Harris, T. (1978). *Social origins of depression: A study of psychiatric disorder in women.* New York: Free Press.

Butzlaff, R. L., & Hooley, J. M. (1998). Expressed emotion and psychiatric relapse: A meta-analysis. *Archives of General Psychiatry, 55,* 547–552.

Cannon, M., Jones, P., Gilvarry, C., Rifkin, L., McKenzie, K., Foerster, A., et al. (1997). Premorbid social functioning in schizophrenia and bipolar disorder: Similarities and differences. *American Journal of Psychiatry, 154,* 1544–1550.

Carlson, G. A., & Goodwin, E. K. (1973). The stages of mania: A longitudinal analysis of the manic episode. *Archives of General Psychiatry, 28,* 221–228.

Carlson, G. A., Kotin, J., Davenport, Y. B., & Adland, M. (1974). Follow-up of 53 bipolar manic–depressive patients. *British Journal of Psychiatry, 124,* 134–139.

Chambers, W. J., Puig-Antich, J., Hirsch, M., Paez, P., Ambrosini, P. J., Tabrizi, M. A., et al. (1985). The assessment of affective disorders in children and adolescents by semi-structured interview: Test–retest reliability. *Archives of General Psychiatry, 42,* 696–702.

Chambless, D. L., & Hollon, S. D. (1998). Defining empirically supported therapies. *Journal of Consulting and Clinical Psychology, 66,* 7–18.

Chang, K. D., Blaser, C., Ketter, T. A., & Steiner, H. (2001). Family environment of children and adolescents with bipolar parents. *Bipolar Disorders, 3,* 73–78.

Chang, K., Steiner, H., & Ketter, T. (2003). Studies of offspring of parents with bipolar disorder. *American Journal of Medical Genetics: C. Seminars in Medical Genetics, 123,* 26–35.

Cohen, M., Baker, G., Cohen, R. A., Fromm-Reichmann, E., & Weigert, V. (1954). An intensive study of 12 cases of manic–depressive psychosis. *Psychiatry, 17,* 103–137.

Colom, F., Vieta, E., Martinez-Aran, A., Reinares, M., Goikolea, J. M., Benabarre, A., et al. (2003). A randomized trial on the efficacy of group psychoeducation in the prophylaxis of recurrences in bipolar patients whose disease is in remission. *Archives of General Psychiatry, 60,* 402–407.

Colom, F., Vieta, E., Tacchi, M. J., Sanchez-Moreno, J., & Scott, J. (2005). Identifying and improving nonadherence in bipolar disorders. *Bipolar Disorders, 7*(5), 24–31.

Coryell, W., Scheftner, W., Keller, M., Endicott, J., Maser, J., & Klerman, G. L. (1993). The enduring psychosocial consequences of mania and depression. *American Journal of Psychiatry, 15,* 720–727.

Coryell, W., Solomon, D., Turvey, C., Keller, M., Leon, A. C., Endicott, J., et al. (2003). The long-term course of rapid-cycling bipolar disorder. *Archives of General Psychiatry, 60,* 914–920.

Coyne, J. C., Downey, G., & Boergers, J. (1992). Depression in families: A systems perspective. In D. Cicchetti &. S. L. Toth (Eds.), *Developmental perspectives on depression* (pp. 211–249). Rochester, NY: University of Rochester Press.

Cutler, N. R., & Post, R. M. (1982). Life course of illness in untreated manic–depressive patients. *Comprehensive Psychiatry, 23,* 101–115.

Decina, P., Kestenbaum, C. J., Farber, S., Kron, L., Gargan, M., Sackheim, H. A., et al. (1983). Clinical and psychological assessment of children of bipolar probands. *American Journal of Psychiatry, 140,* 548–553.

DelBello, M. P., Hanseman, D., Adler, C. M., Fleck, D. E., & Strakowski, S. M. (2007). Twelve month outcome of adolescents with bipolar disorder following first-hospitalization for a manic or mixed episode. *American Journal of Psychiatry, 164*(4), 582–590.

DelBello, M. P., Kowatch, R. A., Adler, C. M., Stanford, K. E., Welge, J. A., Barzman, D. H., et al. (2006). A double-blind randomized pilot study comparing quetiapine and divalproex for adolescent mania. *Journal of the American Academy of Child and Adolescent Psychiatry, 45*(3), 305–313.

Doane, J. A., Goldstein, M. J., Miklowitz, D. J., & Falloon, I. R. H. (1986). The impact of individual and family treatment on the affective climate of families of schizophrenics. *British Journal of Psychiatry, 148,* 279–287.

Doane, J. A., West, K. L, Goldstein, M. J., Rodnick, E. H., & Jones, J. E. (1981). Parental communication deviance and affective style: Predictors of subsequent schizophrenia spectrum disorders in vulnerable adolescents. *Archives of General Psychiatry, 38,* 679–685.

Dohrenwend, B. S., Dohrenwend, B. P., Dodson, M., & Shrout, P. E. (1984). Symptoms, hassles, social supports, and life events: The problem of confounded measures. *Journal of Abnormal Psychology, 93,* 222–230.

Dohrenwend, B. S., Krasnoff, L., Askenasy, A. R., & Dohrenwend, B. P. (1978). Exemplification of a method for scaling life events: The PERI life events scale. *Journal of Health and Social Behavior, 19,* 205–229.

Ehlers, C. L., Frank, E., & Kupfer, D. J. (1988). Social zeitgebers and biological rhythms: A unified approach to understanding the etiology of depression. *Archives of General Psychiatry, 45,* 948–952.

Ehlers, C. L., Kupfer, D. J., Frank, E., & Monk, T. H. (1993). Biological rhythms and depression: The role of zeitgebers and zeitstorers. *Depression, 1,* 285–293.

Ellicott, A., Hammen, C., Gitlin, M., Brown, G., & Jamison, K. (1990). Life events and the course of bipolar disorder. *American Journal of Psychiatry, 147,* 1194–1198.

Fagiolini, A., Kupfer, D. J., Masalehdan, A., Scott, J. A., Houck, P. R., & Frank, E. (2005). Functional impairment in the remission phase of bipolar disorder. *Bipolar Disorders, 7,* 281–285.

Falloon, I. R. H., Boyd, J. L., & McGill, C. W. (1984). *Family care of schizophrenia: A problem-solving approach to the treatment of mental illness.* New York: Guilford Press.

Falloon, I. R. H., Boyd, J. L., McGill, C. W., Williamson, M., Razani, J., Moss, H. B., et al. (1985). Family management in the prevention of morbidity of schizophrenia. *Archives of General Psychiatry, 42,* 887–896.

Findling, R. L., Youngstrom, E. A., McNamara, N. K., Stansbrey, R. J., Demeter, C., Bedoya, D., et al. (2005). Early symptoms of mania and the role of parental risk. *Bipolar Disorders, 7,* 623–634.

First, M. B., Spitzer, R. L., Gibbon, M., & Williams, J. B. W. (1995). *Structured Clinical Interview for DSM-IV Axis I Disorders, Patient Edition.* New York: New York State Psychiatric Institute.

Floyd, F. J., O'Farrell, T. J., & Goldberg, M. (1987). Comparison of marital observational measures: The Marital Interaction Coding System and the Communication Skills Test. *Journal of Consulting and Clinical Psychology, 55*(3), 423–429.

Frank, E. (2005). *Treating bipolar disorder: A clinician's guide to interpersonal and social rhythm therapy.* New York: Guilford Press.

Frank, E., Kupfer, D. J., Thase, M. E., Mallinger, A. G., Swartz, H. A., Fagiolini, A. M., et al. (2005). Two-year outcomes for interpersonal and social rhythm therapy in individuals with bipolar I disorder. *Archives of General Psychiatry, 62*(9), 996–1004.

Fredman, S., Baucom, D. H., Miklowitz, D. J., & Stanton, S. (in press). Observed emotional involvement and overinvolvement in families of bipolar patients. *Journal of Family Psychology.*

Fromm-Reichmann, F. (1950). *Principles of intensive psychotherapy.* Chicago: University of Chicago Press.

Geller, B., Warner, K., Williams, M., & Zimerman, B. (1998). Prepubertal and young adolescent bipolarity versus ADHD: Assessment and validity using the WASH-U-KSADS, CBCL and TRF. *Journal of Affective Disorders, 51,* 93–100.

Gibson, R. W. (1958). The family background and early life experience of the manic–depressive patient. *Psychiatry, 21,* 71–90.

Gitlin, M. J., Swendsen, J., Heller, T. L., & Hammen, C. (1995). Relapse and impairment in bipolar disorder. *American Journal of Psychiatry, 152,* 1635–1640.

Goldberg, J. F. (2004). The changing landscape of psychopharmacology. In S. L. Johnson & R. L. Leahy (Eds.), *Psychological treatment of bipolar disorder* (pp. 109–138). New York: Guilford Press.

Goldstein, M. J., Rodnick, E. H., Evans, J. R., May, P. R. A., & Steinberg, M. R. (1978). Drug and family therapy in the aftercare of acute schizophrenia. *Archives of General Psychiatry, 35,* 1169–1177.

Goodwin, F. K., & Jamison, K. R. (1990). *Manic–depressive illness.* New York: Oxford University Press.

Goodwin, G. M., Bowden, C. L., Calabrese, J. R., Grunze, H., Kasper, S., White, R., et al. (2004). A pooled analysis of 2 placebo-controlled 18-month trials of lamotrigine and lithium maintenance in bipolar I disorder. *Journal of Clinical Psychiatry, 65*(3), 432–441.

Hahlweg, K., Goldstein, M. J., Nuechterlein, K. H., Magana, A. B., Mintz, J., Doane, J. A., et al. (1989). Expressed emotion and patient–relative interaction in families of recent-onset schizophrenics. *Journal of Consulting and Clinical Psychology, 57,* 11–18.

Haley, J. (1987). *Problem-solving therapy* (2nd ed.). San Francisco: Jossey-Bass.

Hamilton, M. (1960). Development of a rating scale for primary depressive illness. *British Journal of Social and Clinical Psychology, 6,* 276–296.

Hammen, C., Burge, D., Burney, E., & Adrian, C. (1990). Longitudinal study of diagnoses in children of women with unipolar and bipolar affective disorder. *Archives of General Psychiatry, 47,* 1112–1117.

Hammen, C., Marks, T., Mayol, A., & deMayo, R. (1985). Depressive self-schemas, life stress, and vulnerability to depression. *Journal of Abnormal Psychology, 94,* 308–319.

Harris, E. C., & Barraclough, B. (1997). Suicide as an outcome for mental disorders: A meta-analysis. *British Journal of Psychiatry, 170,* 205–208.

Hatfield, A. B., Spaniol, L., & Zipple, A. M. (1987). Expressed emotion: A family perspective. *Schizophrenia Bulletin, 13,* 221–226.

Hooley, J. M., & Gotlib, I. H. (2000). A diathesis–stress conceptualization of expressed emotion and clinical outcome. *Applied and Preventive Psychology, 9*, 131–151.

Hooley, J. M., & Richters, J. (1995). Expressed emotion: A developmental perspective. In D. Cicchetti & S. L. Toth (Eds.), *Emotion, cognitions, and representations*. Rochester, NY: University of Rochester Press.

Jacobson, N., & Margolin, G. (1979). *Marital therapy*. New York: Brunner/Mazel.

Jamison, K. R. (1993). *Touched with fire: Manic–depressive illness and the artistic temperament*. New York: Free Press.

Jamison, K. R. (2000). Suicide and bipolar disorder. *Journal of Clinical Psychiatry, 61*(Suppl. 9), 47–56.

Johnson, R. E., & McFarland, B. H. (1996). Lithium use and discontinuation in a health maintenance organization. *American Journal of Psychiatry, 153*, 993–1000.

Johnson, S. L. (2005a). Life events in bipolar disorder: Towards more specific models. *Clinical Psychology Review, 25*, 1008–1027.

Johnson, S. L. (2005b). Mania and dysregulation in goal pursuit. *Clinical Psychology Review, 25*, 241–262.

Johnson, S. L., & Miller, I. (1997). Negative life events and time to recovery from episodes of bipolar disorder. *Journal of Abnormal Psychology, 106*, 449–457.

Johnson, S. L., Sandrow, D., Meyer, B., Winters, R., Miller, I., Solomon, D., et al. (2000). Increases in manic symptoms following life events involving goal-attainment. *Journal of Abnormal Psychology, 109*, 721–727.

Judd, L. L., Akiskal, H. S., Schettler, P. J., Coryell, W., Endicott, J., Maser, J. D., et al. (2003). A prospective investigation of the natural history of the long-term weekly symptomatic status of bipolar II disorder. *Archives of General Psychiatry, 60*, 261–269.

Judd, L. L., Akiskal, H. S., Schettler, P. J., Endicott, J., Maser, J., Solomon, D. A., et al. (2002). The long-term natural history of the weekly symptomatic status of bipolar I disorder. *Archives of General Psychiatry, 59*, 530–537.

Kalbag, A., Miklowitz, D. J., & Richards, J. A. (1999). A method for classifying the course of bipolar I disorder. *Behavior Therapy, 30*, 355–372.

Kaufman, J., Birmaher, B., Brent, D., Rao, U., Flynn, C., Moreci, P., et al. (1997). Schedule for Affective Disorders and Schizophrenia for school-age children—Present and Lifetime version (K-SADS-PL): Initial reliability and validity data. *Journal of the American Academy of Child and Adolescent Psychiatry, 36*, 980–988.

Keck, P. E., Jr., McElroy, S. L., Strakowski, S. M., West, S. A., Sax, K. W., Hawkins, J. M., et al. (1998). Twelve-month outcome of patients with bipolar disorder following hospitalization for a manic or mixed episode. *American Journal of Psychiatry, 155*, 646–652.

Keller, M. B., Lavori, P. W., Coryell, W., Endicott, J., & Mueller, T. I. (1993). Bipolar I: A five-year prospective follow-up. *Journal of Nervous and Mental Disease, 18*, 238–245.

Kessing, L. V., Agerbo, E., & Mortensen, P. B. (2004). Major stressful life events and other risk factors for first admission with mania. *Bipolar Disorders, 6*(2), 122–129.

Klein, D. N., Depue, R. A., & Slater, J. F. (1986). Inventory identification of cyclothymia: IX. Validation in offspring of bipolar I patients. *Archives of General Psychiatry, 43*, 441–445.

Kraepelin, E. (Ed.). (1921). *Manic–depressive insanity and paranoia.* Edinburgh: E & S Livingstone.

Kochman, F. J., Hantouche, E. G., Ferrari, P., Lancrenon, S., Bayart, D., & Akiskal, H. S. (2005). Cyclothymic temperament as a prospective predictor of bipolarity and suicidality in children and adolescents with major depressive disorder. *Journal of Affective Disorders, 85*(1–2), 181–189.

Kupfer, D. J., Frank, E., Grochocinski, V. J., Luther, J. F., Houck, P. R., Swartz, H. A., et al. (2000). Stabilization in the treatment of mania, depression, and mixed states. *Acta Neuropsychiatrica, 12,* 110–114.

Kymalainen, J. A., Weisman, A. G., Rosales, G. A., & Armesto, J. C. (2006). Ethnicity, expressed emotion, and communication deviance in family members of patients with schizophrenia. *Journal of Nervous and Mental Disease, 194,* 391–396.

LaPalme, M., Hodgins, S., & LaRoche, C. (1997). Children of parents with bipolar disorder: A meta-analysis of risk for mental disorders. *Canadian Journal of Psychiatry, 42,* 623–631.

Leff, J., & Vaughn, C. (1985). *Expressed emotion in families: Its significance for mental illness.* New York: Guilford Press.

Leibenluft, E., Cohen, P., Gorrindo, T., Brook, J. S., & Pine, D. S. (2006). Chronic vs. episodic irritability in youth: A community-based, longitudinal study of clinical and diagnostic associations. *Journal of Child and Adolescent Psychopharmacology, 16*(4), 456–466.

Liberman, R. P. (Ed.). (1988). *Psychiatric rehabilitation of chronic mental patients.* Washington, DC: American Psychiatric Press.

Linehan, M. M. (1993). *Cognitive-behavioral treatment of borderline personality disorder.* New York: Guilford Press.

Lish, J. D., Dime-Meenan, S., Whybrow, P. C., Price, R. A., & Hirschfeld, R. M. A. (1994). The National Depressive and Manic–Depressive Association (NDMDA) survey of bipolar members. *Journal of Affective Disorders, 31,* 281–294.

Magana, A. B., Goldstein, M. J., Karno, M., Miklowitz, D. J., Jenkins, J., & Falloon, I. R. H. (1986). A brief method for assessing expressed emotion in relatives of psychiatric patients. *Psychiatry Research, 17,* 203–212.

Malkoff-Schwartz, S., Frank, E., Anderson, B. P., Hlastala, S. A., Luther, J. F., Sherrill, J. T., et al. (2000). Social rhythm disruption and stressful life events in the onset of bipolar and unipolar episodes. *Psychological Medicine, 30,* 1005–1016.

Malkoff-Schwartz, S., Frank, E., Anderson, B., Sherrill, J. T., Siegel, L., Patterson, D., et al. (1998). Stressful life events and social rhythm disruption in the onset of manic and depressive bipolar episodes: A preliminary investigation. *Archives of General Psychiatry, 55,* 702–707.

Manji, H. K., Quiroz, J. A., Payne, J. L., Singh, J., Lopes, B. P., Viegas, J. S., et al. (2003). The underlying neurobiology of bipolar disorder. *World Psychiatry,* 2(3), 136–146.

Marlatt, G. A., & Gordon, J. R. (Eds.). (1985). *Relapse prevention: Maintenance strategies in the treatment of addictive behaviors.* New York: Guilford Press.

Mayo, J. A., O'Connell, R. A., &. O'Brien, J. D. (1979). Families of manic–

depressive patients: Effect of treatment. *American Journal of Psychiatry, 136,* 1535–1539.

Merikangas, K. R., Akiskal, H. S., Angst, J., Greenberg, P. E., Hirschfeld, R. M. A., Petukhova, M., et al. (2007). Lifetime and 12-month prevalence of bipolar spectrum disorder in the National Comorbidity Survey replication. *Archives of General Psychiatry, 64,* 543–552.

Miklowitz, D. J. (2002). *The bipolar disorder survival guide*. New York: Guilford Press.

Miklowitz, D. J. (2004). The role of family systems in severe and recurrent psychiatric disorders: A developmental psychopathology view. *Development and Psychopathology, 16,* 667–688.

Miklowitz, D. J. (2008). Bipolar disorder. In D. H. Barlow (Ed.), *Clinical handbook of psychological disorders* (4th ed., pp. 421–462). New York: Guilford Press.

Miklowitz, D. J., Biuckians, A., & Richards, J. A. (2006). Early-onset bipolar disorder: A family treatment perspective. *Development and Psychopathology, 18*(4), 1247–1265.

Miklowitz, D. J., & Cicchetti, D. (2006). Toward a lifespan developmental psychopathology perspective on bipolar disorder. *Development and Psychopathology, 18*(4), 935–938.

Miklowitz, D. J., & George, E. L. (2008). *The bipolar teen: What you can do to help your child and your family*. New York: Guilford Press.

Miklowitz, D. J., George, E. L., Richards, J. A., Simoneau, T. L., & Suddath, R. L. (2003). A randomized study of family-focused psychoeducation and pharmacotherapy in the outpatient management of bipolar disorder. *Archives of General Psychiatry, 60,* 904–912.

Miklowitz, D. J., & Goldstein, M. J. (1990). Behavioral family treatment for patients with bipolar affective disorder. *Behavior Modification, 14,* 457–489.

Miklowitz, D. J., Goldstein, M. J., Falloon, I. R. H., & Doane, J. A. (1984). Interactional correlates of expressed emotion in the families of schizophrenics. *British Journal of Psychiatry, 144,* 482–487.

Miklowitz, D. J., Goldstein, M. J., & Nuechterlein, K. H. (1995). Verbal interactions in the families of schizophrenic and bipolar affective patients. *Journal of Abnormal Psychology, 104,* 268–276.

Miklowitz, D. J., Goldstein, M. J., Nuechterlein, K. H., Snyder, K. S., & Doane, J. A. (1987). The family and the course of recent-onset mania. In K. Hahlweg & M. J. Goldstein (Eds.), *Understanding major mental disorder: The contribution of family interaction research* (pp. 195–211). New York: Family Process Press.

Miklowitz, D. J., Goldstein, M. J., Nuechterlein, K. H., Snyder, K. S., & Mintz, J. (1988). Family factors and the course of bipolar affective disorder. *Archives of General Psychiatry, 45,* 225–231.

Miklowitz, D. J., Otto, M. W., Frank, E., Reilly-Harrington, N. A., Kogan, J. N., Sachs, G. S., et al. (2007a). Intensive psychosocial intervention enhances functioning in patients with bipolar depression: Results from a 9-month randomized controlled trial. *American Journal of Psychiatry, 164,* 1340–1347.

Miklowitz, D. J., Otto, M. W., Frank, E., Reilly-Harrington, N. A., Wisniewski, S. R., Kogan, J. N., et al. (2007b). Psychosocial treatments for bipolar depression: A 1-year randomized trial from the Systematic Treatment Enhancement Program. *Archives of General Psychiatry, 64,* 419–427.

Miklowitz, D. J., Simoneau, T. L., George, E. L., Richards, J. A., Kalbag, A., Sachs-Ericsson, N., et al. (2000). Family-focused treatment of bipolar disorder: 1-year effects of a psychoeducational program in conjunction with pharmacotherapy. *Biological Psychiatry, 48*, 582–592.

Miklowitz, D. J., & Stackman, D. (1992). Communication deviance in families of schizophrenic and other psychiatric patients: Current state of the construct. In E. F. Walker, R. H. Dworkin, & B. A. Cornblatt (Eds.), *Progress in experimental personality and psychopathology research* (Vol. 15, pp. 1–46). New York: Springer.

Miklowitz, D. J., Velligan, D. I., Goldstein, M. J., Nuechterlein, K. H., Gitlin, M. J., Ranlett, G., et al. (1991). Communication deviance in families of schizophrenic and manic patients. *Journal of Abnormal Psychology, 100*, 163–173.

Miklowitz, D. J., Wendel, J. S., & Simoneau, T. L. (1998). Targeting dysfunctional family interactions and high expressed emotion in the psychosocial treatment of bipolar disorder. *In Session: Psychotherapy in Practice, 4*, 25–38.

Miller, W. R., & Rollnick, S. (1992). *Motivational interviewing*. New York: Guilford Press.

Millett, K. (1990). *The loony-bin trip.* New York: Simon & Schuster.

Monk, T. H., Kupfer, D. J., Frank, E., & Ritenour, A. M. (1991). The social rhythm metric (SRM): Measuring daily social rhythms over 12 weeks. *Psychiatry Research, 36*, 195–207.

Mueser, K. T., & Glynn, S. M. (1995). *Behavioral family therapy for psychiatric disorders.* Boston: Allyn & Bacon.

National Institute for Health and Clinical Excellence. (2006). *The management of bipolar disorder in adults, children and adolescents, in primary and secondary care.* London: Author.

Newman, C., Leahy, R. L., Beck, A. T., Reilly-Harrington, N., & Gyulai, L. (2001). *Bipolar disorder: A cognitive therapy approach*. Washington, DC: American Psychological Association Press.

O'Connell, R. A., Mayo, J. A., Flatow, L., Cuthbertson, B., & O'Brien, B. E. (1991). Outcome of bipolar disorder on long-term treatment with lithium. *British Journal of Psychiatry, 159*, 132–139.

Pavuluri, M. N., Birmaher, B., & Naylor, M. W. (2005). Pediatric bipolar disorder: A review of the past 10 years. *Journal of the American Academy of Child and Adolescent Psychiatry, 44*(9), 846–871.

Perlick, D. A., Hohenstein, J. M., Clarkin, J. F., Kaczynski, R., & Rosenheck, R. A. (2005). Use of mental health and primary care services by caregivers of patients with bipolar disorder: A preliminary study. *Bipolar Disorders, 7*(2), 126–135.

Perlick, D. A., Miklowitz, D. J., Link, B. G., Struening, R., Kaczynski, R., Gonzalez, J., et al. (2007). Perceived stigma and depression among caregivers of patients with bipolar disorder. *British Journal of Psychiatry, 190*, 535–536.

Perlis, R. H., Miyahara, S., Marangell, L. B., Wisniewski, S. R., Ostacher, M., DelBello, M. P., et al. (2004). Long-term implications of early onset in bipolar disorder: Data from the first 1000 participants in the Systematic Treatment Enhancement Program for Bipolar Disorder (STEP-BD). *Biological Psychiatry, 55*, 875–881.

Perlis, R. H., Ostacher, M. J., Patel, J., Marangell, L. B., Zhang, H., Wisniewski, S. R., et al. (2006). Predictors of recurrence in bipolar disorder: Primary outcomes from the Systematic Treatment Enhancement Program for Bipolar Disorder (STEP-BD). *American Journal of Psychiatry, 163*(2), 217–224.

Perris, C. (1966). A study of bipolar (manic–depressive) and unipolar recurrent depressive psychoses: IV. Personality traits. *Acta Psychiatrica Scandinavica, 42*(194), 68–82.

Pitschel-Walz, G., Leucht, S., Bäuml, J., Kissling, W., & Engel, R. R. (2001). The effect of family interventions on relapse and rehospitalization in schizophrenia: A meta-analysis. *Schizophrenia Bulletin, 27*, 73–92.

Podell, R. (1993). *Contagious emotions*. New York: Simon & Schuster.

Post, R. M. (1993). Issues in the long-term management of bipolar affective illness. *Psychiatry Annals, 23*, 86–93.

Post, R. M., & Leverich, G. S. (2006). The role of psychosocial stress in the onset and progression of bipolar disorder and its comorbidities: The need for earlier and alternative modes of therapeutic intervention. *Development and Psychopathology, 18*(4), 1181–1211.

Priebe, S., Wildgrube, C., & Muller-Oerlinghausen, B. (1989). Lithium prophylaxis and expressed emotion. *British Journal of Psychiatry, 154*, 396–399.

Prien, R. F. (1993). Maintenance treatment. In E. S. Paykel (Ed.), *Handbook of affective disorders* (pp. 419–435). New York: Guilford Press.

Rea, M. M., Tompson, M., Miklowitz, D. J., Goldstein, M. J., Hwang, S., & Mintz, J. (2003). Family focused treatment vs. individual treatment for bipolar disorder: Results of a randomized clinical trial. *Journal of Consulting and Clinical Psychology, 71*, 482–492.

Regier, D. A., Farmer, M. E., Rae, D. S., Locke, B. Z., Keith, S. J., Judd, L. L., et al. (1990). Comorbidity of mental disorders with alcohol and other drug abuse: Results from the Epidemiologic Catchment Area (ECA) study. *Journal of the American Medical Association, 264*, 2511–2518.

Rich, B. A., Schmajuk, M., Perez-Edgar, K. E., Fox, N. A., Pine, D. S., & Leibenluft, E. (2007). Different psychophysiological and behavioral responses elicited by frustration in pediatric bipolar disorder and severe mood dysregulation. *American Journal of Psychiatry, 164(2)*, 309–317.

Rosenfarb, I. S., Miklowitz, D. J., Goldstein, M. J., Harmon, L., Nuechterlein, K. H., & Rea, M. M. (2001). Family transactions and relapse in bipolar disorder. *Family Process, 40*(1), 5–14.

Roy, A. (1980). Parental loss in childhood and onset of manic–depressive illness. *British Journal of Psychiatry, 136*, 86–88.

Sachs, G. S., Nierenberg, A. A., Calabrese, J. R., Marangell, L. B., Wisniewski, S. R., Gyulai, L., et al. (2007). Effectiveness of adjunctive antidepressant treatment for bipolar depression. *New England Journal of Medicine, 356*, 1711–1722.

Sachs, G. S., Thase, M. E., Otto, M. W., Bauer, M., Miklowitz, D., Wisniewski, S. R., et al. (2003). Rationale, design, and methods of the systematic treatment enhancement program for bipolar disorder (STEP-BD). *Biological Psychiatry, 53*, 1028–1042.

Schneck, C. D., Miklowitz, D. J., Calabrese, J. R., Allen, M. H., Thomas, M. R., Wisniewski, S. R., et al. (2004). Phenomenology of rapid cycling bipolar disorder: Data from the first 500 participants in the Systematic Treatment Enhancement Program for Bipolar Disorder. *American Journal of Psychiatry, 161*, 1902–1908.

Shaw, J. A., Egeland, J. A., Endicott, J., Allen, C. R., & Hostetter, A. M. (2005). A 10-year prospective study of prodromal patterns for bipolar disorder among Amish youth. *Journal of the American Academy of Child and Adolescent Psychiatry, 44*(11), 1104–1011.

Sheehan, D. V., Lecrubier, Y., Sheehan, K. H., Amorim, P., Janavs, J., Weiller, E., et al. (1998). The Mini-International Neuropsychiatric Interview (M.I.N.I.): The development and validation of a structured diagnostic psychiatric interview for DSM-IV and ICD-10. *Journal of Clinical Psychiatry, 59*(Suppl. 20), 22–33.

Shem, S. (1978). *The house of God.* New York: Dell.

Simoneau, T. L., Miklowitz, D. J., Richards, J. A., Saleem, R., & George, E. L. (1999). Bipolar disorder and family communication: Effects of a psychoeducational treatment program. *Journal of Abnormal Psychology, 108*, 588–597.

Simoneau, T. L., Miklowitz, D. J., & Saleem, R. (1998). Expressed emotion and interactional patterns in the families of bipolar patients. *Journal of Abnormal Psychology, 107*, 497–507.

Smoller, J. W., & Finn, C. T. (2003). Family, twin, and adoption studies of bipolar disorder. *American Journal of Medical Genetics: Part C. Seminars in Medical Genetics, 123*(1), 48–58.

Solomon, D. A., Keitner, G. I., Miller, I. W., Shea, M. T., & Keller, M. B. (1995). Course of illness and maintenance treatments for patients with bipolar disorder. *Journal of Clinical Psychiatry, 56*(1), 5–13.

Solomon, D. A., Leon, A. C., Endicott, J., Coryell, W. H., Mueller, T. I., Posternak, M. A., et al. (2003). Unipolar mania over the course of a 20-year follow-up study. *American Journal of Psychiatry, 160*, 2049–2051.

Strachan, A. M., Feingold, D., Goldstein, M. J., Miklowitz, D. J., &. Nuechterlein, K. H. (1989). Is expressed emotion an index of a transactional process? II. Patient's coping style. *Family Process, 28*, 169–181.

Suppes, T., Baldessarini, R. J., Faedda, G. L., Tondo, L., & Tohen, M. (1993). Discontinuation of maintenance treatment in bipolar disorder: Risks and implications. *Harvard Review of Psychiatry, 1*, 131–144.

Suppes, T., Dennehy, E. B., Hirschfeld, R. M., Altshuler, L. L., Bowden, C. L., Calabrese, J. R., et al. (2005). The Texas implementation of medication algorithms: Update to the algorithms for treatment of bipolar I disorder. *Journal of Clinical Psychiatry, 66*(7), 870–886.

Suppes, T., Leverich, G. S., Keck, P. E., Nolen, W. A., Denicoff, K. D., Altshuler, L. L., et al. (2001). The Stanley Foundation Bipolar Treatment Outcome Network: II. Demographics and illness characteristics of the first 261 patients. *Journal of Affective Disorders, 67*, 45–59.

Thase, M. E. (2006). Pharmacotherapy of bipolar depression: An update. *Current Psychiatry Reports, 8*(6), 478–488.

Tohen, M., Greil, W., Calabrese, J. R., Sachs, G. S., Yatham, L. N., Oerlinghausen, B. M., et al. (2005). Olanzapine versus lithium in the maintenance treatment of bipolar disorder: A 12-month, randomized, double-blind, controlled clinical trial. *American Journal of Psychiatry, 162*, 1281–1290.

Tohen, M., Vieta, E., Calabrese, J., Ketter, T. A., Sachs, G., Bowden, C., et al. (2003). Efficacy of olanzapine and olanzapine-fluoxetine combination in the treatment of bipolar I depression. *Archives of General Psychiatry, 60*, 1079–1088.

Tondo, L., & Baldessarini, R. J. (2000). Reducing suicide risk during lithium maintenance treatment. *Journal of Clinical Psychiatry, 61*(9)(Suppl.), 97–104.

Tondo, L., Baldessarini, R. J., & Floris, G. (2001). Long-term clinical effectiveness of lithium maintenance treatment in types I and II bipolar disorders. *British Journal of Psychiatry, 41*(Suppl.), S184–S190.

Vaughn, C. E., & Leff, J. P. (1976). The influence of family and social factors on the course of psychiatric illness: A comparison of schizophrenia and depressed neurotic patients. *British Journal of Psychiatry, 129,* 125–137.

Velligan, D. I., Goldstein, M. J., Nuechterlein, K. H., Miklowitz, D. J., & Ranlett, G. (1990). Can communication deviance be measured in a family problem-solving interaction? *Family Process, 29,* 213–226.

Weiss, R. D., Griffin, M. L., Kolodziej, M. E., Greenfield, S. F., Najavits, L. M., Daley, D. C., et al. (2007). A randomized trial of integrated group therapy versus group drug counseling for patients with bipolar disorder and substance dependence. *American Journal of Psychiatry, 164*(1), 100–107.

Weissman, M. M., Markowitz, J., & Klerman, G. L. (2000). *Comprehensive guide to interpersonal psychotherapy*. New York: Basic Books.

Wilens, T. E., Biederman, J., Kwon, A., Ditterline, J., Forkner, P., Moore, H., et al. (2004). Risk of substance use disorders in adolescents with bipolar disorder. *Journal of the American Academy of Child and Adolescent Psychiatry, 43*(11), 1380–1386.

Winokur, G., Coryell, W, Akiskal, H. S., Endicott, J., Keller, M., & Mueller, T. (1994). Manic–depressive (bipolar) disorder: The course in light of a prospective ten-year follow-up of 131 patients. *Acta Psychiatrica Scandinavica, 89,* 102–110.

Wynne, L., Singer, M., Bartko, J., & Toohey, M. (1977). Schizophrenics and their families: Recent research on parental communication. In J. M. Tanner (Ed.), *Developments in psychiatric research* (pp. 254–286). London: Hodder & Stoughton.

Yan, L. J., Hammen, C., Cohen, A. N., Daley, S. E., & Henry, R. M. (2004). Expressed emotion versus relationship quality variables in the prediction of recurrence in bipolar patients. *Journal of Affective Disorders, 83,* 199–206.

Yatham, L. N., Kennedy, S. H., O'Donovan, C., Parikh, S., MacQueen, G., McIntyre, R., et al. (2005). Canadian Network for Mood and Anxiety Treatments (CANMAT) guidelines for the management of patients with bipolar disorder: Consensus and controversies. *Bipolar Disorders, 7*(Suppl. 3), 5–69.

Youngstrom, E. A., Findling, R. L., & Calabrese, J. R. (2004). Effects of adolescent manic symptoms on agreement between youth, parent, and teacher ratings of behavior problems. *Journal of Affective Disorders, 82*(Suppl. 1), S5–S16.

Zahn-Waxler, C., McKnew, D. H., Cummings, E. M., Davenport, Y. B., & Radke-Yarrow, M. (1984). Problem behaviors and peer interactions of young children with a manic–depressive parent. *American Journal of Psychiatry, 141,* 236–240.

Zubin, J., & Spring, B. (1977). Vulnerability—A new view of schizophrenia. *Journal of Abnormal Psychology, 86,* 103–126.

Index

"f" following a page number indicates a figure;
"t" following a page number indicates a table.

B

C

D

E

F

I

J

K

L

M

N

O

P

R

S

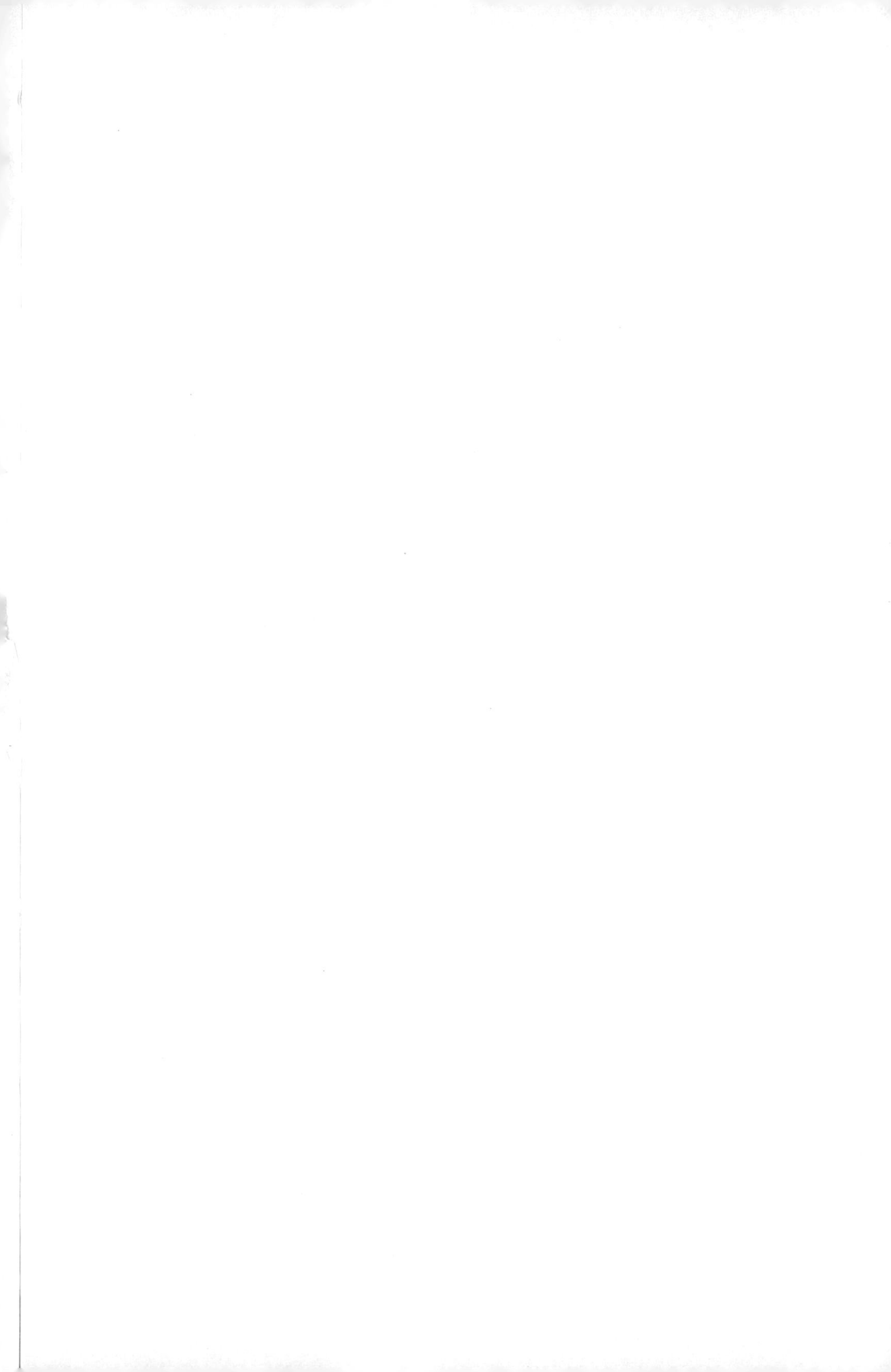